Neuroscience of psychoactive substance use and dependence

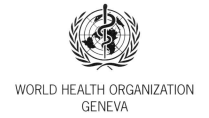

WORLD HEALTH ORGANIZATION
GENEVA

WHO Library Cataloguing-in-Publication Data

Neuroscience of psychoactive substance use and dependence.

1. Psychotropic drugs - pharmacology   2. Substance-related disorders -
physiopathology   3. Psychopharmacology   4. Brain - drug effects
I. World Health Organization.

ISBN 92 4 156235 8   (LC/NLM classification: WM 270)

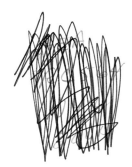

Text design by minimum graphics
Cover design by Tushita Graphic Vision

Printed in Switzerland

Contents

Foreword   ix
Acknowledgements   xi
List of background papers and contributors   xv
Abbreviations   xvii

Chapter 1. Introduction   **1**
     Structure of the report   1
     Psychoactive substances and their sociolegal status   1
     Global use of psychoactive substances   4
         Tobacco   4
         Alcohol   5
         Illicit use of controlled substances   9
     Adverse effects of psychoactive substances and their mechanisms
         of action   10
     Substance dependence in relation to neuroscience   12
     The burden of harm to health from psychoactive substance use   16

Chapter 2. Brain Mechanisms: Neurobiology and Neuroanatomy   **19**
     Introduction   19
     Organization of the brain   19
     The neuron   25
         Cell body   26
         Dendrites   26
         Axon   28
         Terminal buttons   28
     Neurotransmission   29
         Action potential   29
         Neurotransmitter release   30
     Receptors   31
     Neurotransmitters   32
         Acetylcholine   33
         γ-aminobutyric acid   33
         Glutamate   33
         Dopamine   34
         Norepinephrine   34

Serotonin   35
Peptides   35
Genes   35
Cellular and neuronal effects of psychoactive substances   36
    Cellular effects   36
    Neuronal effects   38
Conclusion   39

Chapter 3. Biobehavioural Processes Underlying Dependence   43
Introduction   43
Defining terms   44
    Classical or Pavlovian conditioning   44
    Instrumental or operant conditioning   46
    Reinforcer   47
    Reward   47
    Incentive   47
    Motivation   48
    Incentive-motivational responding   48
Drug reward alone does not explain drug dependence   48
    Drug dependence as a response to incentive-motivation   49
    Drug dependence as a response to drug withdrawal   50
Dopamine and reinforcement learning   50
    Dependence-producing drugs as surrogates of conventional
      reinforcers   51
Dopamine and incentive sensitization   52
    Psychomotor sensitization   53
    Sensitization and drug reward   53
    Sensitization and tolerance   54
    Individual differences   55
Summary   58

**Chapter 4. Psychopharmacology of Dependence for Different
Drug Classes   67**
Introduction   67
Alcohol (ethanol)   69
    Introduction   69
    Behavioural effects   69
    Mechanism of action   70
    Tolerance and withdrawal   70
    Neurobiological adaptations to prolonged use   72
    Pharmacological treatment of alcohol dependence   72
Sedatives and hypnotics   73
    Introduction   73
    Behavioural effects   73
    Mechanism of action   74

Tolerance and withdrawal 74
Neurobiological adaptations to prolonged use 75
Tobacco 75
Introduction 75
Behavioural effects 75
Mechanism of action 76
Tolerance and withdrawal 77
Pharmacological treatment of nicotine dependence 78
Opioids 79
Introduction 79
Behavioural effects 79
Mechanism of action 80
Tolerance and withdrawal 80
Neurobiological adaptations to prolonged use 81
Pharmacological treatment of opioid dependence 81
Cannabinoids 84
Introduction 84
Behavioural effects 85
Mechanism of action 86
Tolerance and withdrawal 87
Neurobiological adaptations to prolonged use 88
Cocaine (hydrochloride and crack) 89
Introduction 89
Behavioural effects 89
Mechanism of action 89
Tolerance and withdrawal 91
Neurobiological adaptations to prolonged use 91
Pharmacological treatment of cocaine dependence 92
Amphetamines 93
Introduction 93
Behavioural effects 94
Mechanism of action 95
Tolerance and withdrawal 95
Neurobiological adaptations to prolonged use 96
Ecstasy 96
Introduction 96
Behavioural effects 99
Mechanism of action 99
Tolerance and withdrawal 100
Neurobiological adaptations to prolonged use 100
Volatile solvents 100
Introduction 100
Behavioural effects 101
Mechanism of action 102

Tolerance and withdrawal 103
Neurobiological adaptations to prolonged use 103
Hallucinogens 104
Introduction 104
Behavioural effects 105
Mechanism of action 105
Tolerance and withdrawal 105
Neurobiological adaptations to prolonged use 106
Summary 106

Chapter 5. Genetic Basis of Substance Dependence **125**
Introduction 125
Family, twin and adoption studies: estimations of heritability 127
Identifying chromosomal locations of interest: linkage studies 127
Candidate gene approach 128
Animal studies 128
Genetics of tobacco dependence 130
Heritability of tobacco dependence 130
Tobacco dependence and linkage studies 131
Candidate genes for tobacco dependence 131
Genetics of alcohol dependence 132
Heritability of alcohol dependence 132
Alcohol dependence and linkage studies 133
Candidate genes for alcohol dependence 134
Genetics of opioid dependence 136
Heritability of opioid dependence 136
Opioid dependence and linkage studies 136
Candidate genes for opioid dependence 136
Genetics of the combined risk of dependence on tobacco, alcohol,
opioids and other psychoactive substances 138
Heritability of substance dependence 138
Linkage studies of substance dependence 139
Candidate genes involved in substance dependence 140
Confounding issues in linkage and candidate gene studies 147
Environment 147
Genetice heterogeneity 147
Phenotype 148
Comorbidity 148
Methodological issues 148
Future directions 149
Social and cultural aspects 150
Risk factors and protective factors for dependence: an overview 150
Summary 151

Chapter 6. Concurrent Disorders **169**
Introduction 169
Hypotheses that may explain the observed comorbidity 170
Schizophrenia 171
    Tobacco smoking and schizophrenia 171
    Psychostimulant (cocaine and amphetamine) dependence and
        schizophrenia 174
    Alcohol use and schizophrenia 176
    Neurobiological interactions between schizophrenia and the effects
        of psychoactive substances 176
Depression 180
    Tobacco smoking and depression 181
    Psychostimulant dependence and depression 182
    Alcohol use and depression 183
    Neurobiological interactions between depression and the effects
        of psychoactive substances 184
Discussion and conclusions 188

Chapter 7. Ethical Issues in Neuroscience Research on Substance
Dependence Treatment and Prevention **209**
Introduction 209
Types of research on neuroscience of substance dependence 209
    Animal experiments 209
    Epidemiological research on substance dependence 209
    Experimental studies in humans 210
    Clinical trials of pharmacotherapy for substance dependence 210
    Trials of pharmacotherapies to prevent substance dependence 211
Approach to ethical analysis 211
    Principles of biomedical ethics 216
    Human rights 217
Ethics of animal experimentation in neuroscience research 218
Ethical principles in human biomedical research 219
    Independent ethical review of risks and benefits 219
    Informed consent 220
    Recruitment of subjects 220
    Privacy and confidentiality 221
Emerging ethical issues in neuroscience research 222
    Research on vulnerable persons 222
    Are substance dependent people vulnerable persons? 223
    Provocation studies 223
Ethical issues in epidemiological research on substance dependence 224
Ethical issues in clinical trials of pharmacological treatments
    for substance dependence 225
    Trial design 225

Distributive justice   226
Conflicts of interest   226
Trials of preventive pharmacological interventions for substance
    dependence   227
Early intervention studies   227
Preventive use of drug immunotherapies   229
Implications of neuroscience research for models of substance
    dependence   231
Implications of neuroscience research for the treatment of substance
    dependence   232
Access to treatment   232
Legally coerced treatment   232
Summary and conclusions   235

Chapter 8. Conclusion and Implications for Public Health Policy   **241**
Introduction   241
Advances in the neuroscience of psychoactive substance use and
    dependence and their implications   241
Potential advances in policy, prevention and treatment   243
Ethical issues in the application of neuroscience findings   244
Implications for public health policy   247
Conclusion   248

Index   **251**

Foreword

Substance use and dependence cause a significant burden to individuals and societies throughout the world. The World Health Report 2002 indicated that 8.9% of the total burden of disease comes from the use of psychoactive substances. The report showed that tobacco accounted for 4.1%, alcohol 4%, and illicit drugs 0.8% of the burden of disease in 2000. Much of the burden attributable to substance use and dependence is the result of a wide variety of health and social problems, including HIV/AIDS, which is driven in many countries by injecting drug use.

This neuroscience report is the first attempt by WHO to provide a comprehensive overview of the biological factors related to substance use and dependence by summarizing the vast amount of knowledge gained in the last 20-30 years. The report highlights the current state of knowledge of the mechanisms of action of different types of psychoactive substances, and explains how the use of these substances can lead to the development of dependence syndrome.

Though the focus is on brain mechanisms, the report nevertheless addresses the social and environmental factors which influence substance use and dependence. It also deals with neuroscience aspects of interventions and, in particular, the ethical implications of new biological intervention strategies.

The various health and social problems associated with use of and dependence on tobacco, alcohol and illicit substances require greater attention by the public health community and appropriate policy responses are needed to address these problems in different societies. Many gaps remain to be filled in our understanding of the issues related to substance use and dependence but this report shows that we already know a great deal about the nature of these problems that can be used to shape policy responses.

This is an important report and I recommend it to a wide audience of health care professionals, policy makers, scientists and students.

LEE Jong-wook
Director General
World Health Organization

Acknowledgements

The World Health Organization acknowledges with thanks the many authors, reviewers, consultants and WHO staff members whose expertise made this report possible. Franco Vaccarino of the Centre for Addiction and Mental Health and the University of Toronto, Toronto, Canada, was the principal editor for the report, with the assistance of Susan Rotzinger from the Centre for Addiction and Mental Health. The opening and closing chapters were written by Robin Room of the Centre for Social Research on Alcohol and Drugs, University of Stockholm, Stockholm, Sweden, with contributions from Isidore Obot and Maristela Monteiro of the Department of Mental Health and Substance Abuse, WHO.

Special acknowledgement is made to the following individuals who contributed reviews that formed the basis for the final report:

Helena M. T. Barros, Federal University of Medical Sciences Foundation, Porto Alegre, Brazil; Lucy Carter, Institute for Molecular Bioscience, University of Queensland, St Lucia, Queensland, Australia; David Collier, Section of Genetics, Institute of Psychiatry, London, England; Gaetano Di Chiara, Department of Toxicology, University of Cagliari, Cagliari, Italy; Patricia Erickson, Centre for Addiction and Mental Health, Toronto, Ontario, Canada; Sofia Gruskin, Department of Population and International Health, Harvard University School of Public Health, Boston, MA, USA; Wayne Hall, Institute for Molecular Bioscience, University of Queensland, St Lucia, Queensland, Australia; Jack Henningfield, Johns Hopkins University School of Medicine, and Pinney Associates, Bethesda, MD, USA; Kathleen M. Kantak, Department of Psychology, Boston University, Boston, MA, USA; Brigitte Kieffer, Ecole Supérieure de Biotechnologie de Strasbourg, Illkirch, France; Harald Klingemann, School of Social Work, University of Applied Sciences, Berne, Switzerland; Mary Jeanne Kreek, Laboratory of the Biology of Addictive Diseases, Rockefeller University, New York, NY, USA; Sture Liljequist, Division of Drug Dependence Research, Karolinska Institute, Stockholm, Sweden; Rafael Maldonado, Laboratory of Neuropharmacology, Pompeu Fabre University, Barcelona, Spain; Athina Markou, Scripps Research Institute, La Jolla, CA, USA; Gina Morato, Federal University of Santa Catarina, Santa Catarina, Brazil; Katherine Morley, Institute for Molecular Bioscience, University of Queensland, St Lucia, Queensland, Australia; Karen Plafker, Department of Population and International Health, Harvard University

School of Public Health, Boston, MA, USA; Andrey Ryabinin, Oregon Health Science University, Portland, OR, USA; Allison Smith, Department of Population and International Health, Harvard University School of Public Health, Boston, MA, USA; Rachel Tyndale, Department of Pharmacology, University of Toronto, Toronto, Ontario, Canada; Claude Uehlinger, Psychosocial Centre of Fribourg, Fribourg, Switzerland; Franco Vaccarino, Centre for Addiction and Mental Health, Toronto, Ontario, Canada; Frank Vocci, National Institute on Drug Abuse, Bethesda, MD, USA; David Walsh, National Institute on Media and the Family, Minneapolis, MN, USA.

Thanks are also due to the international scientific organizations that provided documents reflecting their views on research on and treatment of substance dependence. Notable among these are the College on Problems of Drug Dependence (CPDD) and the International Society of Addiction Medicine (ISAM).

Many individuals participated in the various consultations held to discuss the project. The first such consultation which took place in New Orleans, LA, USA, in 2000 was attended by experts representing several international organizations, including the CPDD, the International Society for Biomedical Research on Alcoholism (ISBRA), the National Institute on Drug Abuse (NIDA), the National Institute of Mental Health (NIMH) and some key scientists in the field (see list below). The second consultation was held in Mexico in June 2002 during which a draft report was presented and discussed extensively. Thanks are due to the following for their various contributions to the report:

Hector Velasquez Ayala, Faculty of Psychology, Universidad Nacional Autonoma de Mexico, Mexico City, Mexico; Floyd Bloom, Scripps Research Institute, La Jolla, CA, USA; Dennis Choi, Department of Neurology, Washington University School of Medicine, St Louis, MO, USA; Patricia Di Ciano, University of Cambridge, Cambridge, England; Linda Cottler, Department of Psychiatry, Washington University, St. Louis, MO, USA; Nady El-Guebaly, Faculty of Medicine, University of Calgary, Calgary, Alberta, Canada; Humberto Estanol, National Council Against Addictions of Mexico, Mexico City, Mexico; Hamid Ghodse, St. George's Hospital Medical School, London, UK; Steven Hyman, National Institute of Mental Health, Bethesda, MD, USA; Mark Jordan, Nyon, Switzerland; Humberto Juarez, National Council Against Addictions of Mexico, Mexico City, Mexico; Michael Kuhar, Division of Pharmacology, Emory University, Atlanta, GA, USA; Stan Kutcher, Canadian Institutes of Health Research, Ottawa, Ontario, Canada; Michel Le Moal, National Institute of Health and Medical Research, Bordeaux, France; Scott MacDonald, Centre for Addiction and Mental Health, Toronto, Ontario, Canada; Guillermina Natera, National Institute of Psychiatry, Mexico City, Mexico; Raluca Popovici, Pinney Associates, Bethesda, MD, USA; Linda Porrino, Wake Forest University School of Medicine, NC, Winston-Salem, USA; David Roberts, Wake Forest University School of Medicine, NC, Winston-Salem, USA; Robin Room, Centre for Social Research on Alcohol and Drugs,

University of Stockholm, Stockholm, Sweden; Christine A. Rose, Pinney Associates, Bethesda, MD, USA; Martin Stafstrom, Malmo University Hospital, Lund University, Lund, Sweden; Julie Staley, Department of Psychiarty, Yale University School of Medicine, New Haven, CT, USA; Howard Stead, Laboratory and Scientific Section, United Nations Office on Drugs and Crime, Vienna, Austria; Boris Tabakoff, University of Colorado School of Medicine, Boulder, CO, USA; Ambros Uchtenhagen, Institute for Research on Addiction, Zurich, Switzerland; George Uhl, Johns Hopkins University School of Medicine, Baltimore, MD, USA; Nora Volkow, Brookhaven National Laboratory, New York, NY, USA; Helge Waal, Oslo, Norway; Roy Wise, National Institute on Drug Abuse, Bethesda, MD, USA. WHO is also grateful to Victor Preedy, King's College, University of London, London, who provided a technical review of the final draft of the document.

Grateful thanks are due to the U.K. Department for International Development (DFID), the Belgian Government, and the Institute of Neurosciences, Mental Health and Addiction of the Canadian Institutes of Health Research for their financial contributions to the project.

The project leading to this report was initiated by Maristela Monteiro, who also directed all activities related to its preparation, review and publication. Isidore Obot coordinated the editing and production of the report. Particular thanks are due to Derek Yach and Benedetto Saraceno who provided leadership for the project and contributed comments on various drafts. Thanks are also due to the following staff of the Department of Mental Health and Substance Abuse for their contributions to the project: Vladimir Poznyak, José Bertolote, and Shekhar Saxena. The report also benefited from the inputs of the following former and current WHO staff who assisted in different capacities: Caroline Allsopp, Alexander Capron, Joann Duffil, Kelvin Khow, Tess Narciso, Mylene Schreiber, Raquel Shaw Moxam, and Tokuo Yoshida.

This report has been produced within the framework of the mental health Global Action Programme (mhGAP) of the Department of Mental Health and Substance Abuse, World Health Organization, under the direction of Dr Benedetto Saraceno.

List of Background Papers and Contributors

Helena M. T. Barros, The basic psychopharmacology of the addictive substances.

David A Collier, The genetics of heroin abuse.

Michael J. Kuhar, Views of the College on Problems of Drug Dependence regarding advances in research on drug abuse.

Gaetano Di Chiara, Psychobiology of drug addiction.

Patricia G Erickson, Responding to substance dependence from an integrated public health perspective.

Wayne Hall and Lucy Carter, Ethical issues in trialing and using cocaine vaccines to treat and prevent cocaine dependence.

Wayne Hall, Lucy Carter and Katherine Morley, Ethical issues in neuroscience research on addiction.

Sofia Gruskin, Karen Plafker & Allison Smith, A human rights framework for preventing psychoactive substance use by youth, in the context of urbanization.

Jack E Henningfield, Neurobiology of tobacco dependence.

Nady El-Guebaly, Views of the International Society of Addiction Medicine (ISAM).

Kathleen M. Kantak, Pre-clinical and clinical studies with the cocaine vaccine.

Brigitte L. Kieffer, Neural basis of addictive behaviours: role of the endogenous opioid system.

Harald Klingemann, Cultural and social aspects of drug dependence.

Mary Jeanne Kreek, The efficacy of methadone and levomethadyl acetate.

Sture Liljequist, The neurochemical basis of craving and abstinence to substance abuse.

Rafael Maldonado, Recent advances in the neurobiology of cannabinoid dependence.

Athina Markou, Comorbidity of drug abuse with mental illness provides insights into the neurobiological abnormalities that may mediate these psychiatric disorders.

Gina Morato, Biological basis for ethanol tolerance in animals and implications for ethanol dependence.

Andrey E. Ryabinin, Genetics and neuroscience of alcohol abuse and dependence: contributions from animal models

Rachel Tyndale, Genetics of alcohol and tobacco use in humans.

Claude Uehlinger, Motivation aux changements de comportements addictifs.

Frank J. Vocci, Buprenorphine as a treatment for opiate dependence.

David Walsh, Slipping under the radar: advertising and the mind.

Abbreviations

2-DG	2-deoxyglucose
ADH	alcohol dehydrogenase
ADHD	attention deficit hyperactivity disorder
AIDS	Acquired Immunodeficiency Syndrome
ALDH2	aldehyde dehydrogenase
AMPA	α-amino3-hydroxy-5-methyl-isoxazole-4-propionate
ASPD	antisocial personality disorder
ATS	amphetamine-type stimulants
cAMP	cyclic adenosine monophosphate
CCK	cholecystokinin
COMT	catechol-O-methyltransferase
CRA	comparative risk analysis
CREB	cAMP response element binding protein
CRF	corticotropin-releasing factor (CRF)
CYP26	Cytochrome P-450 RA1
CYP2D6	Cytochrome P-450 2D6
CYP2E1	Cytochrome P-450 2E1
DALY	disability-adjusted life years
DBH	dopamine beta hydroxylase
DMT	dimethyltryptamine
DNA	deoxyribonucleic acid
DOM	dimethoxy-4-methylamphetamine
DRD1	dopamine receptor D1
DRD3	dopamine receptor D3
DRD4	dopamine receptor D4
DRD5	dopamine receptor D5
DSM-IV	Diagnostic and Statistical Manual of Mental Disorders- Fourth Edition

EMCDDA	European Monitoring Centre for Drugs and Drug Addiction
ESPAD	European School Survey Project on Alcohol and Other Drugs
EEG	electroencephalography
FDA	United States Food and Drug Administration
FDG	fluorodeoxyglucose
fMRI	functional magnetic resonance imaging
GABA	γ-aminobutyric acid
GBD	Global Burden of Disease
HIV	Human Immunodeficiency Virus
ICD-10	Tenth Revision of the International Statistical Classification of Diseases and Related Health Problems
IDU	injecting drug use
LAAM	Levo-alpha-acetyl-methadol
LSA	d-lysergic acid amine
LSD	lysergic acid diethylamide
MAO	monoamine oxidase
MAOI	monoamine oxidase inhibitor
MDA	methylenedioxyamphetamine
MDMA	3,4-methylenedioxymethamphetamine
MET	motivational enhancement therapy
MRI	magnetic resonance imaging
mRNA	messenger ribonucleic acid
nAChR	nicotinic acetylcholine receptor
NHSDA	National Household Survey on Drug Abuse
NIDA	National Institute on Drug Abuse
NMDA	N-methyl-D-aspartate
NPY	neuropeptide Y
PCP	phencyclidine
PET	positron emission tomography
PMA	paramethoxyamphetamine
QTL	quantitative trait loci
SACENDU	South African Community Epidemiology Network on Drug Use
SPECT	single photon emission computed tomography
SSRI	serotonin selective reuptake inhibitors
SUD	substance use disorders

TH	tyrosine hydroxylase
THC	tetrahydrocannabinol
TMA	trimethoxyamphetamine
TPH	tryptophan hydroxylase
UDHR	Universal Declaration of Human Rights
UNDCP	United Nations International Drug Control Programme
UNODC	United Nations Office on Drugs and Crime
UNODCCP	United Nations Office for Drug Control and Crime Prevention
USDHHS	United States Department of Health and Human Services
VTA	ventral tegmental area
WHO	World Health Organization
WMA	World Medical Association

CHAPTER 1

Introduction

This report describes our current understanding of the neuroscience of psychoactive substance use and dependence. It draws on the explosive growth in knowledge in this area in recent decades, which has transformed our understanding of the biochemical action of psychoactive substances, and contributed new insights into why many people use them, and why some use them to the extent of causing harm or of becoming dependent on them.

Structure of the report

The report is divided into eight chapters. The present introductory chapter is intended to provide the context and background for the report. Chapter 2 provides a brief overview of basic neuroanatomy, neurobiology and neurochemistry. Chapter 3 presents the "biobehavioural" view of dependence, which is based on both learning theory and knowledge of the brain's functions. Chapter 4 discusses the pharmacology and behavioural effects of different classes of psychoactive substances, a branch of science also known as psychopharmacology. In Chapters 2–4 we consider neurobiological processes which are to a large extent the common heritage of all human beings. In Chapter 5, we turn to genetic studies, which focus instead on the differentiations that may exist between humans in their genetic heritage. The chapter reviews the evidence for a genetic contribution to substance dependence, and compares the interaction of genetics and environmental factors in the development and maintenance of dependence. Chapter 6 considers the neuroscientific evidence on specific interconnections between substance use and mental disorders, focusing particularly on schizophrenia and depression. The frame of reference changes again in Chapter 7, which is concerned with ethical issues in research, treatment and prevention of substance use disorders, and in particular how these issues may apply to neuroscientific research and its applications. Chapter 8 deals with the public health implications of neuroscience research and ends with specific recommendations for policy.

Psychoactive substances and their sociolegal status

Psychoactive substances, more commonly known as psychoactive drugs, are substances that, when taken, have the ability to change an individual's consciousness, mood or thinking processes. As later chapters will explain, advances in neuroscience have given us a much better understanding of the physical processes by which these substances act. Psychoactive substances act in the brain on mechanisms that exist normally to regulate the functions of mood, thoughts, and motivations. In this report, our emphasis will be on alcohol and other hypnotics and sedatives, nicotine, opioids, cannabis, cocaine, amphetamines and other stimulants, hallucinogens, and psychoactive inhalants.

Use of these substances is defined into three categories according to their sociolegal status. First, many of the substances are used as medications. Western and other systems of medicine have long recognized the usefulness of these substances as medications in relieving pain, promoting either sleep or wakefulness, and relieving mood disorders. Currently, most psychoactive medications are restricted to use under a doctor's orders, through a prescription system. In many countries, as much as one-third of all prescriptions written are for such medications. An example of this is the use of the stimulant methylphenidate to treat childhood attention deficit hyperactivity disorder (ADHD), which will be discussed in Chapter 4. As described in Chapter 6, some of the substances are also often used as "self-medications" to relieve distress from mental or physical disorders, or to alleviate the side-effects of other medications.

A second category of use is illegal, or illicit, use. Under three international conventions (see Box 1.1), most nations have bound themselves to outlaw trade in and non-medical use of opiates, cannabis, hallucinogens, cocaine and many other stimulants, and many hypnotics and sedatives. In addition to this list, countries or local jurisdictions often add their own prohibited substances, e.g. alcoholic beverages and various inhalants.

Despite these prohibitions, illicit use of psychoactive substances is fairly widespread in many societies, particularly among young adults, the usual purpose being to enjoy or benefit from the psychoactive properties of the substance. The fact that it is illegal may also add an attractive *frisson,* and thus strengthen the identification of users with an alienated subculture.

The third category of use is legal, or licit, consumption, for whatever purpose the consumer chooses. These purposes may be quite varied, and are not necessarily connected with the psychoactive properties of the substance. For instance, an alcoholic beverage can be a source of nutrition, of heating or cooling the body, or of thirst-quenching; or it may serve a symbolic purpose in a round of toasting or as a sacrament. However, whatever the purpose of use, the psychoactive properties of the substance inevitably accompany its use.

The most widely used psychoactive substances are the following: caffeine and related stimulants, commonly used in the form of coffee, tea and many soft drinks; nicotine, currently most often used by smoking tobacco cigarettes; and alcoholic beverages, which come in many forms, including beer, wine

BOX 1.1

United Nations drug control conventions

The three major international drug control treaties are mutually supportive and complementary. An important purpose of the first two treaties is to codify internationally applicable control measures in order to ensure the availability of narcotic drugs and psychotropic substances for medical and scientific purposes, and to prevent their diversion into illicit channels. They also include general provisions on illicit trafficking and drug abuse.

Single Convention on Narcotic Drugs, 1961

This Convention recognizes that effective measures against abuse of narcotic drugs require coordinated and international action. There are two forms of intervention and control that work together. First, it seeks to limit the possession, use, trade in, distribution, import, export, manufacture and production of drugs exclusively to medical and scientific purposes. Second, it combats drug trafficking through international cooperation to deter and discourage drug traffickers.

Convention on Psychotropic Substances, 1971

The Convention noted with concern the public health and social problems resulting from the abuse of certain psychotropic substances and was determined to prevent and combat abuse of such substances and the illicit traffic which it gives rise to. The Convention establishes an international control system for psychotropic substances by responding to the diversification and expansion of the spectrum of drugs of abuse, and introduced controls over a number of synthetic drugs according to their abuse potential on the one hand and their therapeutic value on the other.

United Nations Convention against Illicit Traffic in Narcotic Drugs and Psychotropic Substances, 1988

This Convention sets out a comprehensive, effective and operative international treaty that was directed specifically against illicit traffic and that considered various aspects of the problem as a whole, in particular those aspects not envisaged in the existing treaties in the field of narcotic drugs and psychotropic substances. The Convention provides comprehensive measures against drug trafficking, including provisions against money laundering and the diversion of precursor chemicals. It provides for international cooperation through, for example, extradition of drug traffickers, controlled deliveries and transfer of proceedings.

Source: United Nations Office for Drug Control and Crime Prevention (available on the Internet at http://www.odccp.org/odccp/un_treaties_and_resolutions.html).

Note: In October 2002 the United Nations Office for Drug Control and Crime Prevention (ODCCP) changed its name to the United Nations Office on Drugs and Crime (ODC).

and distilled spirits. Because the use of caffeinated substances is relatively unproblematic, it is not further considered in this report. While inhalants are also widely available, they are mostly used for psychoactive purposes by those below the age of easy access to alcohol, tobacco and other psychoactive substances.

While there is a clear rationale for a separate legal status for medications, the rationale for the distinction between substances that are under international control and those that are not is more problematic. The substances which are included in the international conventions reflect historical understandings in particular cultural settings about what should be viewed as uniquely dangerous or alien. Some psychopharmacologists or epidemiologists today, for instance, would argue that alcohol is inherently no less dangerous or harmful than the drugs included in the international conventions. Moreover, as discussed below, dependence on nicotine in tobacco is associated with more death and ill-health than dependence on other psychoactive substances. As will be seen in the chapters which follow, the growing knowledge of the neuroscience of psychoactive substance use has emphasized the commonalities in action which span the three sociolegal statuses into which the substances are divided.

Global use of psychoactive substances

Tobacco

Many types of tobacco products are consumed throughout the world but the most popular form of nicotine use is cigarette smoking. Smoking is a ubiquitous activity: more than 5500 billion cigarettes are manufactured annually and there are 1.2 billion smokers in the world. This number is expected to increase to 2 billion by 2030 (Mackay & Eriksen, 2002; World Bank, 1999). Smoking is spreading rapidly in developing countries and among women. Currently, 50% of men and 9% of women in developing countries smoke, as compared with 35% of men and 22% of women in developed countries. China, in particular, contributes significantly to the epidemic in developing countries. Indeed, the per capita consumption of cigarettes in Asia and the Far East is higher than in other parts of the world, with the Americas and eastern Europe following closely behind (Mackay & Eriksen, 2002).

A conceptual framework for describing the different stages of cigarette smoking epidemics in different regions of the world has been proposed by Lopez, Collishaw & Piha (1994). In this model, there are four stages of the epidemic on a continuum ranging from low prevalence of smoking to a stage in which about one-third of deaths among men in a particular country are attributable to smoking. In Stage 1, less than 20% of the men and a considerably lower percentage of women smoke. Available epidemiological data show that many countries in sub-Saharan Africa fall into this category

4

although smoking is increasing in this region. It has been shown that annual per capita consumption of cigarettes there is less than 100 (Corrao et al., 2000). There is widespread use of other tobacco products (such as snuff and chewing tobacco) in some countries, but the extent of adverse health consequences of use of these forms of tobacco is still not clear.

In Stage 2 of the epidemic, about 50% of the men smoke and there is an increasing percentage of women smokers. This is the case in China and Japan, and in some countries in northern Africa and Latin America. In contrast, Stage 3 describes a situation in which there is a noticeable decrease in smoking among men and women but there is increased mortality from smoking-related diseases. Some countries in Latin America and eastern and southern Europe fall into this category. A final stage is marked by decreasing smoking prevalence, a peaking of deaths from tobacco-related disease among men (accounting for about one-third of the total), and a continued increase in deaths from tobacco-related disease among women. This is currently the case in Australia, Canada, the USA, and western Europe. Table 1.1 shows the rates of smoking for males and females and per capita consumption of cigarettes in selected countries with data from all categories of smokers.

Table 1.1 Prevalence of smoking among adults and youths in selected countries

| Country | Annual per capita consumption of cigarettes | Prevalence of smoking (%) | | | |
| | | Adults | | Youths | |
		Males	Females	Males	Females
Argentina	1495	46.8	34.4	25.7	30.0
Bolivia	274	42.7	18.1	31.0	22.0
Chile	1202	26.0	18.3	34.0	43.4
China	1791	66.9	4.2	14.0	7.0
Ghana	161	28.4	3.5	16.2	17.3
Indonesia	1742	59.0	3.7	38.0	5.3
Jordan	1832	48.0	10.0	27.0	13.4
Kenya	200	66.8	31.9	16.0	10.0
Malawi	123	20.0	9.0	18.0	15.0
Mexico	754	51.2	18.4	27.9	16.0
Nepal	619	48.0	29.0	12.0	6.0
Peru	1849	41.5	15.7	22.0	15.0
Poland	2061	44.0	25.0	29.0	20.0
Singapore	1230	26.9	3.1	10.5	7.5
Sri Lanka	374	25.7	1.7	13.7	5.8
USA	2255	25.7	21.5	27.5	24.2

Source: Mackay & Eriksen, 2002.

Alcohol

Alcohol and tobacco are similar in several ways: both are legal substances, both are widely available in most parts of the world, and both are marketed aggressively by transnational corporations that target young people in advertising and promotion campaigns. According to the Global status report on alcohol (WHO, 1999) and as shown in Fig. 1.1 below, the level of consumption of alcohol has declined in the past twenty years in developed countries but is increasing in developing countries, especially in the Western Pacific Region where the annual per capita consumption among adults ranges from 5 to 9 litres of pure alcohol, and also in countries of the former Soviet Union (WHO, 1999). To a great extent the rise in the rate of alcohol consumption in developing countries is driven by rates in Asian countries. The level of consumption of alcohol is much lower in the African, Eastern Mediterranean, and South-East Asia Regions.

There is a long tradition of research on the epidemiology of alcohol use in developed countries and we have learnt much about the distribution and determinants of drinking in different populations. For many years, researchers focused on average volume of alcohol consumption in determining the level of drinking in a particular country. Using production or sales data from official records has tended to underestimate consumption, especially in developing countries, where unrecorded consumption of locally brewed beverages is significant. In order to improve the measurement of per

Fig. 1.1 Annual per capita alcohol consumption among adults aged 15 years or more

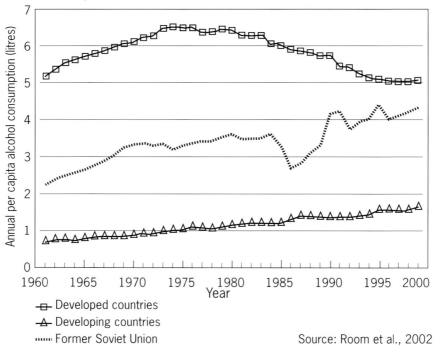

Source: Room et al., 2002

capita consumption, WHO has sponsored research projects in four countries (Brazil, China, India and Nigeria) to determine the level of unrecorded consumption in these countries.

It is expected that more precise estimates of alcohol use will lead to better understanding of the association between use and problems. In this regard the comparative risk analysis (CRA) project of WHO is noteworthy. The CRA uses per capita consumption data together with patterns of drinking to link use to disease burden (Rehm et al., 2002). A patterns approach to alcohol consumption assumes that the way in which alcohol is consumed is closely linked to disease outcome. Drinking during meals, for example, is associated with less risk of problems than drinking during fiestas or drinking in public places. In the CRA analysis, four pattern values have been developed, with 1 as the least hazardous and 4 as the most detrimental. At pattern value 1 there are few occasions of heavy drinking, and drinking is often done with meals, while pattern value 4 is characterized by many heavy drinking occasions and drinking outside meals. Table 1.2 shows the pattern values for different WHO regions, with each region divided into at least two subregions. Values for some regions are based on limited aggregate data and are only indicative of the pattern of drinking in these regions.

In the African Region, there was a steady rise in per capita consumption in the 1970s and a decline beginning from the early 1980s. However, the pattern of drinking has tended towards the higher levels with men in most countries drinking at pattern value 3 of the CRA estimates. This is the case for Gabon, Ghana, Kenya, Lesotho, Senegal, and South Africa, for example. However, it is only in very few countries (e.g. Zambia and Zimbabwe) that the pattern value is 4. The detrimental pattern of drinking in many sub-Saharan countries has been shown in several surveys (e.g. Mustonen, Beukes & Du Preez, 2001; Obot, 2001). In most countries women drink much less than men and in some of these countries the abstention rate for older women is very high.

In the Region of the Americas, heavy drinking (i.e. drinking five or more drinks on at least one occasion in the past month) is a common drinking behaviour among young people. Both alcohol consumption and heavy drinking are reported much more often among males than females in both Mexico and the USA (WHO, 1999; Medina-Mora et al., 2001). Though Mexico has a relatively low per capita consumption of alcohol, the pattern value for that country is 4. This is because there is high frequency of heavy drinking, especially by young people, on fiesta occasions.

Heavy drinking among young people is also common in the Western Pacific Region. Though there has been some decline in the rates of drinking in Australia and New Zealand, 50% of male youths in these countries as well as in South Korea and Japan often drink to intoxication. Table 1.2 shows abstention rates for males and females, annual per capita consumption in the general population and among drinkers, and patterns of drinking in WHO subregions.

Table 1.2 Estimated rate of abstention from alcohol and patterns of hazardous drinking in selected WHO subregions[a]

WHO subregion	Rate of abstention from alcohol (%)		Annual per capita consumption of alcohol in the general population (litres)	Annual per capita consumption of alcohol among drinkers (litres)	Pattern of hazardous drinking[b]
	Males	Females			
African Region – D (e.g. Algeria, Nigeria)	53	73	3.6	9.7	2.3
African Region – E (e.g. Ethiopia, South Africa)	44	70	7.1	16.7	3.2
Region of the Americas – A (e.g. Canada, Cuba, USA)	27	42	9.7	14.8	2.0
Region of the Americas – B (e.g. Brazil, Mexico)	25	47	8.6	12.1	3.1
Region of the Americas – D (e.g. Bolivia, Peru)	26	40	5.8	8.7	3.1
South-East Asia Region – B (e.g. Indonesia, Thailand)	65	91	3.3	15.0	2.5
South-East Asia Region – D (e.g. Bangladesh, India)	74	96	2.0	12.5	3.0
European Region – A (e.g. France, Germany, United Kingdom)	10	19	13.0	15.2	1.3
European Region – B1 (e.g. Bulgaria, Poland, Turkey)	22	43	9.7	14.4	2.9
European Region – B2 (e.g. Armenia, Azerbaijan, Tajikistan)	46	67	4.3	9.9	3.0
European Region – C (e.g. Russian Federation, Ukraine)	11	19	14.8	17.4	3.6
Eastern Mediterranean Region – B (e.g. Iran, Saudi Arabia)	82	96	1.1	10.0	2.0
Eastern Mediterranean Region – D (e.g. Afghanistan, Pakistan)	83	99	0.8	8.9	2.0
Western Pacific Region – A (e.g. Australia, Japan)	13	23	8.7	10.6	1.0
Western Pacific Region – B (e.g. China, Philippines, Viet Nam)	16	75	4.9	8.6	2.1

Source: Based on estimates for the comparative risk assessment within the WHO Global Burden of Disease 2000 Study (see Rehm et al., 2002).

[a] To aid in cause of death analyses, burden of disease analyses, and comparative risk assessment, the 191 Member States of WHO have been divided into five mortality strata on the basis of their levels of child mortality under 5 years of age and mortality among men aged 15–59 years. The mortality strata are defined as follows: A: very low child, very low adult; B: low child, low adult; C: low child, high adult; D: high child, high adult; E: high child, very high adult.

[b] Scored on a level of 1–4, where level 1 is the least hazardous and level 4 is the most detrimental.

Illicit use of controlled substances

Data from the United Nations Office on Drugs and Crime (ODC) show large-scale seizures of cocaine, heroin, cannabis and amphetamine-type stimulants in different parts of the world. Availability of cocaine, heroin and cannabis depends on the level of cultivation in source countries and on the success or failure of trafficking organizations. However, even with increased levels of law enforcement activities, there always seems to be enough drugs available to users.

According to ODC estimates (UNODCCP, 2002), about 185 million people make illicit use of one type of illicit substance or another. Table 1.3 shows that cannabis is consumed by the largest number of illicit drug users, followed by amphetamines, cocaine and the opiates.

Illicit drug use is a predominantly male activity, much more so than cigarette smoking and alcohol consumption. Drug use is also more prevalent among young people than in older age groups. Several national and multi-national surveys have provided data on drug use in different groups. For example, in the USA, the National Household Survey on Drug Abuse (NHSDA) has served as a source of useful information on drug use in the general population, and the Monitoring the Future project provides data on drug use by young people in secondary schools. The European School Survey Project on Alcohol and Other Drugs (ESPAD), an initiative of the Council of Europe, has become a data source on youth drug use for many European countries. The European Monitoring Centre for Drugs and Drug Addiction (EMCDDA) also provides regular data on drug use (including hazardous methods of use, such as injecting drug use (IDU)) in European countries. While national surveys of youth and adults are held on a regular basis in some countries, reliable data on drug use is generally lacking in most developing countries.

Table 1.3 Annual prevalence of global illicit drug use over the period 1998–2001

	All illicit drugs	Cannabis	Amphetamine-type stimulants		Cocaine	All opiates	Heroin
			Amphe-tamines	Ecstasy			
Number of users (in millions)	185.0	147.4	33.4	7.0	13.4	12.9	9.20
Proportion of global population (%)	3.1	2.5	0.6	0.1	0.2	0.2	0.15
Proportion of population 15 years and above (%)	4.3	3.5	0.8	0.2	0.3	0.3	0.22

Source: UNODCCP, 2002.

Projects such as the South African Community Epidemiology Network on Drug Use (SACENDU) and its related regional network have been started to address this lack of information.

The data in Table 1.3 show that 2.5% of the total global population and 3.5% of people 15 years and above had used cannabis at least once in a year between 1998 and 2001. In many developed countries, for example Canada, the USA and European countries, more than 2% of youths reported heroin use and almost 5% reported smoking cocaine in their lifetime. Indeed, 8% of youths in western Europe and more than 20% of those in the USA have reported using at least one type of illicit drug other than cannabis (UNODCCP, 2002). There is evidence of rapid increases in the use of amphetamine-type stimulants among teenagers in Asia and Europe. Injecting drug use is also a growing phenomenon, with implications for the spread of HIV infections in an increasing number of countries.

The nonmedical use of medications (e.g. benzodiazepines, pain killers, amphetamines, etc.) is known to be fairly common but global statistics are lacking.

Adverse effects of psychoactive substances and their mechanisms of action

In the majority of cases, people use psychoactive substances because they expect to benefit from their use, whether through the experience of pleasure or the avoidance of pain. The benefit is not necessarily gained directly from the psychoactive action of the substance. Someone drinking beer with colleagues may be more motivated by the feeling of fellowship this brings than by the psychoactive effect of the ethanol.

However, the psychoactive effect is nevertheless present, and is usually at least peripherally involved in the decision to use.

In spite of the real or apparent benefits, the use of psychoactive substances also carries with it the potential for harm, whether in the short term or long term. Such harm can result from the cumulative amount of psychoactive substance used, for example, the toxic effect of alcohol in producing liver cirrhosis. Harmful effects can also result from the pattern of use, or from the form or medium in which it is taken (see Fig. 1.2). Pattern of use is of obvious importance – for instance, in the case of deaths due to overdose – not only in terms of the amount on a particular occasion, but also in terms of the context of use (e.g. heroin use accompanied by heavy alcohol use). The form or medium of use may also be crucially important. Most of the adverse health effects of tobacco smoking, for instance, come not from the nicotine itself, but from the tars and carbon monoxide which are released when nicotine is taken in cigarette form. Similarly, the adverse effects from taking the drug by injection are evident in the case of heroin use.

The main harmful effects due to substance use can be divided into four categories (see Fig. 1.2). First there are the chronic health effects. For alcohol this includes liver cirrhosis and a host of other chronic illnesses; for nicotine taken in cigarette form, this includes lung cancer, emphysema and other chronic illnesses. Through the sharing of needles, heroin use by injection is a main vector for transmission of infectious agents such as HIV and hepatitis C virus. Second there are the acute or short-term biological health effects of the substance. Notably, for drugs such as opioids and alcohol, these include overdose. Also classed in this category are the casualties due to the substance's effects on physical coordination, concentration and judgement, in circumstances where these qualities are demanded. Casualties resulting from driving after drinking alcohol or after other drug use feature prominently in this category, but other accidents, suicide and (at least for alcohol) assaults are also included. The third and fourth categories of harmful effects comprise the adverse social consequences of the substance use: acute social problems, such as a break in a relationship or an arrest, and chronic social problems, such as defaults in working life or in family roles. These last categories are important in relation to alcohol and many illicit drugs, but are poorly measured and mostly excluded from measurements of health effects such as in the Global Burden of Disease (GBD).

Fig. 1.2   Mechanisms relating psychoactive substance use to health and social problems

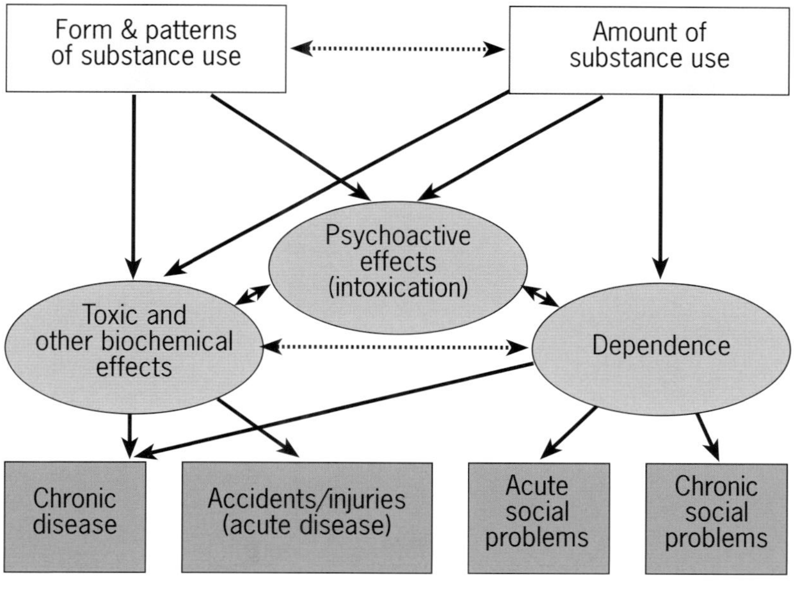

Source: adapted from Babor et al., 2003.

Note that some effects are beneficial rather than toxic, e.g. regular light alcohol use as potentially reducing risk of coronary heart disease.

As earlier noted, the probability of the occurrence of these categories of harmful effects also depends on how much of the substance is used, in what forms, and with what patterns of use. These aspects of use may be thought of as linked to the different kinds of health and social problems by three main mechanisms of action (see Fig. 1.2). One mechanism concerns the direct toxic effects of the substance, either immediate (e.g. poisoning) or cumulative over time (e.g. cirrhosis). A second mechanism concerns the intoxicating or other psychoactive effects of the substance. A traffic accident may result, for instance, from the fact that a car driver is under the influence of sedatives. A retail store employee may be intoxicated at work after using cannabis, and because of this, may be fired by the manager.

The third mechanism concerns dependence on the substance. Substance dependence – or dependence syndrome – is the current technical terminology for the concept of "addiction". At the heart of this concept is the idea that the user's control over and volition about use of the drug has been lost or impaired. The user is no longer choosing to use simply because of the apparent benefits; the use has become habitual, and cravings to reuse mean that the user feels that the habit is no longer under control. The user's dependence is thus seen as propelling further use despite adverse consequences which might have deterred others who are not dependent, from further use.

The link between substance use and harm in a particular case may, of course, involve more than one of the three mechanisms. Benzodiazepines may be involved in a case of suicide, for instance, both through the user's despair over the disruption brought to his or her life by dependence on the drugs, and as the actual means of suicide through overdose. However, the mechanisms can also operate alone. It is important to keep in mind, moreover, that dependence is not the only mechanism potentially linking substance use to health and social harm.

Substance dependence in relation to neuroscience

Social historians have found that the concept of dependence has a specific history, becoming a common idea first in industrialized cultures in the early nineteenth century. The term was initially applied to alcohol and later extended to apply to opioids and other psychoactive substances (Ferentzy, 2001; Room, 2001). In the case of alcohol, the equivalent term became "alcoholism" by the 1950s, while general application of the concept of dependence on tobacco smoking is more recent. While the general idea of dependence is now well established in most of the world, comparative research has found that there is substantial variation between cultures in the applicability and recognition of specific notions and concepts associated with it (Room et al., 1996).

As defined in *The ICD-10 classification of mental and behavioural disorders*, substance use dependence includes six criteria (see Box 1.2); a case which is

---

BOX 1.2

Criteria for substance dependence in ICD-10

Three or more of the following must have been experienced or exhibited together at some time during the previous year:

1. a strong desire or sense of compulsion to take the substance;

2. difficulties in controlling substance-taking behaviour in terms of its onset, termination, or levels of use;

3. a physiological withdrawal state when substance use has ceased or been reduced, as evidenced by: the characteristic withdrawal syndrome for the substance; or use of the same (or a closely related) substance with the intention of relieving or avoiding withdrawal symptoms;

4. evidence of tolerance, such that increased doses of the psychoactive substance are required in order to achieve effects originally produced by lower doses;

5. progressive neglect of alternative pleasures or interests because of psychoactive substance use, increased amount of time necessary to obtain or take the substance or to recover from its effects;

6. persisting with substance use despite clear evidence of overtly harmful consequences, such as harm to the liver through excessive drinking, depressive mood states consequent to heavy substance use, or drug-related impairment of cognitive functioning. Efforts should be made to determine that the user was actually, or could be expected to be, aware of the nature and extent of the harm.

Source: WHO, 1992.

---

positive on at least three of these is diagnosable as "dependent". Some of the criteria are measurable in biological terms, while others are not. The two criteria most easily measured biologically are the third and fourth in Box 1.2: withdrawal – the occurrence of unpleasant physical and psychological symptoms when use of the substance is reduced or discontinued, and tolerance – the idea that increased amounts of the drug are required to achieve the same effect, or that the same amount produces less effect. The other four criteria for dependence include elements of cognition, which are less accessible to biological measurement, but are becoming measurable using improved neuroimaging techniques (see Chapter 3). In the sixth criterion, for instance, the user's knowledge of specific causal connections is to be ascertained, something not accessible to direct biological measurement or to an animal model. The first criterion, "strong desire or sense of compulsion", requires inquiry into the user's self-perceptions, and relates to the idea of craving for the substance. It has proved difficult to agree on a definition of the concept of craving, and the applicability of biological models to the concept remains controversial (Drummond et al., 2000). The criteria for substance dependence in the fourth edition of the *Diagnostic and Statistical Manual (DSM-IV)* of the

---

BOX 1.3

Criteria for substance dependence in DSM-IV

According to the DSM-IV, substance dependence is:

a maladaptive pattern of substance use, leading to clinically significant impairment or distress, as manifested by three (or more) of the following, occurring at any time in the same 12-month period:

1. tolerance, as defined by either of the following:

    (a) a need for markedly increased amounts of the substance to achieve intoxication or desired effect

    (b) markedly diminished effect with continued use of the same amount of the substance

2. withdrawal, as manifested by either of the following:

    (a) the characteristic withdrawal syndrome for the substance

    (b) the same (or a closely related) substance is taken to relieve or avoid withdrawal symptoms

3. the substance is often taken in larger amounts or over a longer period than was intended

4. there is a persistent desire or unsuccessful efforts to cut down or control substance use

5. a great deal of time is spent in activities necessary to obtain the substance (e.g. visiting multiple doctors or driving long distances), use the substance (e.g. chain-smoking), or recover from its effects

6. important social, occupational, or recreational activities are given up or reduced because of substance use

7. the substance use is continued despite knowledge of having a persistent or recurrent physical or psychological problem that is likely to have been caused or exacerbated by the substance (e.g. current cocaine use despite recognition of cocaine-induced depression, or continued drinking despite recognition that an ulcer was made worse by alcohol consumption)

Source: American Psychiatric Association, 1994.

American Psychiatric Association (1994) are similar to those of ICD-10 (Box 1.3), as well as those in many research studies. Other terms used in relation to the use of psychoactive substances are presented in Box 1.4.

A further difficulty is that the diagnostic definition of dependence, as noted above, requires that the case is positive on *any* three of the six criteria. This means that a case can qualify for dependence without being positive on either of the two biologically-measurable criteria; and it means that any case

BOX 1.4

Definitions of terms related to use of psychoactive substances

Harmful use

A pattern of psychoactive substance use that is causing damage to health. The damage may be physical or mental.

Hazardous use

A pattern of psychoactive substance use that increases the risk of harmful consequences for the user.

Intoxication

A condition that follows the administration of a psychoactive substance and results in disturbances in the level of consciousness, cognition, perception, affect, or behaviour, or other psychophysiological functions and responses. The disturbances are related to the acute pharmacological effects of, and learned responses to, the substance and resolve with time, with complete recovery, except where tissue damage or other complications have arisen. Complications may include trauma, inhalation of vomitus, delirium, coma and convulsions, and other medical complications. The nature of these complications depends on the pharmacological class of substance and mode of administration.

Substance abuse

Persistent or sporadic drug use inconsistent with or unrelated to acceptable medical practice. A maladaptive pattern of substance use leading to clinically significant impairment or distress, as manifested by one (or more) of the following: failure to fulfil major role obligations at home, school or work; substance use in situations in which it is physically hazardous; recurrent substance-related legal problems; continued substance use despite having persistent or recurrent social or interpersonal problems exacerbated by the effects of the substance.

Source: adapted from *Lexicon of alcohol and drug terms*, WHO (1994).

qualifying as dependent must be positive on at least one criterion which is not fully biologically measurable.

Thus a continuing difficulty in the neuroscience of psychoactive substances is that, while most of their effects shown in Fig. 1.2 are directly measurable, drug dependence is not, both as it is currently technically defined and as it is generally understood in the wider society.

However, as will be discussed later in the report, neuroscientists have made a number of advances in understanding why humans find using these substances attractive in the first place, what the mechanisms of psychoactivity are, and the neurobiological changes which occur with repeated heavy use of a substance.

The burden of harm to health from psychoactive substance use

No global assessments are available for social harm from substance use (as shown in Fig. 1.2). However, there is now a developing tradition of estimating the contribution of alcohol, tobacco and illicit drug use to the global burden of disease. The first significant attempt at this was in the earlier WHO project on global burden of disease and injury (Murray & Lopez, 1996). Based on a standard of measurement known as disability-adjusted life years (DALYs), estimates of the burden imposed on society due to premature death and years lived with disability were assessed. The global burden of disease (GBD) project showed that tobacco and alcohol were major causes of mortality and disability in developed countries, with the impact of tobacco expected to increase in other parts of the world.

The reliability of the GBD and other estimates of deaths and disease depends on the quality of the data they are based upon. Data used in these analyses were mostly from studies conducted in developed countries (especially the USA and European countries) and a few, often non-representative, surveys in developing countries. The inherent difficulty of assessing the prevalence of substance use and the association between use and problems also means that the burden estimates were highly approximate. However, the GBD provided for the first time a set of global data on the burden of alcohol and other drug use/dependence and there are continuing efforts to come up with more precise estimates of death and disease burden associated with licit and illicit substances.

The 2002 *World health report* (WHO, 2002) includes a new set of estimates for the year 2000 of the burden attributable to tobacco, alcohol and other drugs. These estimates are based on data that are significantly more complete and on more defensible methodologies, and there is no doubt that they will be improved further in future years. Table 1.4 shows the results from the estimates for 2000, in terms of the mortality attributable to each class of substances, as well as a measure of the years of life lost or impaired due to disability (DALYs). Note that estimated protective effects for heart disease from moderate drinking have been subtracted to yield the net negative burden for alcohol (this accounts for the negative number in the table).

Among the 10 leading risk factors in terms of avoidable burden, tobacco was fourth and alcohol fifth for 2000, and both remain high on the list in the projections for 2010 and 2020. The estimated attributable burden in 2000 was 59 million DALYs for tobacco, 58 million for alcohol, and 11 million for illicit drugs. In other words, tobacco and alcohol accounted for 4.1% and 4.0%, respectively, of the burden of ill-health in 2000, while illicit drugs accounted for 0.8%. The burdens attributable to tobacco and alcohol are particularly acute among males in developed countries (mainly North America and Europe), where tobacco, alcohol and illicit drugs account for 17.1%, 14.0% and 2.3%, respectively of the total burden (see Table 1.4).

Table 1.4 Percentage of total global mortality and DALYs attributable to tobacco, alcohol and illicit drugs, 2000

Risk factor	High mortality developing countries		Low mortality developing countries		Developed countries		Worldwide
	Males	Females	Males	Females	Males	Females	
Mortality							
Tobacco	7.5	1.5	12.2	2.9	26.3	9.3	8.8
Alcohol	2.6	0.6	8.5	1.6	8.0	−0.3	3.2
Illicit drugs	0.5	0.1	0.6	0.1	0.6	0.3	0.4
DALYs							
Tobacco	3.4	0.6	6.2	1.3	17.1	6.2	4.1
Alcohol	2.6	0.5	9.8	2.0	14.0	3.3	4.0
Illicit drugs	0.8	0.2	1.2	0.3	2.3	1.2	0.8

Source: WHO, 2002.

Table 1.4 offers ample evidence that the burden of ill-health from use of psychoactive substances, taken together, is substantial: 8.9% in terms of DALYs. However, GBD findings re-emphasize that the main global health burden is due to licit rather than illicit substances.

The primary emphasis in this report, however, is not on the harmful consequences which can result from substance use (except as they occur in the body's nervous system) and neither is it primarily on the toxic qualities of the substances. Rather the emphasis is on patterns of substance use, and on the mechanisms of psychoactivity and of dependence (as indicated in Fig. 1.2). Since dependence refers to mechanisms by which use is sustained over time – thereby multiplying the probabilities of harmful consequences of use – special attention is given in this report to the neuroscience of dependence.

References

American Psychiatric Association (1994) *Diagnostic and statistical manual of mental disorders, 4th ed. (DSM-IV)*. Washington, DC, American Psychiatric Association.

Babor T et al. (forthcoming) *No ordinary commodity: alcohol and public policy*. Oxford, Oxford University Press.

Corrao MA et al., eds. (2000) *Tobacco control: country profiles*. Atlanta, GA, The American Cancer Society.

Degenhardt L et al. (2002) *Comparative risk assessment: illicit drug use*. Geneva, World Health Organization, unpublished manuscript.

Drummond DC et al. (2000) Craving research: future directions. *Addiction*, **95**(Suppl. 2):S247–S258.

Ferentzy P (2001) From sin to disease: differences and similarities between past and current conceptions of chronic drunkenness. *Contemporary Drug Problems*, **28**:363–390.

Lopez AD, Collishaw NE, Piha T (1994) A descriptive model of the cigarette epidemic in developed countries. *Tobacco Control*, **3**:242–247.

Mackay J, Eriksen M (2002) *The tobacco atlas*. Geneva, World Health Organization.

Medina-Mora E et al. (2001) Patterns of alcohol consumption and related problems in Mexico: results from two general population surveys. In: Demers A, Room R, Bourgault C, eds. *Surveys of drinking patterns and problems in seven developing countries*. Geneva, World Health Organization:13-32.

Murray CJ, Lopez AD (1996) *Global health statistics. Global burden of disease and injury series. Vol. 2*. Geneva, World Health Organization.

Mustonen H, Beukes L, Du Preez V (2001) Alcohol drinking in Namibia. In: Demers A, Room R, Bourgault C, eds. *Surveys of drinking patterns and problems in seven developing countries*. Geneva, World Health Organization:45-62.

Obot IS (2001) Household survey of alcohol use in Nigeria: the Middlebelt Study. In: Demers A, Room R, Bourgault C, eds. *Surveys of drinking patterns and problems in seven developing countries*. Geneva, World Health Organization: 63-76.

Rehm J et al. (2002) *Alcohol as a risk factor for burden of disease*. Geneva, World Health Organization, unpublished manuscript.

Room R (2001) Governing images in public discourse about problematic drinking. In: Heather N, Peters TJ, Stockwell T, eds. *Handbook of alcohol dependence and alcohol-related problems*. Chichester, Wiley:33–45.

Room R et al. (1996) WHO cross-cultural applicability research on diagnosis and assessment of substance use disorders: an overview of methods and selected results. *Addiction*, **91**:199–220.

Room R et al. (2002) *Alcohol and the developing world: a public health perspective*. Helsinki, Finnish Foundation for Alcohol Studies.

UNODCCP (2002) *Global illicit drug trends 2002*. New York, NY, United Nations Office for Drug Control and Crime Prevention.

World Bank (1999) *Curbing the epidemic: governments and the economics of tobacco control*. Washington, DC, World Bank.

WHO (1992) *The ICD-10 classification of mental and behavioural disorders: clinical descriptions and diagnostic guidelines*. Geneva, World Health Organization.

WHO (1999) *Global status report on alcohol*. Geneva, World Health Organization.

WHO (1994) *Lexicon of alcohol and drug terms*. Geneva, World Health Organization.

WHO (2002) *The world health report 2002*. Geneva, World Health Organization.

CHAPTER 2

Brain Mechanisms: Neurobiology and Neuroanatomy

Introduction

Substance dependence is a disorder that involves the motivational systems of the brain. As with any disorder specific to an organ or system, one must first understand the normal function of that organ or system to understand its dysfunction. Because the output of the brain is behaviour and thoughts, disorders of the brain can result in highly complex behavioural symptoms. The brain can suffer many types of disease and traumas, from neurological conditions such as stroke and epilepsy, to neurodegenerative diseases such as Parkinson disease and Alzheimer disease, to infections or traumatic brain injuries. In each of these cases, the behavioural output is recognized as being part of the disorder.

Similarly, with dependence, the behavioural output is complex, but is mostly related to the effects of drugs on the brain. The tremors of Parkinson disease, the seizures of epilepsy, even the melancholy of depression are widely recognized and accepted as symptoms of an underlying brain pathology. Dependence has not previously been recognized as a disorder of the brain, in the same way that psychiatric and mental illnesses were not previously viewed as being a result of a disorder of the brain. However, with recent advances in neuroscience, it is clear that dependence is as much a disorder of the brain as any other neurological or psychiatric illness. New technologies and research provide a means to visualize and measure changes in brain function from the molecular and cellular levels to changes in complex cognitive processes, that occur with short-term and long-term substance use.

This chapter reviews basic principles of brain anatomy and function to provide a framework within which the neuroscience of dependence can be discussed.

Organization of the brain

The nervous system is the body's major communication system, and is divided into central and peripheral regions. The central nervous system consists of the brain and spinal cord, and the peripheral nervous system consists of all nerves outside of this. The spinal cord controls reflex actions, and relays sensory and motor information between the body and the brain, so that the organism can respond appropriately to its environment.

The region of the brain where it meets the spinal cord is called the rhombencephalon or hindbrain, and is composed of the myelencephalon (medulla) and metencephalon (pons and cerebellum) (Fig. 2.1). The medulla is vital to sustaining life, and controls processes such as breathing, heartbeat and blood flow. The medulla also contains receptors for the opioid drugs, such as heroin and morphine, which is why these drugs can cause respiratory depression and death. The pons is a relay station for signals being carried from the cortex to the cerebellum, which is involved in body movements and coordination.

Fig. 2.1 Central nervous system

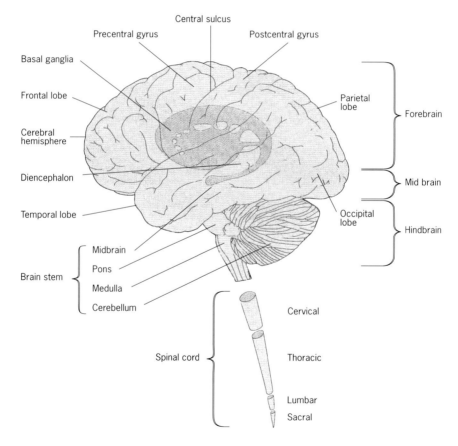

Source: Reproduced from Kandel, Schwartz, & Jessell, 1995, with permission from the publishers.

Above the hindbrain is the mesencephalon or midbrain (Fig. 2.1), which contains two areas that are very important in substance dependence. The ventral tegmental area (VTA) is rich in dopamine cell bodies, and projects to the limbic system and forebrain regions. The VTA is involved in signalling the importance of stimuli that are critical to survival such as those associated with feeding and reproduction. However, many psychoactive drugs also have powerful effects on this brain area, which contributes to the development of dependence by signalling to the brain that psychoactive substances are very important from a motivational perspective. The dopaminergic projection from the VTA to the nucleus accumbens (discussed below) is known as the mesolimbic dopamine system, and is the neurotransmitter system that is most strongly implicated in the dependence-producing potential of psychoactive drugs (Wise, 1998). This key concept will be discussed in more detail in Chapters 3 and 4. Another important midbrain structure is the substantia nigra, which also has dopaminergic projections to the forebrain, but these pathways are involved in coordinating and executing movements of the body. Degeneration of neurons in the substantia nigra leads to the characteristic symptoms of Parkinson disease.

Finally, there is the prosencephalon or forebrain, which is composed of the diencephalon and the telencephalon (cerebral hemispheres) (Fig. 2.1). Important areas of the diencephalon (Fig. 2.2) are the thalamus, the hypothalamus, and the posterior lobe of the pituitary gland. The hypothalamus is critical for regulating hormonal signals and basic bodily

Fig. 2.2 Diencephalon
The figure shows the location of the two lobes of the thalamus, joined by the massa intermedia. Beneath the thalamus lies the hypothalamus and posterior pituitary gland, which regulate autonomic, endocrine and visceral functions.

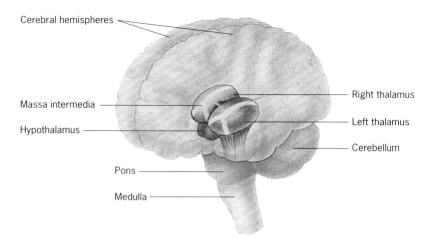

Source: Reproduced from Pinel, 1990, with permission from the publishers.

functions – concerning, for example, water balance, body temperature and reproductive hormones – as well as for responding to changes in these functions. The hypothalamus also secretes hormones that travel to the nearby posterior lobe of the pituitary gland. The thalamus functions as a relay station for sensory and motor information going to and from the cortex to other areas of the brain and body.

The telencephalon of the forebrain is the most highly developed area of the brain, and is composed of two cerebral hemispheres separated by the longitudinal fissure (Fig. 2.3). The outermost layer of the brain is the cortex, which is made up of layers of nerve cells or neurons, and has a highly folded organization that increases its surface area and the number of neurons that it contains. Beneath the cortex run millions of axons that interconnect the neurons and allow the different areas of the brain to communicate and to coordinate behaviour.

Each hemisphere of the brain is divided into four lobes: frontal, parietal, temporal, and occipital (Fig. 2.3). Different areas of the cortex are specialized for different functions (Fig. 2.4). The motor association cortex, for example, is involved in coordinating movements of the body, and the primary motor

Fig. 2.3 Cerebral hemispheres
The telencephalon is composed of two cerebral hemisphere separated by the medial longitudinal fissure. Each hemisphere is subdivided into four lobes: frontal, parietal, occipital, and temporal.

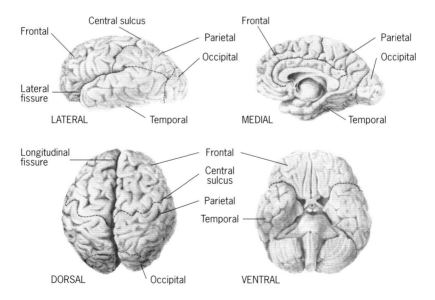

Source: Reproduced from Kolb & Whishaw, 1996, with permission from the publishers.

Fig. 2.4   Structural and functional regions of the cerebral cortex

The cerebral cortex is structurally differentiated into four lobes. The cerebral cortex can also be differentiated into functionally specialized areas.

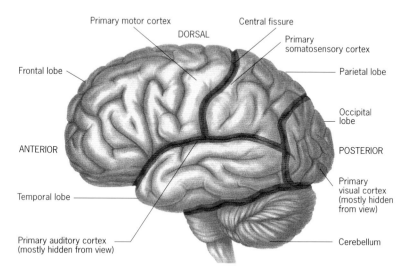

Source: Reproduced from Carlson, 1988, with permission from the publishers.

cortex is involved in executing this function. Similarly, there is a primary sensory cortex that receives information from each of these sense organs. Information from the primary sensory areas goes to sensory association areas of the cortex, which are involved in perception and memory connected with the sense organs. Here information from several sense organs can be combined to form complex perceptions (Fig. 2.5). The cortex is involved in many aspects of substance dependence, from the primary effects of psychoactive drugs on sensations and perceptions, to the complex behaviours and thoughts involved in drug craving and uncontrolled substance use. Neuroimaging techniques such as positron emission tomography (PET) have shown changes in areas of the cortex following both short-term and long-term substance use (see Box 2.1 and Chapter 4 for details).

Beneath the cortex are several other important structures. The basal ganglia (Fig. 2.6) are structures involved in voluntary motor behaviour and consist of the caudate, putamen, globus pallidus and amygdala (the amygdala is also part of the limbic system, and will be discussed in the next section). The caudate and putamen together are known as the striatum. Just below the striatum is a key area for substance dependence and motivation, known as the nucleus accumbens, which is made up of core and shell regions. (Note: clusters of neurons with similar structure and function make up "nuclei" of the brain, not to be confused with the nuclei of individual cells). The nucleus

Fig. 2.5   The relation between different functional brain regions
Information received from primary sensory cortices is integrated in sensory
association areas, which are involved in perception and memories.

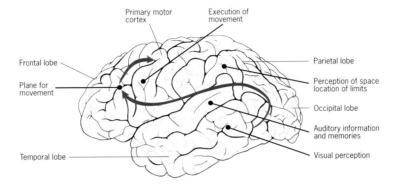

Source: Reproduced from Carlson, 1988, with permission from the publishers.

Fig. 2.6   Basal ganglia
The basal ganglia are shown, comprised of a number of structures involved
in the performance of voluntary motor responses.

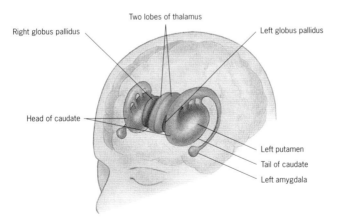

Source: Reproduced from Pinel, 1990, with permission from the publishers.

accumbens is a very important brain area involved in motivation and
learning, and signalling the motivational value of stimuli (Robbins & Everitt,
1996; Cardinal et al., 2002). Psychoactive substances increase the production
of dopamine in the nucleus accumbens, which is thought to be an important
event in drug reinforcement. This will be discussed further in Chapters 3
and 4.

Another region relevant to the neuroscience of dependence is the limbic system (Fig. 2.7). This is an interconnected series of structures that are important in relation to emotion, motivation and learning. The limbic system plays a vital role in the development of dependence, and interacts with the cortex and nucleus accumbens. Important structures of the limbic system are the hippocampus, which plays an important role in memory, and the amygdala, which is critical in emotional regulation. All of these areas receive sensory information from other brain areas to help coordinate the appropriate emotional and behavioural response to external stimuli.

The neuron

Communication in the brain takes place between nerve cells or neurons. Psychoactive substances alter many aspects of communication between neurons, as will be discussed below. Neurons are highly specialized cells that exist in many shapes, sizes and varieties. However, they share the following basic structural regions: cell body or soma, dendrites, axon, and terminal buttons (Fig. 2.8) (Carlson, 1988).

Fig. 2.7   Major structures of the limbic system

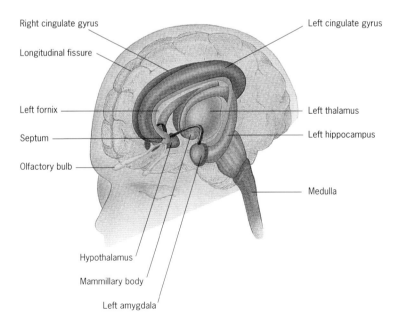

Source: Reproduced from Pinel, 1990, with permission from the publishers.

Fig. 2.8   Structure of a neuron

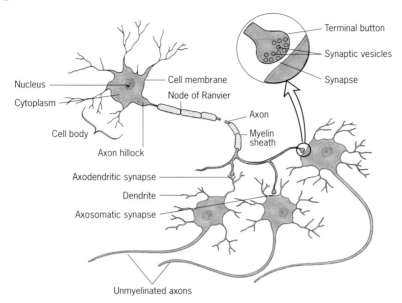

Source: Reproduced from Pinel, 1990, with permission from the publishers.

Cell body

The cell body, or soma, is the metabolic centre of the neuron, and contains the nucleus and other structures that sustain the neuron. A specialized membrane that helps to regulate the internal environment of the cell surrounds the cell body. It is selectively permeable in that it allows only certain molecules into or out of the cell body, in order to maintain the proper functioning of the cell.

By definition, the cell body is the part of the neuron that contains the nucleus (Fig. 2.9). The nucleus contains the genetic material deoxyribonucleic acid (DNA). DNA is used in cell division and growth, but also plays a role in mature neurons, where it is used to synthesize proteins in response to a wide variety of stimuli. Psychoactive substances can affect the expression of DNA, resulting in short-term or long-term changes in neuronal function, and ultimately, behaviour. This will be discussed in more detail at the end of the chapter.

Dendrites

Dendrites are highly branched processes extending from the cell body of the neuron, that receive chemical messages from other neurons (see Fig. 2.8). This branching, and the presence of dendritic spines (small swellings on the

26

Fig. 2.9 **Synthesis of proteins**

Portions of DNA in the nucleus of a neuron are encoded into messenger RNA. Ribosomes in the cell body use messenger RNA to synthesize proteins.

Step 1. Strands of mRNA duplicate portions of the genetic code from DNA in the nucleus and carry it into the cytoplasm.

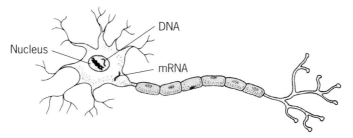

Step 2. In the cytoplasm, the strands of mRNA bind to ribosomes.

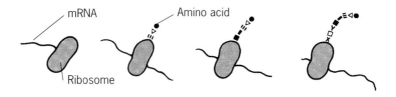

Step 3. The ribosomes move along the strands of mRNA reading the genetic code, and create the appropriate chain of amino acids from the amino acids in the cytoplasm.

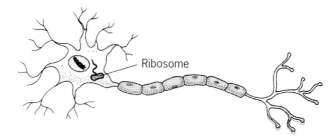

Step 4. The proteins are released into the cytoplasm.

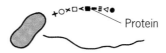

Source: Reproduced from Pinel, 1990, with permission from the publishers.

surface of a dendrite with which a terminal button from another neuron forms a synapse), allows many different neurons to converge on a single nerve cell, facilitating the coordination and integration of many complex messages. The number of dendritic spines can increase or decrease following exposure to psychoactive substances (Sklair-Tavron et al., 1996; Robinson & Kolb, 1999; Eisch et al., 2000), thus altering communication between neurons, and most likely contributing to the behavioural and neurological effects of the substances. This will also be discussed in more detail at the end of the chapter.

Axon

The axon is a long slender process extending from the cell body, that carries information from the cell body to the terminal buttons (see Fig. 2.8). Certain chemicals such as neurotransmitters are transported along the axon, and it also propagates nerve impulses (see below). The area where the axon leaves the cell body is known as the axon hillock.

Terminal buttons

The terminal buttons are the bulbous structures found at the end of axons (see Figs 2.8 and 2.10). At the terminal button, chemical signalling molecules (which will be discussed more in the section on neurotransmission) are stored in small packages, or vesicles. When an appropriate signal arrives at the terminal button, neurotransmitter is released into the synapse or synaptic cleft, the space between the terminal button and the membrane of the next cell or dendrite with which it is communicating. The membrane of the terminal button that is transmitting the message is known as the presynaptic

Fig. 2.10 A terminal button and synapse

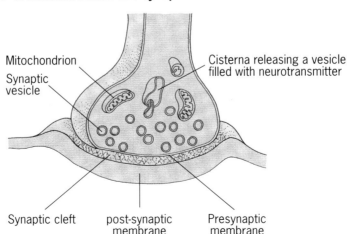

Mitochondrion

Synaptic vesicle

Cisterna releasing a vesicle filled with neurotransmitter

Synaptic cleft

post-synaptic membrane

Presynaptic membrane

Source: Reproduced from Pinel, 1990, with permission from the publishers.

Fig. 2.9 Synthesis of proteins

Portions of DNA in the nucleus of a neuron are encoded into messenger RNA. Ribosomes in the cell body use messenger RNA to synthesize proteins.

Step 1. Strands of mRNA duplicate portions of the genetic code from DNA in the nucleus and carry it into the cytoplasm.

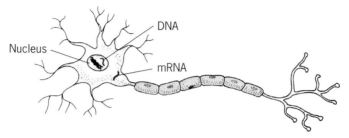

Step 2. In the cytoplasm, the strands of mRNA bind to ribosomes.

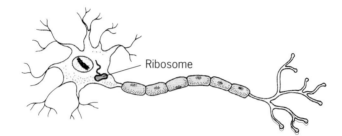

Step 3. The ribosomes move along the strands of mRNA reading the genetic code, and create the appropriate chain of amino acids from the amino acids in the cytoplasm.

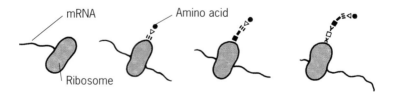

Step 4. The proteins are released into the cytoplasm.

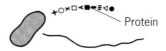

Source: Reproduced from Pinel, 1990, with permission from the publishers.

surface of a dendrite with which a terminal button from another neuron forms a synapse), allows many different neurons to converge on a single nerve cell, facilitating the coordination and integration of many complex messages. The number of dendritic spines can increase or decrease following exposure to psychoactive substances (Sklair-Tavron et al., 1996; Robinson & Kolb, 1999; Eisch et al., 2000), thus altering communication between neurons, and most likely contributing to the behavioural and neurological effects of the substances. This will also be discussed in more detail at the end of the chapter.

Axon

The axon is a long slender process extending from the cell body, that carries information from the cell body to the terminal buttons (see Fig. 2.8). Certain chemicals such as neurotransmitters are transported along the axon, and it also propagates nerve impulses (see below). The area where the axon leaves the cell body is known as the axon hillock.

Terminal buttons

The terminal buttons are the bulbous structures found at the end of axons (see Figs 2.8 and 2.10). At the terminal button, chemical signalling molecules (which will be discussed more in the section on neurotransmission) are stored in small packages, or vesicles. When an appropriate signal arrives at the terminal button, neurotransmitter is released into the synapse or synaptic cleft, the space between the terminal button and the membrane of the next cell or dendrite with which it is communicating. The membrane of the terminal button that is transmitting the message is known as the presynaptic

Fig. 2.10 A terminal button and synapse

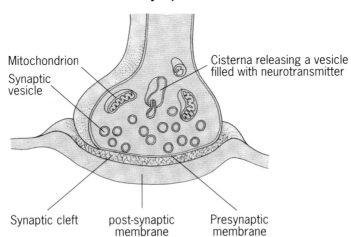

Mitochondrion
Synaptic vesicle
Cisterna releasing a vesicle filled with neurotransmitter

Synaptic cleft   post-synaptic membrane   Presynaptic membrane

Source: Reproduced from Pinel, 1990, with permission from the publishers.

membrane, and the membrane of the receiving neuron is known as the postsynaptic membrane. The synaptic cleft contains extracellular fluid through which chemical substances can diffuse to interact with a variety of membrane proteins known as receptors.

Changes in the release or reuptake of neurotransmitters play an important role in the mechanism of action of many psychoactive substances. Cocaine and amphetamine, for example, block the reuptake of the neurotransmitters dopamine and norepinephrine, thereby prolonging the actions of these transmitters. These mechanisms will be examined in more detail in Chapter 4.

Neurotransmission

Action potential

Neurons communicate with each other through a highly specialized, precise and rapid method. The action potential is a brief electrical impulse that travels along an axon and allows one neuron to communicate with another through the release of neurotransmitter. The action potential is possible because of the selectively permeable membrane that maintains a chemical and electrical gradient across the membrane known as the membrane potential. The membrane at rest is polarized; however, it can become depolarized if diffusion

Fig.2.11 The action potential
During an action potential, voltage-sensitive sodium channels open causing a rapid influx of sodium and resulting depolarization of the cell. The cell is repolarized by the opening of potassium channels that permit the efflux of potassium from the cell and restore the resting membrane potential. Active ion pumps later exchange sodium for potassium within the cell.

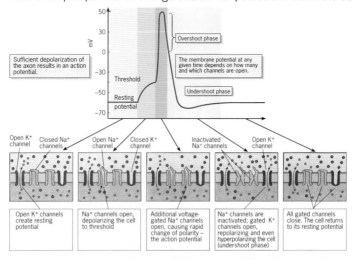

Source: Reproduced from Rosenzweig, Leiman, & Breedlove, 1999, with permission from the publishers.

of ions is allowed to occur, which is what happens during an action potential (Fig. 2.11).

An ion channel is a pore in the membrane through which ions can pass under certain circumstances (e.g. there are Na^+, K^+, and Ca^{2+} channels). There are channels that only open under certain circumstances, such as at a particular membrane voltage (known as voltage-gated ion channels). Depolarization in a local area of a neuron changes the voltage in that area, and if it is of sufficient strength, may cause voltage-sensitive ion channels to open, allowing ionic diffusion. Thus, adjacent areas become sequentially depolarized, allowing propagation of the signal. This signal can be propagated along an axon extremely rapidly. An action potential is an "all-or-none" event, in that if the depolarizing stimulus is sufficient to reach a threshold value, the action potential will be initiated and will travel without decrement to the end of the axon.

After depolarization, the membrane rapidly becomes repolarized by the opening of voltage-dependent K^+ channels that are also opened by depolarization, but only after a slight delay (approximately 1 millisecond). Na^+ channels also, do not stay open, but are inactivated after a certain period of time. These factors enable rapid transmission and termination of messages.

Neurotransmitter release

Action potentials allow a message to be propagated along an axon within one neuron. However, for communication to be complete, this message must be transmitted between neurons. This is accomplished at the synapses of the terminal buttons, through the release of neurotransmitter. Neurotransmitters are chemical substances that are released from one neuron and that interact with receptors on another neuron to affect a change in that neuron. They will be discussed in further detail below.

The terminal buttons contain small structures known as vesicles, which are packages of neurotransmitter that have been transported to the cell body. When an action potential arrives at the terminal button, voltage-sensitive Ca^{2+} channels open, allowing Ca^{2+} to flow into the terminal button and activate a number of processes that cause the release of neurotransmitter into the synaptic cleft. Once in the cleft, neurotransmitters diffuse across and bind to postsynaptic receptors.

The chemical message needs a means of termination, and this occurs by several mechanisms. One is by enzymatic degradation of the neurotransmitter in the cleft, and another is by active reuptake of the neurotransmitter by the presynaptic membrane. One of cocaine's primary mechanisms of action is to block the reuptake of neurotransmitters, thereby increasing their concentration in the synaptic cleft, and increasing their effects. Amphetamine acts by reversing the uptake mechanism, so that neurotransmitter is released into the synaptic cleft independently of action potentials. These mechanisms will be discussed in more detail in Chapter 4.

When the neurotransmitter binds to its receptors on the postsynaptic cell, the postsynaptic cell can either become more or less excitable, and thus more or less likely to fire an action potential. These are known as excitatory and inhibitory postsynaptic potentials, respectively.

Receptors

Receptors are protein complexes that are located in distinct regions of the cell membrane, and that neurotransmitters bind with to initiate the communication of a signal between neurons. There are specific receptors for each specific neurotransmitter found in the brain. Psychoactive substances are able to bind to these receptors, interfering with normal transmitter function. Different classes of substances bind with distinct receptors, thus giving the characteristic effects of each substance class – e.g. opioids such as heroin and morphine bind to opioid receptors, cannabinoids bind to cannabinoid receptors, and nicotine binds to nicotinic receptors in the brain – and have powerful effects on behaviour. These and other mechanisms will be discussed in more detail in Chapter 4.

There are two basic mechanisms of signal transduction that are important when considering the actions of psychoactive substances. Binding of neurotransmitters to receptors can cause the opening of ion channels directly, through ligand-gated ion channels (Fig. 2.12). Binding of a ligand to the receptor opens the ion channel, allowing rapid changes in the postsynaptic membrane. An example of this type of channel is the γ-aminobutyric acid (GABA)-A receptor, to which benzodiazepines and barbiturates can bind to increase the opening of this channel. Alternatively, binding of the ligand can

Fig. 2.12 Two types of chemical synapses
The first diagram shows binding to and opening of a ligand-gated ion channel. The second diagram demonstrates activation of a G protein-coupled receptor resulting in the opening of an ion channel via a second messenger.

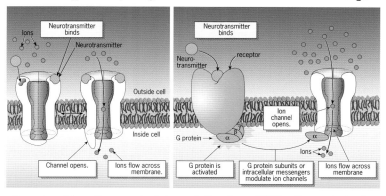

Source: Reproduced from Rosenzweig, Leiman, & Breedlove, 1999, with permission from the publishers.

result in the propagation of a signal through the generation of second messengers. The second messenger can either open an ion channel, or can initiate a series of biochemical reactions leading to longer-term changes in neuronal function in the postsynaptic cell. There are many different second messenger pathways; this increases the diversity of signals that can be sent, and the consequences of those signals. An example of this type of receptor is called a G protein-coupled receptor. Dopamine receptors are G protein-coupled receptors, and depending upon the subtype of dopamine receptor, ligand binding can either stimulate or inhibit the production of cyclic adenosine monophosphate (cAMP). Psychoactive substances can have long-term effects on cAMP function, as will be discussed in more detail at the end of this chapter.

Receptors play a role not only in the immediate, reinforcing effects of psychoactive substances, but also in the processes of tolerance and withdrawal. Specific examples will be discussed in Chapter 4, but as one example, tolerance to benzodiazepines and barbiturates develops through changes in GABA-A receptor structure. The receptor adapts to the presence of the substance, leading to tolerance. Thus, higher doses are required to have an effect. When the substance is removed, withdrawal symptoms appear, because of these structural changes which have occurred to accommodate the presence of the substance.

Neurotransmitters

A neurotransmitter can be defined as a chemical substance that is released synaptically from one neuron and that affects another cell in a specific manner (Kandel & Schwartz, 1985). A neurotransmitter must also meet the following criteria:

— synthesized in the neuron;

— present in the presynaptic neuron;

— released in sufficient quantity to have a postsynaptic effect;

— has the same effect whether released by natural means (endogenously) or whether applied as a drug (exogenously).

It must also have a specific mechanism for its removal from the synaptic cleft.

Many types of neurotransmitters have been discovered so far, but in general there are three categories: amino acid neurotransmitters, amino acid-derived neurotransmitters, and peptides, which are chains of amino acids. The amino acid transmitters include glutamate, GABA, glycine and aspartate. The monoamines (norepinephrine and dopamine (catecholamines) and serotonin (indoleamine) are derived from amino acids. Large molecule peptide neurotransmitters are generally synthesized in the cell body, and transported along the axons to the terminal buttons. Small molecule neurotransmitters can be synthesized in the terminals.

32

There are distinct regions of the brain where cell bodies for a specific neurotransmitter exist, and other regions or "projection areas" where the axons from those cell bodies project to, and where the neurotransmitter is ultimately released. Thus, not every neurotransmitter is released in every area of the brain. This allows certain areas of the brain to perform specific functions. Some of the more important neurotransmitters with respect to the neuroscience of dependence are discussed below.

Acetylcholine

Acetylcholine is a neurotransmitter formed from choline, which is derived from the diet. It is formed by an enzymatic reaction with coenzyme A. Acetylcholine plays an important role in learning and memory, and is thought to be involved in Alzheimer disease. Neurons that synthesize and release acetylcholine are called cholinergic neurons. The cell bodies are located in the basal nucleus, but they project widely throughout the cortex. Acetylcholine receptors are ligand-gated cation channels, and there are two main subtypes, nicotinic and muscarinic, named on account of their responsiveness to nicotine and muscarine respectively. Receptors for acetylcholine have been implicated in nicotine dependence and may also contribute to the effects of cocaine and amphetamine.

γ-aminobutyric acid

GABA is widely distributed throughout the nervous system, and is an amino acid formed from the amino acid glutamate. GABA is an inhibitory neurotransmitter that acts through two distinct receptor subtypes, named GABA-A and GABA-B. The GABA-A receptors form a chloride ion channel. The binding of GABA to GABA-A receptors opens this channel resulting in the rapid diffusion of chloride ions into the cell, thus hyperpolarizing the cell and making it less likely to fire an action potential. The sedative, anxiety-reducing effects of benzodiazepines, barbiturates and alcohol are derived from their effects on the GABA-A receptor. Anti-epileptic medications also act to facilitate the function of the GABA-A receptor, and blocking the effects of GABA can lead to seizures. This is why withdrawal from benzodiazepines or alcohol can be associated with seizures. The GABA-B receptors are G protein-coupled receptors, and binding of GABA to the GABA-B receptor opens a potassium channel.

Glutamate

Glutamate is an excitatory amino acid neurotransmitter found throughout the brain. It is derived from proteins in the diet and is produced by the metabolic processes of the cells. Glutamate acts at four receptor subtypes; NMDA, AMPA, kainate, and metabotropic glutamate receptors. Some of the glutamate receptors are coupled to sodium channels and therefore can mediate rapid (approximately 1 millisecond) actions, whereas other receptors are coupled to potassium channels through a G protein, and therefore take approximately 1 second for response. Glutamate is important for learning and plays an essential role in the hippocampus. Hallucinogens, such as phencyclidine (PCP) act at the NMDA subtype of glutamate receptor. In addition, it is thought that glutamate pathways play a very important role in modulating neural responses to many other psychoactive substances.

Dopamine

Dopamine is a neurotransmitter that is derived from the amino acid tyrosine, and is structurally related to norepinephrine. Dopamine produces inhibitory postsynaptic potentials. It is involved in movement, learning and motivation. Dopamine plays a paramount role in the neurobiology of dependence, and will be discussed in more detail in Chapters 3 and 4. Dopamine receptor genes have also been highly implicated in substance dependence in general, as well as in nicotine and alcohol dependence. There are two major dopamine projections in the brain. One, the mesolimbic pathway, projects from the VTA to the nucleus accumbens. This pathway appears to be directly or indirectly activated by most known psychoactive substances. Closely associated with this is the mesocortical dopamine pathway, which projects from the VTA to regions of the cortex. The second major dopamine pathway projects from the substantia nigra to the striatum, which is known as the nigrostriatal pathway. In Parkinson disease, this pathway undergoes degeneration leading to the characteristic movement disorders. Excessive dopamine function in the mesolimbic and mesocortical dopamine systems is thought to underlie the delusions and hallucinations of schizophrenia. It is interesting to note here that certain substances such as cocaine and amphetamine can, in high doses, mimic some of the features of schizophrenia and bipolar disorders through the same basic actions on the dopamine system.

Norepinephrine

Norepinephrine is another catecholamine that is derived from tyrosine. Norepinephrine-synthesising cell bodies are found in the locus coeruleus, and project widely throughout the brain. Norepinephrine is involved in arousal and stress responses. Cocaine and amphetamine affect the transmission of norepinephrine by increasing its concentration in the synaptic cleft. This increase in synaptic norepinephrine contributes to the stimulatory and rewarding effects of cocaine and amphetamine, and also to the feelings of nervousness and anxiety that can accompany the use of these substances.

Serotonin

Serotonin, like dopamine and norepinephrine, is a monoamine. It is an indoleamine that is derived from the amino acid tryptophan. It is involved in regulation of mood, arousal, impulsivity, aggression, appetite and anxiety. Serotonin-synthesizing cell bodies are found in the midbrain in a region called the raphe nuclei. These neurons project to many areas of the brain such as the cortex, hypothalamus and limbic system. There are many subtypes of serotonin receptor. In the body, serotonin is found in the gastrointestinal tract, platelets and spinal cord. Most antidepressant drugs work by increasing the action of serotonin in the brain. Serotonin is also involved in the primary actions of some psychoactive drugs such as lysergic acid diethylamide (LSD) and ecstasy, and is also implicated in the effects of cocaine, amphetamine, alcohol and nicotine.

Peptides

Peptides are chains of two or more amino acids linked by peptide bonds. There are many peptides that are widely distributed throughout the nervous system, and at least 200 identified neuropeptides to date. Some are hormones that cause the release of other hormones, such as corticotrophin-releasing hormone and growth hormone-releasing hormone. There are pituitary peptides such as adrenocorticotropin, prolactin and growth hormone, and there are a wide variety of peptides that were originally discovered in the gut, but that also have actions in the brain, such as cholecystokinin, substance P and vasoactive intestinal polypeptide. The endogenous opioids are also an important class of peptide neurotransmitters. Substances such as heroin and morphine bind to the receptors used by the endogenous opioids. Peptides control a wide variety of functions in the body, from food intake and water balance, to modulating anxiety, pain, reproduction and the pleasurable effects of food and drugs. Although the opioids are widely recognized as being involved in substance dependence, it has been shown that other peptides also play a role (Kovacs, Sarnyai & Szabo, 1998; McLay, Pan & Kastin, 2001; Sarnyai, Shaham & Heinrichs, 2001).

Genes

Inside the nucleus of the cell are the chromosomes, which are made up of strands of DNA. The chromosomes are made up of distinct sets of instructions, or genes, that "code" for proteins. Messenger ribonucleic acid (mRNA) makes copies of sections of DNA, and transports it into the cytoplasm. In the cytoplasm, the mRNA binds to ribosomes, which "read" the genetic code and assemble the appropriate proteins from amino acids in the cytoplasm (Fig. 2.9). These proteins are then used to carry out the functions of the cell.

Genes can be turned on or off at different times during the entire life of an organism. Some genes are turned on or "expressed" only during development. Others are expressed in response to certain stimuli. Eating certain foods, for example, can increase the expression of genes that code for the enzymes that will break down constituents of that food. Being out in the sun can stimulate the expression of other genes that cause the skin to become more pigmented. Similarly, drugs of all kinds can cause changes in gene expression in the brain. Changes in gene expression cause changes in protein synthesis that can have both short-term and long-term consequences on behaviour. This concept will be covered in more detail below.

There are both genetic commonalities and differences among all humans. The basic mechanisms of drug action are common to all. However, there is considerable individual variation in the response to these drugs, the particular forms of certain genes, and the way in which these genes interact with the full complement of genes and with the environment in which that individual lives. The main genetic differences currently known to be relevant to dependence will be discussed in Chapter 5.

Cellular and neuronal effects of psychoactive substances

Cellular effects

Psychoactive substances have immediate effects on neurotransmitter release or second messenger systems, but there are also many changes that occur at the cellular level, both in the short-term and long-term, following single or repeated substance use.

The primary sites of action for most psychoactive substances are the cell membrane receptors, and their associated cascade of signal transduction processes. The long-term effects brought about during the process of substance dependence are usually mediated by alterations in gene transcription, which leads to altered gene expression and subsequent changes in the proteins synthesised. Since these proteins affect the function of the neurons, such changes are ultimately manifested in altered behaviour of the individual. Among the best-established molecular changes following chronic substance use is the compensatory upregulation or superactivation of the cyclic AMP (cAMP) pathway. Cyclic AMP is an intracellular second messenger that can initiate a wide variety of changes in the postsynaptic cell.

The ability of chronic exposure to opioids to upregulate the cAMP pathway has been known for decades (Sharma, Klee & Nirenberg, 1975). In addition to opioids, upregulation of the cyclic AMP pathway has been observed in response to chronic use of alcohol and cocaine (Unterwald et al., 1993; Lane-Ladd et al., 1997). When a system that has been upregulated by chronic substance use is acutely exposed to the substance, the acute effects are diminished, representing cellular tolerance. In the absence of the substance, the upregulated system contributes to symptoms of withdrawal (Nestler & Aghajanian, 1997). Effects of an upregulated cAMP system have been demonstrated in many of the relevant brain regions, such as the nucleus accumbens, striatum, VTA, locus coeruleus and periaqueductal gray (Cole et al., 1995; Lane-Ladd et al., 1997; Nestler & Aghajanian, 1997).

Role of cyclic AMP response element binding protein (CREB)

Cyclic AMP stimulates the expression of cAMP response element binding protein (CREB), which is a transcription factor. Gene transcription and expression in neurons are regulated by numerous transcription factors. Transcription factors are proteins that bind to regions of genes to increase or decrease their expression. It has been shown that the functions of several transcription factors are altered by substance use and therefore are implicated in dependence.

Alterations in the CREB-regulated pathways are among the best-characterized adaptations related to chronic exposure to psychoactive substances and there is evidence for upregulation and sensitization of the cAMP/CREB-linked mechanisms (Nestler, 2001).

Role of transcriptional regulator Fos

Other transcription factors induced by exposure to psychoactive substances belong to the Fos protein family of immediate early genes. The products of these genes are induced very rapidly (hence the name) and play important roles in transducing receptor-mediated signals into changes in gene expression. These changes in gene expression affect neuronal protein expression and function. Single administrations of a substance cause transient increases in several members of the Fos protein family but with chronic use, a modified variant of FosB, ΔFosB, which is more stable, accumulates and persists in the nucleus accumbens (Hope et al., 1994). DFosB, once generated, has an unusually prolonged half-life resulting in persistently elevated levels (Keltz & Nestler, 2000). The accumulation of ΔFosB has been shown to occur following chronic use of cocaine, opioids, amphetamine, nicotine, phencyclidine and alcohol (Keltz & Nestler, 2000). This occurs in the nucleus accumbens and dorsal striatum, and constitutes a process specific for psychoactive drugs (Moratalla et al., 1996; Keltz & Nestler, 2000). The elevated ΔFosB can then continue to affect the expression of many other genes within the same neurons, which in turn by alterations in synaptic transmission will be able to affect many neuronal functions locally and in other areas of brain, to which these neurons project. This provides some insight into the nature of the long-lasting changes in neuronal composition that occur and persist well beyond the time frame of the acute drug effects.

Role of receptor systems targeted by drugs

Repeated stimulation of receptors by drugs can lead to alterations in receptor number and function. For example, long-term exposure to nicotine increases the number of nicotinic acetylcholine receptors in the brain (Wonnacott, 1990; Marks et al., 1992).

The development of tolerance and dependence to morphine and other opioids has some unique features. When the μ-opioid receptor is activated by endogenous opioids in the brain, the receptor is internalized into the cell, as a means of turning off the activation signal (Pak et al., 1996; Law, Wong & Loh, 2000). This process of receptor desensitization is a highly conserved mechanism for G protein-coupled receptors. In contrast, activation of the μ-opioid receptor by morphine (Matthes et al., 1996) does not induce receptor internalization (or does so very slowly), and there is abnormal prolongation of the cell surface activation signal without desensitization (Whistler et al., 1999). This unique property of morphine is fundamental to its ability to induce tolerance and withdrawal.

Neuronal effects

Since substance dependence induces long-lasting and near permanent alterations in behaviour, the likelihood of persistent changes in neural circuitry is high, brought about by remodelling and restructuring of neurons, as a consequence of the molecular changes induced.

Synaptic plasticity

The reorganization of neural circuitry by psychoactive substances can occur via changes in neurotransmitter release, the status of the neurotransmitter receptors, receptor-mediated signalling, or the number of ion channels regulating neuronal excitability. The mechanisms that mediate compulsive drug-seeking and drug-taking appear to mimic the physiological mechanisms for learning and memory (Hyman & Malenka, 2001; Nestler, 2001). There are many parallels between the processes mediating learning and memory and substance dependence, which will be examined in more detail in Chapter 3.

Alterations in synaptic structure

Structural changes in several brain regions as a consequence of substance use have been shown. Neurons typically have multiply-branched processes called dendrites, and following the activation of particular neurons, the increase in dendritic spines is indicative of the activated state. Cocaine administration has been associated with a marked increase in the number of dendritic spines of the neurons of the nucleus accumbens and the prefrontal cortex (Robinson & Kolb, 1999). In contrast, there is relative loss of the dendrites in some areas such as the hippocampus, in response to chronic use of morphine (Sklair-Tavron et al., 1996; Eisch et al., 2000). Some of the long-lasting behavioural changes seen in chronic substance use will no doubt relate to such structural changes. Many of the synaptic changes are thought to be mediated by processes similar to those discovered for learning and memory (Hyman & Malenka, 2001).

Conclusion

This chapter has provided an overview of normal brain function, and of the many distinct processes that interact to produce behaviour. Alterations in any one of the steps in the process (generation of action potentials, changes in electrical activity or chemical conductance, neurotransmitter release, neurotransmitter reuptake, changes in second messenger function, altered gene expression, altered synaptic connectivity) can alter the function of other interacting processes, which ultimately can affect behaviour. As will be seen in the following chapters, psychoactive substances can profoundly alter neuronal processes, leading to the behaviours characteristic of dependence.

The immediate psychoactive and rewarding effects of substance use can be explained by understanding the mechanism of action of these substances at the pharmacological level. Further, the development of tolerance and withdrawal, and the long-term effects of substance use can also be understood through knowledge of a drug's mechanism of action. The effects of psychoactive substances on more complex processes such as motivation can also be understood through the knowledge of their effects on the brain. Their effects on motivational systems in the brain will be discussed further in Chapter 3. The specific effects of the major psychoactive substances will be explored in Chapter 4.

BOX 2.1

Neuroimaging techniques
Magnetic Resonance Imaging

Magnetic resonance imaging (MRI) uses magnetic fields and radio waves to produce high-quality two- or three-dimensional images of brain structures without injecting radioactive tracers. The brain can be imaged with a high degree of detail. Although MRI gives only static pictures of brain anatomy, functional MRI (fMRI) can provide functional information by comparing oxygenated and deoxygenated blood, which provides information on changes in brain activity in specific brain regions in response to various stimuli such as drugs, sounds, pictures, etc. An fMRI scan can produce images of brain activity as fast as every second, whereas positron emission tomography (PET) usually takes 40 seconds or much longer to produce images of brain activity. Thus, with fMRI, there is greater temporal precision. fMRI has the advantages of having the highest spatial resolution among imaging techniques, and does not require the use of ionizing radiation, thus it provides increased experimental safety and the ability to retest subjects multiple times. Magnetic resonance spectroscopy is used to gather information on the chemical composition of a discrete brain region.

Positron emission tomography

Positron emission tomography (PET) is a technique for viewing the activity in different regions in the brain. PET scans provide information about the metabolic activity in a certain brain region. Most commonly, the person is injected with a radioactive compound that can be followed through the bloodstream in the brain. This is usually labelled 2-deoxyglucose (2-DG), which is taken up by active neurons due to its similarity in structure to glucose. Thus, areas that are more metabolically active will take up more glucose and 2-DG. Unlike glucose, 2-DG is not metabolized, and therefore accumulates in the neurons. This can be visualized as two- or three-dimensional images, with different colours on a PET scan indicating different levels of radioactivity (blues and greens indicating areas of lower activity, and yellows and reds indicating areas of higher activity). Using different compounds, PET scans can be used to show blood flow, oxygen and glucose metabolism, and drug concentrations in the tissues of the living brain. Regional cerebral blood flow can be measured using PET imaging using a "flow tracer" such as [^{15}O] water to look at blood flow in a given area. Selective labelling of radiotracers allows highly selective biochemical specificities at low concentrations of tracers.

Single photon emission computed tomography

Similar to PET, single photon emission computed tomography (SPECT) uses radioactive tracers and a scanner to record data that a computer uses to construct two- or three-dimensional images of active brain regions. However, SPECT tracers are more limited than PET tracers in the kinds of brain activity they can monitor, and the SPECT tracers also deteriorate more slowly than many PET tracers, which means that SPECT studies require longer test and retest periods than PET studies. However, because SPECT tracers are longer lasting, they do not require an onsite cyclotron to produce them. SPECT studies also require less technical and medical staff support than PET studies do. While PET is more versatile than SPECT and produces more detailed images with a higher degree of resolution, particularly of deeper brain structures, SPECT is considerably less expensive than PET and can address many of the same drug dependence research questions that PET can.

Electroencephalography

Electroencephalography (EEG) uses electrodes placed on the scalp to detect and measure patterns of electrical activity emanating from the brain due to the communication between neurons. EEG can determine the relative strengths and positions of electrical activity in different brain regions within fractions of a second after a stimulus has been administered. However, the spatial resolution of EEG is not as good as with other imaging techniques. As a result, EEG images of brain electrical activity are often used in combination with other techniques such as MRI scans to better pinpoint the location of the activity within the brain.

Sources: Aine CJ, 1995; National Institute on Drug Abuse , 1996; Volkow et al., 1997; Gatley & Volkow, 1998.

References

Aine CJ (1995) A conceptual overview and critique of functional neuro-imaging techniques in humans. I. MRI/fMRI and PET. *Critical Reviews in Neurobiology*, **9**:229–309.

Cardinal RN et al. (2002) Emotion and motivation: the role of the amygdala, ventral striatum, and prefrontal cortex. *Neuroscience and Biobehavioral Reviews*, **26**:321–352.

Carlson NR (1988) *Foundations of physiological psychology*. Boston, MA, Allyn & Bacon.

Cole RL et al. (1995) Neuronal adaptation to amphetamine and dopamine: molecular mechanisms of prodynorphin gene regulation in rat striatum. *Neuron*, **14**:813–823.

Eisch AJ et al. (2000) Opiates inhibit neurogenesis in the adult rat hippocampus. *Proceedings of the National Academy of Science of the United States of America*, **97**:7579–7584.

Gatley SJ, Volkow ND (1998) Addiction and imaging of the living human brain. *Drug and Alcohol Dependence*, **51**:97–108.

Hope BT et al. (1994) Induction of a long-lasting AP-1 complex composed of altered Fos-like proteins in brain by chronic cocaine and other chronic treatments. *Neuron*, **13**:1235–1244.

Hyman SE, Malenka RC (2001) Addiction and the brain: the neurobiology of compulsion and its persistence. *Nature Reviews: Neuroscience*, **2**:695–703.

Kandel ER, Schwartz JH, eds (1985) *Principles of neural science*, 2nd ed. New York, NY, Elsevier.

Kandel ER, Schwartz JH, Jessell TM, eds (1995) Essentials of neural science and behavior. Norwalk, CT, Appleton & Lange.

Keltz MB, Nestler EJ (2000) ΔFosB: a molecular switch underlying long-term neural plasticity. *Current Opinion in Neurology*, **13**:715–720.

Kolb B, Whishaw IQ (1996) *Fundamentals of human neuropsychology*, 4th ed. San Francisco, CA, WH Freeman.

Kovacs GL, Sarnyai Z, Szabo G (1998) Oxytocin and addiction: a review. *Psychoneuroendocrinology*, **23**:945–962.

Lane-Ladd SB et al. (1997) CREB in the locus coeruleus: biochemical, physiological and behavioral evidence for a role in opiate dependence. *Journal of Neuroscience*, **17**:7890–7901.

Law PY, Wong YH, Loh HH (2000) Molecular mechanisms and regulation of opioid receptor signaling. *Annual Review of Pharmacology and Toxicology*, **40**:389–430.

Marks MJ et al. (1992) Nicotine binding and nicotinic receptor subunit RNA after chronic nicotine treatment. *Journal of Neuroscience*, **12**:2765–2784.

Matthes HW et al. (1996) Loss of morphine-induced analgesia, reward effect and withdrawal symptoms in mice lacking the μ-opioid receptor gene. *Nature*, **383**:819–823.

McLay RN, Pan W, Kastin AJ (2001) Effects of peptides on animal and human behavior: a review of studies published in the first twenty years of the journal *Peptides*. *Peptides*, **22**:2181–2255.

Moratalla R et al. (1996) D1-class dopamine receptors influence cocaine-induced persistent expression of Fos-related proteins in striatum. *Neuroreport*, **8**:1–5.

Nestler EJ (2001) Molecular basis of long-term plasticity underlying addiction. *Nature Reviews: Neuroscience*, **2**:119–128.

Nestler EJ, Aghajanian GK (1997) Molecular and cellular basis of addiction. *Science*, **278**:58–63.

National Institute on Drug Abuse (1996) Special report: brain imaging research. *NIDA Notes*, November/December. http://165.112.78.61/NIDA_Notes/NN96Index.html#Number5.

Pak Y et al. (1996) Agonist-induced functional desensitization of the mu-opioid receptor is mediated by loss of membrane receptors rather than uncoupling from G protein. *Molecular Pharmacology*, **50**:1214–1222.

Pinel JPJ (1990) *Biopsychology*. Boston, MA Allyn & Bacon.

Robbins TW, Everitt BJ (1996) Neurobehavioural mechanisms of reward and motivation. *Current Opinion in Neurobiology*, **6**:228–236.

Robinson TE, Kolb B (1999) Alterations in the morphology of dendrites and dendritic spines in the nucleus accumbens and prefrontal cortex following repeated treatment with amphetamine or cocaine. *European Journal of Neuroscience*, 11:1598–1604.

Rosenzweig MR, Leiman AL, Breedlove SM (1999) *Biological psychology*, 2nd ed. Sunderland, MA, Sinauer Associates.

Sarnyai Z, Shaham Y, Heinrichs SC (2001) The role of corticotropin-releasing factor in drug addiction. *Pharmacological Reviews*, **53**:209–293.

Sharma SK, Klee WA, Nirenberg N (1975) Dual regulation of adenylate cyclase accounts for narcotic dependence and tolerance. *Proceedings of the National Academy of Science of the United States of America*, **72**:3092–3096.

Shepherd GM (1994) *Neurobiology*. New York, NY, Oxford University Press.

Sklair-Tavron L et al. (1996) Chronic morphine induces visible changes in the morphology of mesolimbic dopamine neurons. *Proceedings of the National Academy of Science of the United States of America*, 93:11202–11207.

Unterwald EM et al. (1993) Chronic repeated cocaine administration alters basal and opioid-regulated adenylyl cyclase activity. *Synapse*, **15**:33–38.

Volkow ND, Rosen B, Farde L (1997) Imaging the living human brain: magnetic resonance imaging and positron emission tomography. *Proceedings of the National Academy of Sciences of the United States of America*, **94**:2787–2788.

Whistler J et al. (1999) Functional dissociation of μ-opioid receptor signaling and endocytosis: implications for the biology of opiate tolerance and addiction. *Neuron*, 23:737–746.

Wise RA (1998) Drug-activation of brain reward pathways. *Drug and Alcohol Dependence*, **51**:13–22.

Wonnacott S (1990) The paradox of nicotinic acetylcholine receptor upregulation by nicotine. *Trends in Neuroscience*, **11**:216–218.

CHAPTER 3

Biobehavioural Processes Underlying Dependence

Introduction

This chapter focuses on specific brain processes that are involved in the rewarding effects of psychoactive substance use, reinforcement and the development of dependence. Biological systems that have evolved to guide and direct behaviour towards stimuli that are critical to survival are recruited and abnormally strengthened by repeated use of psychoactive substances, leading to the cycle of behaviours characteristic of dependence.

The chapter also describes the current hypotheses and evidence on the biological basis of the behavioural and psychological factors that contribute to substance dependence. Dependence is the result of a complex interaction of the physiological effects of drugs on brain areas associated with motivation and emotion, combined with "learning" about the relationship between drugs and drug-related cues, all of which have a biological basis. These learning processes are critically dependent upon the same motivational and emotional systems in the brain that are acted upon by psychoactive substances (Hyman & Malenka, 2001).

Although each class of psychoactive substances has its own unique pharmacological mechanism of action (see Chapter 4), all psychoactive substances activate the mesolimbic dopamine system (Fig. 3.1). The current chapter focuses on mechanisms that are common to all psychoactive substances and that are responsible for the cluster of symptoms characteristic of substance dependence. The mesolimbic dopamine system, in particular, will be highlighted because of its key role in learning and motivational processes. In all cases, individual differences in biology and environment will affect the neurobiological effects of psychoactive substances; however, this chapter presents basic mechanisms that may underlie the development of dependence from a biobehavioural perspective.

The first section of this chapter provides an overview of learning theory and terminology as it relates to dependence. The next section explains how the unique properties of psychoactive substances can lead to dependence through sensitization of the incentive value of drugs. The processes of withdrawal and tolerance are also considered. Finally, individual differences in responses to psychoactive substances are discussed.

Fig. 3.1   Mesolimbic dopamine pathway

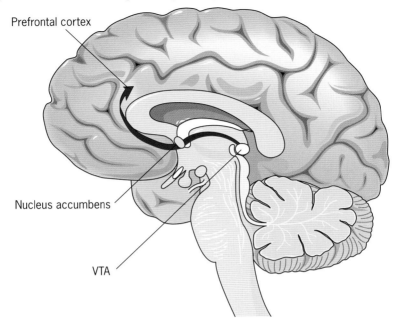

Source: National Institute on Drug Abuse (NIDA) website http://www.drugabuse.gov/pubs/teaching/largegifs/slide-9.gif

Defining terms

Behavioural science is concerned with studying those aspects of behaviour that can be objectively viewed and verified, and describing behaviour in terms of stimuli and responses to those stimuli. The development of dependence can be seen as part of a learning process, in the sense that enduring changes in behaviour result from interactions with drugs and drug-related environments. Psychoactive substances cause profound activation of specific areas of the brain involved in motivation, namely the mesolimbic dopamine system (see Fig. 3.1). Through associative learning processes, this may eventually lead to the classic symptoms of dependence following repeated exposure.

Basic principles of learning have been studied for decades, and have been applied to the field of drug dependence. Two major theories of learning and behaviour are relevant: (a) classical or Pavlovian conditioning and (b) instrumental or operant conditioning.

Classical or Pavlovian conditioning

Classical or Pavlovian conditioning is based on simple stimulus–response relationships as illustrated in Figure 3.2.

(a) A stimulus, such as the appearance of a light, normally elicits no particular response, i.e. it is a neutral stimulus.

(b) When a puff of air is blown into the eye, it reliably elicits a response: the eye blinks. The puff of air is the unconditioned stimulus and the eye blink is the unconditioned response. The unconditioned response occurs in response to the unconditioned stimulus.

(c) The unconditioned stimulus (puff of air) is repeatedly paired with the neutral stimulus (light).

(d) Eventually the light alone is able to elicit the same response (eye blink) as the puff of air on the assumption that a puff of air will follow. The light is now known as a conditioned stimulus and the response to it is the conditioned response.

This type of conditioning can occur for even complex behaviours such as emotional responses and drug craving. Advertisements for alcohol and tobacco products generally try to pair their products with images that create a positive emotional response. This leads to an association being formed in the brain between the product and the emotional response evoked by the advertisement. To an individual with substance dependence, the sight of drug paraphernalia (e.g. syringes, smoking devices) or exposure to environments in which drugs have previously been used can induce craving for drugs and relapse to substance use through classical conditioning processes. As discussed later in this chapter, the neurobiological basis of these associations with respect to psychoactive substance dependence appears to be dopamine signals in the nucleus accumbens.

Fig. 3.2 Classical or Pavlovian conditioning (see text)

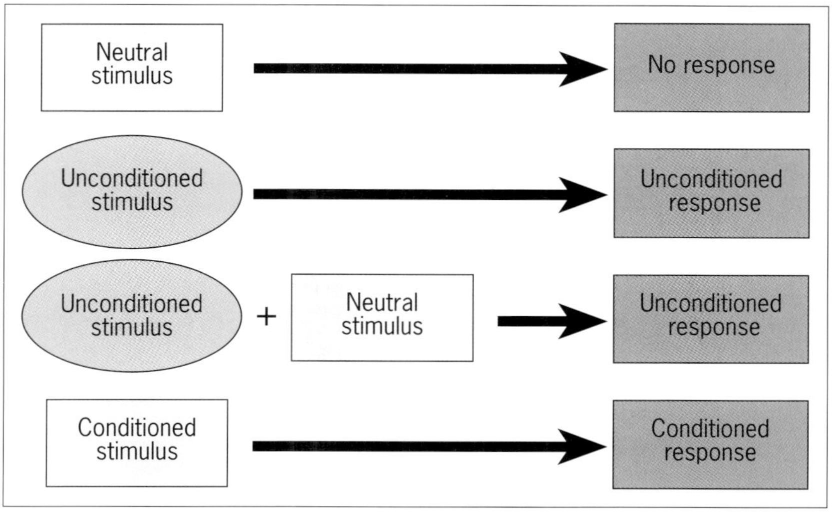

Instrumental or operant conditioning

Instrumental or operant conditioning is different from classical or Pavlovian conditioning in that in the latter the organism has no control over the presentation of the stimulus. For example, when the conditioned stimulus (light) appears, the conditioned response (eye blink) occurs. In contrast, in instrumental conditioning, the organism's behaviour produces the stimulus. That is, the behaviour occurs because of the consequences that it produces; it is instrumental in producing the consequences. This is often referred to as "goal-directed behaviour". There are three main categories of instrumental conditioning as illustrated in Figure 3.3: positive reinforcement, negative reinforcement and punishment. In positive reinforcement, a behaviour brings about a pleasurable stimulus, which reinforces the repetition of the behaviour. For example, animals can be trained to press a lever to obtain a food pellet. Thus, the behaviour produces the food, which is the stimulus. If the animal wants food, it learns to press the lever to obtain it. In negative reinforcement, a behaviour eliminates or prevents an aversive stimulus, which again reinforces the behaviour, or increases the likelihood of that behaviour occurring again. In punishment, the behaviour elicits an aversive stimulus. In this case, the behaviour is less likely to occur again. Instrumental

Fig. 3.3   Examples of instrumental conditioning (see text)

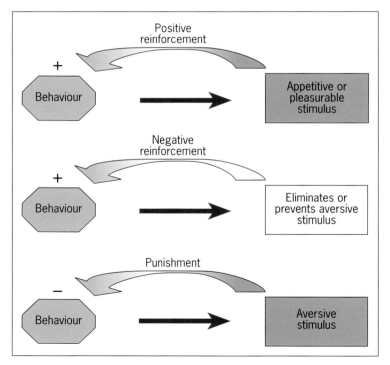

conditioning is important in substance use and dependence, since a person performs an operant response when choosing to acquire and use a psychoactive substances to experience its effects. Mesolimbic dopamine systems are also thought to be important in instrumental learning about the effects of psychoactive substances.

The following sections will examine aspects of learning theory as they relate to dependence.

Reinforcer

A reinforcer is commonly defined as a stimulus that strengthens responses upon which it is contingent (i.e. which it reliably follows). Thus, if one puts money in a vending machine to obtain a bar of chocolate, the chocolate acts as a reinforcer for the behaviour of putting money into the machine.

Reward

Reward is a term frequently used in the psychobiology of substance dependence, to describe the pleasurable or enjoyable effects of a drug. In general, rewards are stimuli that provide positive motivation for behaviour.

A fundamental feature of rewards is that of transferring their motivational properties to stimuli that predict their occurrence, and of strengthening responses upon which they are contingent. For this reason, rewards are reinforcers. Although many drugs are taken for their pleasure-producing or "rewarding" properties, this alone cannot account for the entire range of behavioural processes involved in substance dependence (Robinson & Berridge, 2000). Many stimuli can serve as rewards, but few take on the profound, all-consuming value that psychoactive substances do, such that they can lead to the symptoms and behaviours characteristic of dependence (see Chapter 1).

Incentive

The term incentive was originally used to refer to the ability of certain stimuli to elicit species-specific response patterns such as orienting, approaching or exploring (Bindra, 1974). This term implies that responding is a consequence of the stimuli (incentives). Accordingly, while reinforcers act as consequences of responding, incentives act as premises. An example of an incentive is a stimulus associated with food, such as smell, the sight of a restaurant, or an advertisement for food. These stimuli may elicit certain responses that direct attention and behaviour towards the acquisition of the food, and activate the motivational circuits in the brain in order to acquire the food. This example illustrates that incentives have two properties. One is a directional property that promotes responses directed towards the incentive, and towards the reward to which the incentive has been conditioned. The second is an activational property that promotes a state of motivational arousal. These two properties have their biological roots in the mesolimbic dopamine system, and act together to direct behaviour towards goals.

Motivation

Motivation is the allotment of attentional and behavioural resources to stimuli in relation to their predicted consequences. Motivation therefore involves learning of predictive relationships (contingencies) between neutral stimuli and biologically meaningful ones, and between responses and their outcomes. Learning of these contingencies enables the subject to act in ways that lead to the most desirable outcomes.

Incentive-motivational responding

Incentive-motivational responding is responding based on the motivation aroused by an external stimulus. Responding is a function of the perceived value of the stimulus to the organism. The basis for this form of motivated responding is hard-wired by evolution in the brain of organisms, including humans. Thus, certain stimuli such as the taste of a sweet or the cry of a predator, evoke responses that, depending on the stimulus, involve approaching or avoiding the object or organism from which they originate. Incentive-motivational responding is, however, subject to conditioning principles, and therefore stimuli associated with the primary unconditioned stimuli can take on incentive-motivational properties. Thus, individuals with substance dependence may seek out people or environments previously associated with drug use.

As an example of incentive-motivational responding, consider the earlier example of the sight or smell of food. If a person is not hungry, this may have little incentive-motivational value and hardly any attention will be paid to the food, with no attempt to obtain it. If the person is hungry, the incentive of food may cause him or her to orient towards the food, to begin to salivate, and prepare to eat. If extremely hungry, the incentive-motivational value of the food will be very high, and may cause the person to focus specifically on the food to the exclusion of other stimuli, to become preoccupied with the food, and possibly to engage in risky behaviour in order to obtain it. Similarly, as described in the following sections, once drugs become conditioned reinforcers, their incentive-motivational value can become higher than all other competing motivations.

Drug reward alone does not explain drug dependence

The self-administration of drugs for non-therapeutic and non-medical use is probably as old as human culture and civilization, and testifies that drugs serve as positive reinforcers (Johanson & Uhlenhuth, 1978). Additionally, the property of eliciting pleasurable feelings also indicates that drugs are indeed rewarding. Rewarding properties of drugs do not necessarily consist of sheer sensations of pleasure like the "high" or the "rush" typical of amphetamine and heroin or of inhaled crack (cocaine base) but can take milder forms of hedonia, such as relief of tension, reduction of fatigue, increased arousal, or improvement of performance. These positive sensations can explain why drugs are used, but not necessarily why they can produce the behavioural repertoire characteristic of dependence. In particular, drug reward alone cannot account for drug dependence, a condition characterized by compulsive, relapsing drug use and focusing of motivated behaviour on drugs to the exclusion of alternative goals and in the face of familiar, social and medical problems.

Clearly, the rewarding properties of drugs, at least as we understand them from their comparison with conventional rewards, do not fully explain the behavioural abnormalities associated with their use.

In the context of dependence, it is important to remember that over a lifespan many people experiment with a variety of potentially dependence-producing drugs, but most do not become dependent. Therefore, the question specifically becomes:

— what is the process by which drug-taking behaviour, in certain individuals, evolves into compulsive patterns of drug-seeking and drug-taking behaviour that take place at the expense of most other activities?

— what accounts for the inability of some compulsive drug users to stop using drugs?

A complex interplay of psychological, neurobiological and individual factors appears to be responsible. This section will cover some of the general principles concerning effects of psychoactive substances on learning and motivational processes that may come into effect during the development of dependence. Clearly, an individual's genetic and environmental background will influence the ultimate behavioural expression of these influences. These factors will be considered separately in other sections of this report. The following discussion is intended to provide information on how substance use interacts with motivational systems in the brain to contribute to the development of dependence.

Drug dependence as a response to incentive-motivation

While not sufficient, the rewarding properties of drugs are nonetheless necessary for their dependence-producing effects for at least two reasons. First, drug reward, by promoting drug self-administration, is necessary for repeated drug exposure. Secondly, the rewarding properties of drugs are necessary for attributing – by an associative learning mechanism – positive motivational value to stimuli that predict drug availability and act as powerful incentives of drug-seeking behaviour.

Because psychoactive drugs have strongly reinforcing properties, and because these reinforcing properties can increase the motivational value of drugs and drug-associated stimuli (e.g. environments where drugs are taken, the presence of drug dealers or drug users, the sight of drug paraphernalia) through repeated pairings, the incentive-motivational responding towards drugs and drug-associated stimuli is increased. (Wikler, 1973; Goldberg, 1976; Stewart, de Wit & Eikelboom, 1984; Childress et al., 1988; O'Brien et al., 1992; Robinson & Berridge, 1993; Di Chiara, 1998). Thus, the drug is used, it has rewarding effects, and this reinforces the drug-using behaviour and associated stimuli. The question is then: why are psychoactive substances such powerful reinforcers that they can lead to the development of dependence?

Drug dependence as a response to drug withdrawal

In addition to understanding drug dependence in terms of incentive theories, it can also be seen as a response to withdrawal reactions. Early theories of drug dependence, for example, placed major emphasis on the physical effects of withdrawal as a factor of drug dependence (Himmelsbach, 1943). In this regard, the adverse physical consequences of withdrawing from a drug's effects are viewed as a key motivational determinant of sustained drug taking through negative reinforcement mechanisms (see Fig. 3.3). However, it is possible to have dependence without withdrawal and withdrawal without dependence. For example, it is possible to have cocaine or alcohol dependence, but not to experience withdrawal symptoms between episodes of use. There can also be withdrawal symptoms in the absence of dependence, such as following long-term medical use of benzodiazepines or morphine. These factors are recognized in diagnostic criteria, where withdrawal is not necessary or sufficient for a diagnosis of dependence (see Chapter 1). For these reasons, more recent theories of dependence have moved the emphasis away from physical withdrawal, and towards motivational dependence produced in part by withdrawal-induced negative moods such as anhedonia and dysphoria. This state, by a negative reinforcing mechanism, would maintain drug self-administration because the drug removes the negative emotional state of withdrawal (Koob et al., 1989, 1997). The advantage of this modern version over early physical dependence theories is that motivational dependence has properties that are common to different classes of psychoactive substances while the properties of physical dependence differ widely from one class to another.

Dopamine and reinforcement learning

The role of dopamine in response-reinforcement learning is at the root of current models of instrumental responding (Montague, Dayan & Sejnowski,

1996; Schultz, Dayan & Montague, 1997). This is why, although different classes of psychoactive substances have different primary pharmacological mechanisms of action, dopamine is important to the development of dependence for all classes because of its critical role in response-reinforcement learning. Almost all psychoactive substances with reinforcing properties activate mesolimbic dopamine, either directly or indirectly. According to these models, dopamine is released in response to an unexpected reward. This leads to a strengthening of the synaptic connections in neural pathways that led to the behaviour that was associated with the reward. Although psychoactive substances act through a wide variety of primary pharmacological mechanisms, almost all eventually influence mesolimbic dopamine function, which is why dopamine is such an important neurochemical in the neuroscience of dependence. Dopamine is released in response to all unexpected rewards, thus reinforcing the behaviours that led to the occurrence of that reward.

Dependence-producing drugs as surrogates of conventional reinforcers

Drug and non-drug (e.g. stimuli associated with food, water, sex) reinforcers share behavioural and neurochemical similarities. For example, drug and non-drug reinforcers share the property of activating dopamine transmission preferentially in a region of the nucleus accumbens known as the "shell" (Pontieri, Tanda & Di Chiara, 1995; Robbins & Everitt, 1996; Bassareo & Di Chiara, 1997; Tanda, Pontieri & Di Chiara, 1997; Bassareo & Di Chiara, 1999). Therefore, dependence-producing drugs reproduce certain central neurochemical effects of conventional reinforcers (Di Chiara et al., 1993), thereby obtaining motivational significance in the brain.

Dependence-producing drugs, however, differ from conventional reinforcers in that their stimulant effects on dopamine release in the nucleus accumbens are significantly greater than natural reinforcers such as food. Whereas food increased dopamine levels in the nucleus accumbens by 45%, amphetamine and cocaine increased dopamine levels by 500% (Hernandez and Hoebel, 1988). The mesolimbic dopamine system reinforces behaviours and signals that are associated with stimuli that are critical to survival, such as feeding and reproduction. Because psychoactive substances also activate this circuit so powerfully and reliably, the drug-taking behaviour and stimuli associated with it are registered in the brain as being critically important. The repetitive, profound stimulation of dopamine transmission induced by drugs in the nucleus accumbens abnormally strengthens stimulus–drug associations (Pavlovian incentive learning). By this mechanism stimuli that are associated with or predictive of drugs are attributed great motivational value, thus becoming capable of facilitating behaviour that is instrumental to the self-administration of the drug.

Relapse to substance use is known to be triggered by cues previously paired with substance use, by stress, or by the presence of the drug itself (Stewart,

2000). All of these phenomena are mediated by increased mesolimbic dopamine. Thus, activity in these circuits can mediate not only the primary rewarding effects of the drugs, but also the conditioning of secondary stimuli, and the subsequent ability of these stimuli to trigger cravings and relapse.

Functional brain imaging techniques (see Chapter 2) are beginning to revolutionize the study of previously obscure concepts such as craving, which can now be "visualized" in discrete brain regions. For example, activation of the mesolimbic dopamine system and other brain regions by cocaine (Breiter et al., 1997), heroin (Sell et al., 1999), alcohol (Wang et al., 2000), nicotine (Volkow et al., 1999), or any other psychoactive substance, can be observed using functional imaging techniques. Moreover, brain responses to predictors of the drugs, or cues associated with drug use can also be measured. This is very important in terms of studying craving and relapse. When visual or verbal cues associated with heroin and cocaine are presented to people who use these substances, they result in metabolic activation in brain regions associated with expectancy of reward and learning (Childress et al., 1999; Sell et al., 1999; Wang et al., 1999; Sell et al., 2000). These studies also found that self-reports of "craving" and "urge to use" strongly correlated with metabolic changes in specific brain regions. This indicates that previously unmeasurable concepts such as craving are now beginning to be quantifiable, measurable phenomena associated with specific brain regions. In addition, the conditioning of secondary stimuli with drug effects can also be measured.

Dopamine and incentive sensitization

Dopamine was originally thought to mediate the rewarding or hedonic properties of drug and non-drug reinforcers (Wise, 1982). However, evidence obtained subsequently suggested that dopamine was affecting the motivation to respond for reward, rather than the experience of reward itself (Phillips & Fibiger, 1979; Gray & Wise, 1980). On this basis it was hypothesized that dopamine mediates the incentive-motivational properties of both primary reinforcers (rewards) and secondary reinforcers (Gray & Wise, 1980).

The above hypothesis has been further modified to distinguish between the rewarding properties of drugs, and the response-eliciting properties of drugs. Mesolimbic dopamine has been assigned a role in response-eliciting but not in rewarding (Robinson and Berridge 1993; Berridge 1996; Berridge & Robinson 1998; Robinson & Berridge, 2000). In other words, the reasons that people enjoy the primary effects of psychoactive substances may have to do with their effects on several different neurotransmitter systems, but the desire to repeat using the drugs comes from the activation of the brain mesolimbic dopamine system that guides motivated behaviour. Because psychoactive substances activate the mesolimbic dopamine system, and because the mesolimbic dopamine system has a primary role in guiding motivated behaviour, the repeated exposure of the brain to psychoactive substances leads to strong associations being formed. The mechanism by which dopamine exerts this function has been termed "incentive sensitization". Thus, the brain becomes more sensitive, or "sensitized" to the motivational and rewarding effects of psychoactive substances.

It is hypothesized that this process of incentive sensitization produces compulsive patterns of drug-seeking behaviour. Through associative learning, the enhanced incentive value becomes focused specifically on drug-related stimuli, leading to more and more compulsive patterns of drug-seeking and drug-taking behaviour.

Psychomotor sensitization

Most laboratory studies showing that the repeated administration of psychoactive substances can produce sensitization of the mesolimbic dopamine system involve two measures: measures of levels of dopamine and its metabolites in the nucleus accumbens, and measures of the psychomotor-activating effects of drugs, such as their ability to enhance locomotor activity in laboratory animals. Studies on the psychomotor-activating effects of drugs are relevant to dependence because the mesolimbic dopamine system controls both locomotion and behaviour, and locomotion is an easily observable behavioural assay of nucleus accumbens function (Wise & Bozarth, 1987).

There is now considerable evidence that the repeated intermittent administration of psychomotor-stimulant substances results in a progressive increase in their psychomotor- activating effects. Psychomotor sensitization has been shown for amphetamine, cocaine, methylphenidate, fencamfamin, morphine, phencyclidine, ecstasy, nicotine and ethanol (Robinson & Berridge, 1993).

Sensitization is remarkably persistent, and animals that have been sensitized may remain hypersensitive to the psychomotor-activating effects of drugs for months or years (Robinson & Becker, 1986; Paulson, Camp & Robinson, 1991). It is important to note that sensitization can develop even after a drug has been self-administered (Hooks et al., 1994; Phillips & DiCiano, 1996; Marinelli, Le Moal & Piazza, 1998), and therefore, that the experimental models of sensitization are valid models of human substance use.

Sensitization and drug reward

Studies show that sensitization results from the psychomotor-activating effects as well as the rewarding effects of psychoactive drugs (Schenk & Partridge, 1997). Thus, upon repeated exposure to drugs *over time*, their subjective rewarding effects are increased. (Note that this is in contrast to the short-term tolerance that may occur within a single session of drug intake. Sensitization develops over days to weeks to months). It is thought that the shift from substance use to substance dependence may be closely related to the phenomenon of sensitization (Deroche, Le Moal & Piazza, 1999).

There is a large body of data showing that sensitization is associated with marked changes in the mesolimbic dopamine system. There are both presynaptic changes (increased dopamine release) and postsynaptic changes (changes in receptor sensitivity). In addition, structural changes in output neurons in the nucleus accumbens and prefrontal cortex have also been seen following sensitization to amphetamine and cocaine (Robinson & Kolb, 1997; 1999).

Sensitization and tolerance

It is important at this point to emphasize again that this discussion focuses on sensitization of the mesolimbic dopamine system, i.e. the increase in dopamine in the nucleus accumbens that is observed on repeated drug presentations, and that has been reported for psychoactive substances of all classes.

Tolerance can be defined as a given drug producing a decreasing effect with repeated dosing, or when larger doses must be administered to produce the same effect (Jaffe, 1985, 1990). There is differential tolerance to psychomotor stimulants, meaning that tolerance develops to some of the drug effects, but not to others. Indeed, as will be discussed, some drug effects are *increased* upon repeated drug use. In humans, rapid tolerance develops to the anorexic effects and the lethal effects of amphetamine and cocaine (Angrist & Sudilovsky, 1978; Hoffman & Lefkowitz, 1990). However, no tolerance or change in sensitivity of behavioural responses was observed after repeated daily oral doses of 10 mg of D-amphetamine (Johanson, Kilgore & Uhlenhuth, 1983). Similarly, no tolerance developed to the subjective "high" after repeated daily oral doses of 10 mg of methamphetamin, but tolerance did develop to the cardiovascular effects with repeated daily dosing (Perez-Reyes et al., 1991). Some acute tolerance appears to develop to the cardiovascular effects of cocaine even over a 4-hour infusion period (Ambre et al., 1988). Subjective, behavioural and cardiovascular effects also decline after sequential oral doses of D-amphetamine, despite substantial plasma levels, also suggesting acute tolerance (Angrist et al., 1987). Tolerance does not develop to the stereotyped behaviour and psychosis induced by stimulants, and in fact these behavioural effects appear to show sensitization or an increase with repeated administration (Post et al., 1992). Similar results have been observed in animal studies, with tolerance developing to the anorexic and lethal effects of amphetamine but not to stereotyped behaviour (Lewander, 1974). The same is also true of tolerance to nicotine, alcohol and benzodiazepines, which develops to some drug effects but not others. Tolerance to specific classes of psychoactive substances will be discussed further in Chapter 4.

Tolerance can also develop as a result of metabolic enzyme induction, i.e. enzymes that are involved in the metabolism of a drug can increase their activity in the presence of increasing concentrations of the drug. The metabolism of alcohol and nicotine by the cytochrome P450 enzymes in the liver can be increased in this way, thus larger doses are needed for the drug to achieve the same effects as it had prior to enzyme induction. Tolerance can also develop due to changes in receptor number or sensitivity. These concepts will be further discussed in Chapter 4.

Although tolerance and sensitization to different aspects of a drug's effects can coexist (Hyman & Malenka, 2001), sensitization and tolerance are essentially separate phenomena.

Sensitization occurs in connection with the rewarding effects of psycho-active substances, and appears to be very important in the acquisition of persistent substance use (Schenk & Partridge, 1997). Pre-exposure to a drug can reduce the latency period for experimental animals to acquire self-administration, and also can result in lower than expected doses of a drug having reinforcing effects (Schenk & Partridge, 1997). This sensitization can occur either through pre-exposure or from environmental factors such as stress (Antelman et al., 1980; Cador et al., 1992; Deroche et al., 1992; Henry et al., 1995; Badiani, Oates & Robinson, 2000). A key feature of sensitization is that it is long-lasting (Robinson & Becker, 1986). Conversely, tolerance to the behavioural effects of a drug appears to be more transient, and associated with high frequency of drug use in a short period of time (Schenk & Partridge, 1997). Again, it is important to emphasize that tolerance and sensitization can coexist in respect to different aspects of the drug's effects (Hyman & Malenka, 2001), and that tolerance can have both acute and chronic aspects.

Individual differences

There are individual differences in biology and environmental factors that mediate the reinforcing effects of psychoactive substances. Individual differences in response to first drug use can determine who will be more likely to use the drug again (Davidson, Finch & Schenk, 1993). In animal models, there are clear behavioural differences that can predict which animals are more likely to develop sensitization and learn to self-administer drugs more quickly (Piazza et al., 1990; Hooks et al. 1992; De Sousa, Bush & Vaccarino, 2000; Sutton, Karanian & Self, 2000). These behavioural factors are related to increased mesolimbic dopamine in susceptible animals, both at baseline and following food and drug rewards (Sills & Crawley, 1996; Sills, Onalaja & Crawley, 1998). These findings have led to suggestions that there may be a behavioural phenotype associated with mesolimbic dopamine function in humans that can predict those who are more susceptible to developing substance dependence (Zuckerman, 1984; Bardo, Donohew & Harrington, 1996; Dellu et al., 1996; Depue & Collins, 1999).

To summarize, dependence-producing substances share the ability to produce persistent changes in brain regions that are involved in the process of incentive- motivation and reward, and such changes make these regions hypersensitive (sensitized). There is a wealth of evidence to support this claim.

BOX 3.1

Definitions

Classical conditioning

Also called Pavlovian conditioning after Pavlov's experiments with dogs, in which stimuli such as the sound of a bell, repeatedly paired with food presentation, eventually came to elicit salivation in the dogs in the absence of the food. Classical conditioning is the simplest form of learning to make new responses to stimuli and to learn about relationships between stimuli. It is a form of learning in which a previously neutral stimulus (conditioned stimulus) gains power over behaviour through association with a biologically relevant stimulus (unconditioned stimulus), and can elicit the same behavioural or physiological response (unconditioned response) as the unconditioned stimulus. The response to the conditioned stimulus is called the conditioned response.

Conditioned response

In classical (or Pavlovian) conditioning, a response elicited by a previously neutral stimulus, which occurs as a result of pairing the neutral stimulus with an unconditioned stimulus.

Conditioned stimulus

In classical conditioning, the previously neutral stimulus which comes to elicit a conditioned response.

Cognition

The process of knowing, including attending, remembering, reasoning etc., as well as the content of these processes, such as concepts and memories.

Craving

Drug craving is the desire for the previously-experienced effects of a psychoactive substance. This desire can become compelling and can increase in the presence of both internal and external cues, particularly with perceived substance availability. It is characterized by an increased likelihood of drug-seeking behaviour and, in humans, of drug-related thoughts.

Dependence

A cluster of cognitive, behavioural, and physiological symptoms indicating that the individual continues the use of the substance despite significant substance-related problems.

Emotion

A complex phenomenon, including physiological arousal, feelings, cognitive processes, and behavioural reactions, made in response to a situation perceived to be personally significant.

Habit

A behaviour performed automatically in response to specific stimuli, independently from its outcome.

Habituation

A decrease in the ability of a stimulus to elicit a response.

Incentive-motivation

Motivation due to stimuli that elicit responses on the basis of their contingency with other stimuli (Pavlovian principle).

Learning

A process that results in a relatively permanent change in behaviour or behavioural potential based on experience.

Memory

The mental capacity to store and later recognize or recall events that were previously experienced.

Reinforcement

The increase in the probability that a behaviour will occur because of the consequences of that behaviour.

Reinforcer

A stimulus that strengthens responses upon which it is contingent (i.e. which it reliably follows).

Reward

A primary, unconditioned stimulus that utilizes sensory modalities (e.g. gustatory, tactile, thermic), and provides feelings of pleasure or well-being.

Sensitization

An increase in the effect of a drug following repeated use. It may be expressed as behavioural sensitization, and is presumably the result of neural sensitization. (An increase in the ability of a stimulus to elicit a response).

Stimulus

Any event in the environment that is detected by the sense organs could be a stimulus.

Tolerance

A decrease in the effect of the same dose of a drug following repeated use.

Withdrawal

A maladaptive behavioural change, with physiological and cognitive concomitants, that occurs when blood or tissue concentrations of a substance decline in an individual who had maintained prolonged heavy use of the substance.

Persistence of neural sensitization may leave dependent individuals susceptible to relapse long after discontinuation of substance use. Relapse can occur following stress, exposure to the drug or a similar drug or to drug cues. Individual differences in genetics and environmental factors, however, will have mitigating effects on the primary rewarding effects of psychoactive substances.

Summary

Substance dependence may be viewed as the result of the action of various factors. In the early stages of substance use, as a result of curiosity, peer pressure, social marketing factors, ubiquity of exposure, personality traits, and other related factors, the subject comes into contact with a drug with dependence-producing effects. The reinforcing properties of the drug, together with the individual's own biological make-up and environmental background, may facilitate further exposure to the drug. Associative learning properties related to release of dopamine in the nucleus accumbens also strengthen the reinforcing effects of the drug and of the environment and emotions associated with its use. In this stage the subject responds to the drug and to drug-related stimuli in a manner not dissimilar from normal motivated responding. Through activation of emotional and motivational centres of the brain, learning processes are invoked. It is important to note here that exposure to psychoactive substances and substance use in everyday life and through the media, particularly when presented in a positive environment, can create pleasurable emotions. An individual can easily become conditioned to associate these emotions with substance use, resulting in learning, focused attention, facilitated memory, and the development of attitudes surrounding substance use that guide motivation. These factors all interact with individual, biological, social, and cultural factors to determine whether or not substance use is repeated, and whether that repeated substance use results in the cluster of symptoms known as dependence.

With repeated drug exposure, there is the repeated association of drug reward and drug-related stimuli parallel to the stimulation of dopamine transmission in the nucleus accumbens, resulting in the attribution of motivational value to drug-associated stimuli. This is the stage of incentive sensitization. In this stage the person can still control drug intake in the absence of drug-related stimuli and is not dependent, but can experience health and social consequences of his or her substance use. This stage is often called hazardous substance use.

The stage of dependence is clinically defined by at least three of the following:

— a strong desire or sense of compulsion to take the substance;

— difficulties in controlling substance-taking behaviour in terms of its onset, termination or levels of use;

— a physiological state of withdrawal;

— evidence of tolerance;

— progressive neglect of alternative pleasures or interests;

— persistent use despite clear evidence of overtly harmful consequences.

Compulsive drug-seeking and craving are elicited by the presence of drugs or associated stimuli (see Chapter 1).

Neuroscience focuses on the events that occur to bring about each of these symptoms. However, some behaviours are more easily studied than others. Tolerance and withdrawal have been relatively easier to define and measure in laboratory animals, which has led to a greater understanding of the effects of drugs on health and the long-term consequences of substance use. Concepts such as craving, loss of control and persistent use have been harder to study in the laboratory. However, modern neuroimaging studies of the human brain are helping researchers to understand these processes in greater detail than ever before, and are for the first time giving objective, measurable images of previously uncharacterizable phenomena such as "craving".

It is also interesting to relate these biobehavioural learning processes to the behavioural therapies that are sometimes employed in treating substance dependence (see Box 3.2). Motivational and cognitive therapies are designed to work on the same motivational systems in the brain as those that are affected by substance dependence. These therapies try to replace the motivation to use drugs with the motivation to engage in other behaviours. Note that these therapies rely on the same principles of learning and motivation that are used to describe the development of dependence. Contingency management, for example, uses the principles of positive reinforcement and punishment to manage behaviour. Cognitive behavioural therapies and relapse prevention help the person develop new stimulus–response associations that do not involve substance use or craving. These principles are employed in an attempt to "unlearn" the dependence-related behaviour and to learn more adaptive responses. Similar neurobiological mechanisms are involved in the development of dependence, as are involved in learning to overcome dependence.

BOX 3.2

Types of psychotherapies/behavioural interventions

Cognitive behavioural therapies

Cognitive behavioural therapies focus on (a) altering the cognitive processes that lead to maladaptive behaviours of substance users, (b) intervening in the behavioural chain of events that lead to substance use, (c) helping patients deal successfully with acute or chronic drug craving, and (d) promoting and reinforcing the development of social skills and behaviours compatible with remaining drug free. The foundation of cognitive therapy is the belief that by identifying and subsequently modifying maladaptive thinking patterns, patients can reduce or eliminate negative feelings and behaviour (e.g. substance use).

Relapse prevention

An approach to treatment in which cognitive behavioural techniques are used in an attempt to help patients develop greater self-control in order to avoid relapse. Specific relapse prevention strategies include discussing ambivalence, identifying emotional and environmental triggers of craving and substance use, and developing and reviewing specific coping strategies to deal with internal or external stressors.

Contingency management

A behavioural treatment based on the use of predetermined positive or negative consequences to reward abstinence or punish (and thus deter) drug-related behaviours. Rewards have included vouchers – awarded for producing drug-free urine samples – that can be exchanged for mutually agreed-upon on items (e.g. cinema tickets) or 'community reinforcement,' in which family members or peers reinforce behaviours that demonstrate or facilitate abstinence (e.g. participation in positive activities). Negative consequences for returning to substance use may include notification of courts, employers or family members.

Motivational enhancement therapy (MET)

This brief treatment modality is characterized by an empathetic approach in which the therapist helps to motivate the patient by asking about the pros and cons of specific behaviours, by exploring the patient's goals and associated ambivalence about reaching these goals, and by listening reflectively. Motivational enhancement therapy has demonstrated substantial efficacy in the treatment of substance dependence.

Source: The American Journal of Psychiatry, 1995.

References

Ambre JJ et al. (1988) Acute tolerance to cocaine in humans. *Clinical Pharmacology and Therapeutics*, **44**:1–8.

Angrist B, Sudilovsky A (1978) Central nervous system stimulants: historical aspects and clinical effects. In: Iversen LL, Iversen SD, Snyder SH, eds. *Handbook of psychopharmacology. Vol. 11. Stimulants*. New York, NY, Plenum Press:99–165.

Angrist B et al. (1987) Early pharmacokinetics and clinical effects of oral D-amphetamine in normal subjects. *Biological Psychiatry*, **22**:1357–1368.

Antelman SM et al. (1980) Interchangeability of stress and amphetamine in sensitization. *Science*, **207**:329–331.

Badiani A, Cabib S, Puglisi-Allegra S (1992) Chronic stress induces strain-dependent sensitization to the behavioral effects of amphetamine in the mouse. *Pharmacology, Biochemistry and Behavior*, **43**:53–60.

Badiani A, Anagnostaras SG, Robinson TE (1995) The development of sensitization to the psychomotor stimulant effects of amphetamine is enhanced in a novel environment. *Psychopharmacology*, **117**:443–452.

Badiani A, Oates MM, Robinson TE (2000) Modulation of morphine sensitization in the rat by contextual stimuli. *Psychopharmacology*, **151**:273–282.

Bardo MT, Donohew RL, Harrington NG (1996) Psychobiology of novelty-seeking and drug-seeking behavior. *Behavioural Brain Research*, **77**:23–43.

Bassareo V, Di Chiara G (1997) Differential influence of associative and non-associative learning mechanisms on the responsiveness of prefrontal and accumbal dopamine transmission to food stimuli in rats fed ad libitum. *Journal of Neuroscience*, **17**:851–861.

Bassareo V, Di Chiara G (1999) Differential responsiveness of dopamine transmission to food stimuli in nucleus accumbens shell/core compartments. *Neuroscience*, **89**:637–641.

Berridge KC (1996) Food reward: brain substrates of wanting and liking. *Neuroscience and Biobehavioral Reviews*, **20**:1–25.

Berridge KC, Robinson TE (1998) What is the role of dopamine in reward: hedonic impact, reward learning, or incentive salience? *Brain Research Reviews*, **28**:309–369.

Bindra D (1974) A motivational view of learning, performance, and behavior modification. *Psychological Reviews*, **81**:199–213.

Breiter HC et al. (1997) Acute effects of cocaine on human brain activity and emotion. *Neuron*, **19**:591–611.

Cador M et al. (1992) Behavioral sensitization induced by psychostimulants or stress: search for a molecular basis and evidence for a CRF-dependent phenomenon. *Annals of the New York Academy of Sciences*, **654**:416–420.

Childress AR et al. (1988) Classically conditioned responses in opioid and cocaine dependence: a role in relapse? *NIDA Research Monograph*, **94**:25–43.

Childress AR et al. (1999) Limbic activation during cue-induced cocaine craving. *American Journal of Psychiatry*, **156**:11–18.

Davidson ES, Finch JF, Schenk S (1993) Variability in subjective response to cocaine: initial experiences of college students. *Addictive Behaviors*, **18**:445–453.

Dellu F et al. (1996) Novelty-seeking in rats: biobehavioral characteristics and possible relationship with the sensation-seeking trait in man. *Neuropsycho-biology*, **34**:136–145.

Depue RA, Collins PF (1999) Neurobiology of the structure of personality: dopamine, facilitation of incentive motivation, and extraversion. *Behavioral Brain Science*, **22**:491–517.

Deroche V, Le Moal M, Piazza PV (1999) Cocaine self-administration increases the incentive motivational properties of the drug in rats. *European Journal of Neuroscience*, **11**:2731–2736.

Deroche V et al. (1992) Stress-induced sensitization to amphetamine and morphine psychomotor effects depend on stress-induced corticosterone secretion. *Brain Research*, **598**:343–348.

De Sousa NJ, Bush DEA, Vaccarino FJ (2000) Self-administration of intravenous amphetamine is predicted by individual differences in sucrose feeding in rats. *Psychopharmacology*, **148**:52–58.

Di Chiara G (1998) A motivational learning hypothesis of the role of dopamine in compulsive drug use. *Journal of Psychopharmacology*, **12**:54–67.

Di Chiara G et al. (1993) On the preferential release of dopamine in the nucleus accumbens by amphetamine: further evidence obtained by vertically implanted concentric dialysis probes. *Psychopharmacology*, **112**:398–402.

Goldberg SR (1976) Stimuli associated with drug injections as events that control behavior. *Pharmacological Reviews*, **27**:325–340.

Gray T, Wise RA (1980) Effects of pimozide on lever pressing behavior maintained on an intermittent reinforcement schedule. *Pharmacology, Biochemistry and Behavior*, **12**:931–935.

Henry C et al. (1995) Prenatal stress in rats facilitates amphetamine-induced sensitization and induces long-lasting changes in dopamine receptors in the nucleus accumbens. *Brain Research*, **685**:179–186.

Hernandez L, Hoebel BG (1988) Food reward and cocaine increase extracellular dopamine in the nucleus accumbens as measured by microdialysis. *Life Sciences*, **42**:1705–1712.

Himmelsbach CK (1943) Morphine, with reference to physical dependence. *Federation Proceedings*, **2**:201–203.

Hoffman BB, Lefkowitz RJ (1990) Catecholamines and sympathomimetic drugs. In: Gilman AG et al., eds. *Goodman and Gilman's: The pharmacological basis of therapeutics*, 8th ed. New York, NY, Pergamon Press:187–220.

Hooks MS et al. (1992) Individual differences in amphetamine sensitization: dose-dependent effects. *Pharmacology, Biochemistry and Behavior*, **41**:203–210.

Hooks MS et al. (1994) Behavioral and neurochemical sensitization following cocaine self-administration. *Psychopharmacology*, **115**:265–272.

Hyman SE, Malenka RC (2001) Addiction and the brain: the neurobiology of compulsion and its persistence. *Nature Reviews: Neuroscience*, **2**:695–703.

Jaffe JH (1985) Drug addiction and drug abuse. In: Gilman AG, Goodman LS, Rall TW, eds. *Goodman and Gilman's: The pharmacological basis of therapeutics*, 7th ed. New York, NY, MacMillan:522–573.

Jaffe JH (1990) Drug addiction and drug use. In: Gilman AG et al., eds. *Goodman and Gilman's: The pharmacological basis of therapeutics*, 8th ed. New York, NY, Pergamon Press: 522–573.

Johanson CE, Uhlenhuth EH (1978) Drug self-administration in humans. *NIDA Research Monograph*, **20**:68–85.

Johanson CE, Kilgore K, Uhlenhuth EH (1983) Assessment of dependence potential of drugs in humans using multiple indices. *Psychopharmacology*, **81**:144–149.

Koob GF et al. (1989) Opponent process theory of motivation: neurobiological evidence from studies of opiate dependence. *Neuroscience and Biobehavioral Reviews*, **13**:135–140.

Koob GF et al. (1997) Opponent process model and psychostimulant addiction. *Pharmacology, Biochemistry and Behavior*, **57**:513–521.

Lewander T (1974) Effect of chronic treatment with central stimulants on brain monoamines and some behavioral and physiological functions in rats, guinea pigs, and rabbits. In: Usdin E, ed. *Advances in biochemical psychopharmacology. Vol. 12. Neuropsychopharmacology of monoamines and their regulatory enzymes*. New York, NY, Raven Press:221–239.

Marinelli M, Le Moal M, Piazza PV (1998) Sensitization to the motor effects of contingent infusions of heroin but not of kappa agonist RU 51599. *Psychopharmacology* (Berlin), **139**:281–285.

Montague PR, Dayan P, Sejnowski TJ (1996) A framework for mesencephalic dopamine systems based on predictive Hebbian learning. *Journal of Neuroscience*, **16**:1936–1947.

O'Brien CP et al. (1992) Classical conditioning in drug-dependent humans. *Annals of the New York Academy of Sciences*, **654**:400–415.

Paulson PE, Camp DM, Robinson TE (1991) Time course of transient behavioral depression and persistent behavioral sensitization in relation to regional brain monoamine concentrations during amphetamine withdrawal in rats. *Psychopharmacology* (Berlin), **103**:480–492.

Perez-Reyes M et al. (1991) Clinical effects of daily methamphetamine administration. *Clinical Neuropharmacology*, **14**:352–358.

Phillips AG, Fibiger HC (1979) Decreased resistance to extinction after haloperidol: implications for the role of dopamine in reinforcement. *Pharmacology, Biochemistry and Behavior*, **10**:751–760.

Phillips AG, Di Ciano P (1996) Behavioral sensitization is induced by intravenous self-administration of cocaine by rats. *Psychopharmacology* (Berlin), **124**:279–281.

Piazza PV et al. (1990) Individual reactivity to novelty predicts probability of amphetamine self-administration. *Behavioural Pharmacology*, **1**:339–345.

Pontieri FE, Tanda G, Di Chiara G (1995) Intravenous cocaine, morphine and amphetamine preferentially increase extracellular dopamine in the "shell" as compared with the "core" of the rat nucleus accumbens. *Proceedings of the National Academy of Science of the United States of America*, **92**:12 304–12 308.

Post RM et al. (1992) Conditioned sensitization to the psychomotor stimulant cocaine. *Annals of the New York Academy of Sciences.* **654**:386–399.

Robbins TW, Everitt BJ (1996) Neurobehavioural mechanisms of reward and motivation. *Current Opinion in Neurobiology*, **6**:228–236.

Robinson TE, Becker JB (1986) Enduring changes in brain and behavior produced by chronic amphetamine administration: a review and evaluation of animal models of amphetamine psychosis. *Brain Research Reviews*, **11**:157–198.

Robinson TE, Berridge KC (1993) The neural basis of drug craving: an incentive-sensitization theory of addiction. *Brain Research Reviews*, **18**:247–291.

Robinson TE, Kolb B (1997) Persistent structural modifications in nucleus accumbens and prefrontal cortex neurons produced by previous experience with amphetamine. *Journal of Neuroscience*, **17**:8491–8497.

Robinson TE, Kolb B (1999) Alterations in the morphology of dendrites and dendritic spines in the nucleus accumbens and prefrontal cortex following repeated treatment with amphetamine or cocaine. *European Journal of Neuroscience*, **11**:1598–1604.

Robinson TE, Berridge KC (2000) The psychology and neurobiology of addiction: an incentive-sensitization view. *Addiction*, **95**(Suppl 2):S91–S117.

Schenk S, Partridge B (1997) Sensitization and tolerance in psychostimulant self-administration. *Pharmacology, Biochemistry and Behavior*, **57**:543–550.

Schultz W, Dayan P, Montague PR (1997) A neural substrate of prediction and reward. *Science*, **275**:1593–1599.

Sell LA et al. (1999) Activation of reward circuitry in human opiate addicts. *European Journal of Neuroscience*, **11**:1042–1048.

Sell LA et al. (2000) Neural responses associated with cue evoked emotional states and heroin in opiate addicts. *Drug and Alcohol Dependence*, **60**:207–216.

Sills TL, Crawley JN (1996) Individual differences in sugar consumption predict amphetamine-induced dopamine overflow in nucleus accumbens. *European Journal of Pharmacology*, **303**:177–181.

Sills TL, Onalaja AO, Crawley JN (1998) Mesolimbic dopaminergic mechanisms underlying individual differences in sugar consumption and amphetamine hyperlocomotion in Wistar rats. *European Journal of Neuroscience*, **10**:1895–1902.

Stewart J (2000) Pathways to relapse: the neurobiology of drug- and stress-induced relapse to drug-taking. *Journal of Psychiatry and Neuroscience*, **25**:125–136.

Stewart J, de Wit H, Eikelboom R (1984) Role of unconditioned and conditioned drug effects in the self-administration of opiates and stimulants. *Psychological Reviews*, **91**:251–268.

Sutton MA, Karanian DA, Self DW (2000) Factors that determine a propensity for cocaine-seeking behavior during abstinence in rats. *Neuropsychopharmacology*, **22**:626–641.

Tanda G, Pontieri FE, Di Chiara G (1997) Cannabinoid and heroin activation of mesolimbic dopamine transmission by a common µl opioid receptor mechanism. *Science*, **276**:2048–2050.

The American Journal of Psychiatry (1995) Practice guidelines for the treatment of patients with substance use disorders: alcohol, cocaine, opioids. *The American Journal of Psychiatry,* **152**(Suppl):S1–S59.

Volkow ND et al. (1999) Imaging the neurochemistry of nicotine actions: studies with positron emission tomography. *Nicotine and Tobacco Research*, **1**(Suppl 2):S127–S132.

Wang GJ et al. (1999) Regional brain metabolic activation during craving elicited by recall of previous drug experiences. *Life Sciences*, **64**:775–784.

Wang GJ et al. (2000) Regional brain metabolism during alcohol intoxication. *Alcoholism: Clinical and Experimental Research*, **24**:822–829.

Wikler A (1973) Dynamics of drug dependence: implications of a conditioning theory for research and treatment. *Archives of General Psychiatry,* **28**:611–616.

Wise RA (1982) Neuroleptics and operant behavior: the anhedonia hypothesis. *Behavioral and Brain Sciences*, **5**:39–87.

Wise RA, Bozarth MA (1987) A psychomotor stimulant theory of addiction. *Psychological Reviews*, **94**:469–492.

Zuckerman M (1984) Sensation seeking: a comparative approach to a human trait. *Behavioral and Brain Sciences*, **7**:413–471.

CHAPTER 4

Psychopharmacology of Dependence for Different Drug Classes

Introduction

The purpose of this chapter is to provide an overview of the major classes of psychoactive substances, and their individual and common effects in the brain. The previous chapter introduced the biobehavioural concepts that explain how a substance[1] with rewarding properties can be reinforcing, causing the self-administration of that substance to be repeated, and how this can lead to sensitization of motivational circuits in the brain, and ultimately to dependence. This chapter will discuss each class of psychoactive substances, its mechanism of action, behavioural effects, development of tolerance and withdrawal, long-term neuropsychological consequences, and potential pharmacological treatments (see Tables 4.1 and 4.2). Finally, common neurobiological and cellular effects of psychoactive substances will be presented. By understanding the acute and chronic effects of drug action, targeted therapies can be developed, and questions concerning how and why some drugs can be used by certain individuals without leading to dependence, whereas others lead to chronic dependence and relapse, can be better understood.

At all times, it is important to remember that individual differences in genetics, biology, and social and cultural factors influence the effects of a substance on a person and the outcome of substance use. This chapter presents the commonly known effects of drugs from research on large groups of people and on experimental animals.

The pharmacology of the common psychoactive substances is considered: alcohol, sedative/hypnotics, nicotine, opioids, cannabis, cocaine, amphetamines, ecstasy, volatile solvents, and hallucinogens. For each one of those, a brief review is provided of:

— behavioural manifestations of acute and chronic use of a drug in humans and in animal models;

— molecular and biochemical mechanism of action in the main brain areas involved with acute effects;

---

[1] The terms substance, drug, psychoactive substance or psychoactive drug, are used interchangeably in this report, and may refer to nicotine, alcohol or other drugs.

— development of tolerance and withdrawal;

— neurological adaptations (direct effects and indirect effects) due to prolonged use;

— information on pharmacological treatment approaches for each drug class where available.

Animal models are frequently employed in order to better understand the biological basis of drug use and drug action. The following animal models show reliability when used to study selective aspects of human dependence and substance use:

— self-administration;

— intracerebral self-stimulation;

— place preference;

— drug discrimination.

There are several different procedures within each one of these models, as extensively reviewed by Koob (1995). The reinforcing properties of the drugs will cause animals from different species to perform operant tasks to self-administer drugs. This is considered to model the dependence-producing potential of the drugs, and is also widely used for preclinical assessment of new therapies. Self-stimulation of certain brain areas activates brain circuits that are probably activated by natural reinforcers. Psychoactive substances are tested in this paradigm to verify whether they decrease the reward threshold and if they influence in the reward and reinforcement processes. Place preference uses a Pavlovian conditioning procedure to evaluate reinforcement by a drug. One assumes that an animal that chooses to spend more time in an area that has been paired with a certain drug state expresses the positive reinforcement experience in that location. The last model, i.e. drug discrimination, relies on the assumption that the discriminative stimulus of a drug in animals is a reflection of the subjective effects of the drug in humans. These drug effects would serve as an internal cue that induces effects similar to the effects of a well-known psychoactive drug.

Research into dependence has been difficult for neuroscientists for the reason that dependence is made up of many behavioural and physiological components, some of which can be readily measured, such as withdrawal symptoms, while others are more difficult to study experimentally, such as craving and loss of control.

Animal models have been very useful for studying substance use, and the short-term and long-term physical effects of substance use. Other components of dependence are more difficult to study, or are uniquely human, such as craving, social consequences of substance use, and feelings of loss of control over substance use. However, developments in neuroscience over the past several years have greatly enhanced the ability to study changes in human brain function and composition, using functional magnetic resonance imaging (MRI), regional cerebral blood flow, and positron emission tomography (PET).

Major advances in the understanding and treatment of dependence have come from understanding the basic mechanisms of drug action and long-term health consequences. There have been some successful treatments, such as methadone for heroin dependence, nicotine patches for nicotine dependence, and various pharmacotherapies for alcohol dependence.

The development of treatments and medications is promising, but brings with it a host of ethical issues which need to be addressed (see Chapter 7). However, it is important to first understand the biology behind these new approaches to treatment, as well as the research and animal models used to gain insight into the effects of psychoactive substance use.

Alcohol (ethanol)

Introduction

Beverage alcohol (ethyl alcohol or ethanol) is consumed throughout the world for recreational and religious purposes (Jacobs & Fehr, 1987). It is produced by fermentation and distillation of agricultural products.

Ethanol is almost always taken orally, and absorbed quickly from the small intestine into the bloodstream. Delays in gastric emptying, caused by, for example, the presence of food, will slow its absorption. First-pass metabolism by gastric, and consequently hepatic alcohol dehydrogenase, decreases the bioavailability of ethanol while gender and genetic diversity may account for individual differences in blood alcohol levels. Very small amounts of ethanol may be excreted unchanged in urine, sweat and breath while most of it is metabolized to acetyldehyde by alcohol dehydrogenase, catalase and microsomal P450 enzymes largely in the liver. Subsequently, acetaldehyde is converted to acetate by hepatic aldehyde dehydrogenase. As discussed in Chapter 5 the effects of ethanol differ widely between individuals because of genetic variation in these metabolic enzymes. This may contribute to the fact that some people are more prone than others to the development of alcohol dependence.

Behavioural effects

In humans, the acute behavioural effects of ethanol vary between individuals according to many factors such as dose, rate of drinking, gender, body weight, blood alcohol level and the time since the previous dose. Ethanol has biphasic behavioural effects. At low doses, the first effects that are observed are heightened activity and disinhibition. At higher doses, cognitive, perceptual and motor functions become impaired. Effects on mood and emotions vary greatly from person to person (Jacobs & Fehr, 1987).

Ethanol is self-administered orally by animals. Rats selectively bred for high preference for ethanol will reliably self-administer ethanol by free-choice drinking and will operantly respond to oral ethanol in amounts that produce pharmacologically meaningful blood alcohol concentrations. Compared with non-preferring rats, alcohol-preferring rats are less sensitive to the sedative/ hypnotic effects of ethanol, develop tolerance more quickly to high doses of ethanol, and show signs of physical dependence after withdrawal (McBride & Li, 1998). Ethanol increases the sensitivity of animals to brain stimulation reward, (Kornetsky et al., 1988), place preference conditioning (Grahame et al., 2001), and drug discrimination (Hodge et al., 2001).

Mechanism of action

Ethanol increases the inhibitory activity mediated by GABA-A receptors and decreases the excitatory activity mediated by glutamate receptors, especially the NMDA receptors. These two mechanisms of action may be related to the general sedative effect of alcohol and impairment of memory during periods of intoxication. GABA-A receptors are sensitive to ethanol in distinct brain regions and are clearly involved in the acute effects of ethanol, ethanol tolerance and dependence, and ethanol self-administration (Samson & Chappell, 2001; McBride, 2002). GABA-A receptor activation mediates many of the behavioural effects of ethanol including motor incoordination, anxiolysis and sedation (Grobin et al., 1998).

The reinforcing effects produced by ethanol are probably related to increased firing rate of ventral tegmental area (VTA) dopamine neurons (Gessa et al., 1985), and dopamine release in the nucleus accumbens (Di Chiara & Imperato, 1988a), probably as a secondary consequence of activation of the GABA system or stimulation of endogenous opioids (O´Brien, 2001). The increase in dopamine activity occurs only while blood concentration of ethanol is rising. The increase in mesolimbic dopamine is critical to the reinforcing effects of psychoactive substances (see Chapter 3).

Imaging studies of brain metabolism show that alcohol decreases metabolic activity in occipital brain regions and increases metabolism in the left temporal cortex (Wang et al., 2000; Fig. 4.1)

Tolerance and withdrawal

Ethanol induces diverse types of tolerance. Among them is behavioural tolerance which refers to adaptive learning to overcome some of the effects of ethanol (Vogel-Sprott & Sdao-Jarvie, 1989). Both operant and associative learning can play a major role in the development of tolerance to alcohol and cross-tolerance to other drugs. Most of the neural mechanisms related to learning and memory are now known to be involved in the development and retention of tolerance (Kalant, 1998). Metabolic tolerance also occurs, and is a function of the upregulation of metabolic enzymes in the liver, with the result that an increased dose or more frequent use of alcohol is required to obtain the desired psychopharmacological effects.

Fig. 4.1   Fluorodeoxyglucose (FDG)-PET images of normal subject after placebo (diet soda) and ethanol (0.75 g/kg)

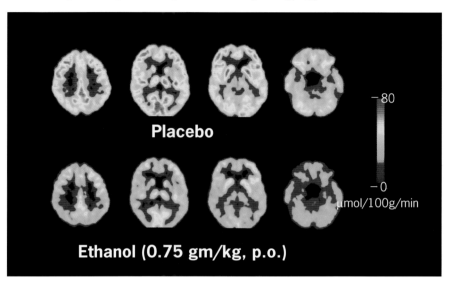

Source: Wang et al., 2000. Reproduced with permission of the publisher.

Of particular clinical importance is the development of adaptive changes in synaptic function in response to ethanol's action on ion channels (see Chapter 2), which also contribute to tolerance. Ethanol tolerance and dependence may be explained, in part, by changes in the function of GABA(A) receptors. Cross-tolerance and sensitization (see Chapter 3) have also been intensely researched during the past few years. Sensitization to the neuroactive steroids – endogenous modulators of the GABA-A receptors – influences ethanol dependence and withdrawal and may explain gender differences in the molecular effects of ethanol (Grobin et al., 1998). Animal models of ethanol dependence have identified GABA-A receptor genes as likely mediators of the behavioural adaptations associated with ethanol dependence and withdrawal (Grobin et al., 1998).

A withdrawal syndrome that may be severe enough to be fatal characterizes ethanol withdrawal. The severity of this syndrome is a function of the amount of ethanol consumed, frequency of use, and the duration of drinking history. Early signs of withdrawal are severe shaking, sweating, weakness, agitation, headache, nausea and vomiting, and rapid heart rate. Within 24 hours after stopping drinking, seizures may start to appear (Jacobs & Fehr, 1987). The alcohol withdrawal can be complicated by the state that is known as delirium tremens, and is characterized by severe agitation, autonomic hyperactivity, hallucinations and delusions. Untreated, the withdrawal syndrome lasts 5 to 7 days. Benzodiazepines are usually used to lessen the severity of alcohol withdrawal, because of their actions on the GABA-A receptors.

Neurobiological adaptations to prolonged use

Chronic alcohol consumption can induce alterations in most if not all brain systems and structures. In animals and humans, specific alterations occur in the function and morphology of the diencephalon, medial temporal lobe structures, basal forebrain, frontal cortex and cerebellum, while other subcortical structures, such as the caudate nucleus, seem to be relatively unaffected (see Chapter 2). The neuropathological alterations in mesencephalic and cortical structures are correlated with impairments in cognitive processes. In people who are dependent on alcohol, the prefrontal cortex seems particularly vulnerable to the effects of ethanol. Due to the role of these cortical structures in cognitive functions and in the control of motivated behaviour, functional alterations in this area of the brain may have an important part to play in the onset and development of alcohol dependence (Fadda & Rossetti, 1998). There is a loss in brain volume and impairment of function that worsens with continued alcohol consumption, but may be partially reversed after a period of complete abstinence. After prolonged use of alcohol, impairment of pre-frontal cortex functions, due to neuronal lesion, may compromise decision-making and emotion, inducing a lack of judgement and loss of control in reducing alcohol use (Pfefferbaum et al., 1998). These cognitive impairments need to be readdressed during alcohol dependence treatment.

Pharmacological treatment of alcohol dependence

Acamprosate (calcium acetyl-homotaurine) is a synthetic drug with structural similarity to a naturally occurring amino acid. Acamprosate acts centrally and appears to restore the normal activity of glutaminergic neurons, which become hyperexcited as a result of chronic exposure to alcohol. Acamprosate has been available on prescription in France since 1989 and is now available in many other countries throughout the world. Overall, patients treated with acamprosate exhibit a significant increase in rate of completion of treatment, time to first drink, abstinence rate and/or cumulative duration of abstinence, than patients treated with placebo (Mason, 2001).

The opioid antagonist naltrexone is also effective in reducing relapse and in helping people to remain abstinent and to decrease alcohol consumption (Streeton & Whelan, 2001).

Disulfiram is known as a "deterrent" medication because it makes the ingestion of alcohol unpleasant by altering the body's normal metabolism of alcohol. Disulfiram inhibits aldehyde dehydrogenase, the enzyme that converts acetaldehyde to acetate, thus reducing the clearance of acetaldehyde from the body. High acetaldehyde levels produce an unpleasant reaction (see

Chapter 5) that is intended to render the consumption of alcohol aversive (Kranzler, 2000). The efficacy of disulfiram is not clear, and is confounded by the need to carefully titrate the dose, and by the need for a high degree of compliance (Kranzler, 2000). Some people are thought to be naturally protected from alcohol dependence because, due to a genetic alteration, they lack a functional enzyme that metabolizes acetaldehyde (see Chapter 5) and, therefore, have an aversive reaction (known as "flushing reaction") when they drink.

Sedatives and hypnotics

Introduction

Although alcohol falls under the category of sedatives and hypnotics, it has been considered separately in this report since there is such a large body of research on alcohol, and since its use is so prevalent. In this section, other sedatives/hypnotics and minor tranquillizers will be discussed.

The most common minor tranquillizers are sleeping pills (benzodiazepines and barbiturates) (Jacobs & Fehr, 1987). Many solvents produce similar effects to sedatives/hypnotics when inhaled, but they will be considered separately in the section on volatile solvents. The sedatives/hypnotics cause a slowing of the functions of the brain and other parts of the nervous system.

Behavioural effects

The effects of sedatives/hypnotics range from mild sedation to general anaesthesia, and, in the case of severe overdose, death. These drugs are generally used for their intoxicating and inhibition-releasing properties. Sleeping pills also become habit-forming, and tolerance readily develops to these drugs (Jacobs & Fehr, 1987). The most common symptoms of sedative/hypnotic use are drowsiness, mild to moderate motor incoordination, and some clouding of mental functions (Jacobs & Fehr, 1987). These effects are related to the role of the GABA-A receptor, discussed below. With higher doses, these effects become more pronounced and lead to general impairment of motor function, increased reaction times, and impairments in cognitive function and memory. Eventually, sleep is induced in severe cases, and death can occur from respiratory depression. Hangover effects of fatigue, headache and nausea also occur.

Benzodiazepines and barbiturates show strong reinforcing properties in animal models, and are self-administered by monkeys (Meisch, 2001; Munzar et al., 2001; Gomez, Roach & Meisch, 2002) and rodents (Davis, Smith & Smith, 1987; Szostak, Finlay & Fibiger, 1987; Naruse & Asami, 1990). Benzodiazepines have reward-consistent effects on brain self-stimulation (Carden & Coons, 1990), induce conditioned place preferences (Spyraki, Kazandjian & Varonos, 1985), and show discriminative stimulus effects (Wettstein & Gauthier, 1992).

Mechanism of action

Benzodiazepines act by binding to a specific binding site on the GABA-A receptor complex, which facilitates the effects of GABA on the opening of the chloride channel (Haefely, 1978). Barbiturates also bind to a separate specific site on the GABA-A receptor and directly open the chloride channel (Nutt & Malizia, 2001). Benzodiazepines do not directly open the channel, but they modulate the ability of GABA to do so, thus less GABA than usual is required to open the channel (Barnard et al., 1998). The effects of benzodiazepines on endogenous GABA function makes them safer in large doses than the barbiturates and alcohol. The latter directly open the chloride channel and therefore can have effects in excess of the naturally occurring effects of GABA.

The increase in chloride conductance following opening of the chloride channel hyperpolarizes the cell, making it less likely to fire an action potential (see Chapter 2). Because GABA controls neuronal excitability in all brain regions, increasing GABA function is the mechanism by which sedatives and hypnotics have their characteristic effects of sedation, amnesia and motor incoordination (Nutt & Malizia, 2001).

Like other dependence-producing drugs, there is also evidence that sedatives and hypnotics affect the mesolimbic dopamine system (Feigenbaum & Yanai, 1983), leading to their reinforcing effects and enhancing the motivation to repeat their use.

Similarly to alcohol, the benzodiazepine lorazepam decreases metabolic activity in the occipital cortex, increases activity in the temporal cortex, and also decreases thalamic metabolism, as measured by positron emission tomography (Wang et al., 2000).

Tolerance and withdrawal

Tolerance to the effects of sedatives/hypnotics develops rapidly, and increased doses are required to maintain the same level of effect. Tolerance develops to the pleasurable and sedative effects, as well as to the effects of benzodiazepines and barbiturates on motor coordination. Tolerance to the anticonvulsant effects does not appear to occur (Jacobs & Fehr, 1987). There is also a high degree of cross-tolerance between sedatives/hypnotics, including alcohol.

Upon withdrawal of sedatives and hypnotics, certain effects are observed which are opposite to those of the drug. Thus, increased arousal, anxiety, restlessness, insomnia and excitability are characteristic withdrawal symptoms (Nutt & Malizia, 2001). In severe cases, seizures can occur.

There is evidence that chronic treatment with benzodiazepines alters the composition of GABA-A receptor subunits (Holt, Bateson & Martin, 1996), which may also be due to changes in receptor coupling and function. This results in tolerance in the presence of benzodiazepines, and withdrawal symptoms when benzodiazepines are removed.

Neurobiological adaptations to prolonged use

Dependence on sedatives and hypnotics may develop with chronic use, regardless of how often these drugs are used, or their doses. For example, people may feel an overwhelming urge or craving for the drug only under specific circumstances, such as social gatherings or times of increased stress (Jacobs & Fehr, 1987).

It is important to note that many individuals require long-term therapy with benzodiazepines or barbiturates for epilepsy, brain injuries or other disorders. This use may lead to tolerance to some of the effects of the drugs, and withdrawal effects upon cessation of their use. The use of benzodiazepines or barbiturates for medical purposes may or may not lead to dependence, even if tolerance and withdrawal are present (see Table 4.1). Problems are more often related to the non-medical use of benzodiazepines by polydrug users, and their chronic use by some patients. These include impairment of memory, risk of accidents, falls and hip fractures in the elderly, a withdrawal syndrome, brain damage, and oversedation when combined with alcohol or other drugs (which can lead to coma, overdose and death) (Griffiths & Weerts, 1997). Treatment of sedative dependence involves slowly tapering off drug use, together with behavioural therapy (see Chapter 3 for types of behavioural therapies).

Tobacco

Introduction

Although tobacco contains thousands of substances, nicotine is the one most frequently associated with dependence because it is the component that is psychoactive and causes observable behavioural effects, such as mood changes, stress reduction and enhancement of performance. The behavioural effects associated with nicotine delivered during smoking include arousal, increased attention and concentration, enhancement of memory, reduction of anxiety and suppression of appetite.

The average half-life of nicotine is approximately 2 hours but is about 35% longer in persons with a particular form of a gene (i.e. an allele) for the enzyme (CYP2A6) that inhibits the primary metabolic pathway of nicotine (Benowitz et al., 2002). Preliminary studies suggest that the CYP2A6 allele frequency is more common in Asians than in Africans or Caucasians, and that this difference partially accounts for the lower daily consumption of cigarettes and lower risk of lung cancer in Asians as compared to Africans and Caucasians (Ahijevych, 1999; Tyndale & Sellers, 2001; Benowitz et al., 2002). This is discussed further in Chapter 5.

Behavioural effects

Nicotine is a potent and powerful agonist of several subpopulations of nicotinic receptors of the cholinergic nervous system (Henningfield, Keenan

& Clarke, 1996; Vidal, 1996; Paterson & Nordberg, 2000). Acute doses can produce alteration of mood, although daily users are substantially less sensitive to such effects than non-users, suggesting that tolerance develops to some of the effects (Soria et al., 1996; Taylor, 1996; Foulds et al., 1997; US DHHS, 1988). In brief, nicotine produces dose-related psychoactive effects in humans that are similar to those of stimulants, and it elevates scores on standardized tests for liking and euphoria that are relied upon by WHO for assessing dependence potential (Henningfield, Mizasato & Jasinsk, 1985; US DHHS, 1988; Jones, Garrett & Griffiths, 1999; Royal College of Physicians, 2000).

The potential for dependence associated with smoking seems to equal or surpass that of other psychoactive substances. In animal models, nicotine can serve as a potent and powerful reinforcer, it induces intravenous self-administration, facilitates intracranial self-stimulation and conditioned place preference and has discriminative stimulus properties (Goldberg et al., 1983; Goldberg & Henningfield, 1988; Corrigall, 1999; Di Chiara, 2000). Patterns of self-administration are more similar to those of stimulants than of other drug classes (Griffiths, Bigelow & Henningfield, 1980).

Mechanism of action

At the cellular level, nicotine binds to nicotinic acetylcholine receptors (nAChRs). There are a variety of subtypes of neuronal nAChRs. Cloning techniques have revealed several different neuronal nAChR subunits in mammals (Lukas et al., 1999). The receptors are composed of five subunits around an ion channel. Agonist (e.g. nicotine) binding causes the resting conformation of the subunits to change to the open conformation and allows sodium ion inflow, which causes cell depolarization (Miyazawa et al., 1999; Corringer, Le Novere & Changeux, 2000).

In the brain, nicotinic receptors are situated mainly in presynaptic terminals and modulate neurotransmitter release; therefore, nicotine effects may be related to various neurotransmitter systems (reviewed in Dani & De Biasi, 2001; Kenny & Markou, 2001; Malin, 2001). Nicotine is known to promote dopamine synthesis by increasing tyrosine hydroxylase expression and release through activation of somatodendritic nAChRs in both nigrostriatal and mesolimbic dopamine pathways (Clarke & Pert , 1985; Panagis et al., 2000).

Nicotine increases dopamine output in the nucleus accumbens, and blocking dopamine release reduces nicotine self-administration in rats (Schilstrom et al., 1998; Dani & De Biasi, 2001). Nicotine stimulates dopamine transmission in specific brain areas and in particular, in the shell of the nucleus accumbens and in areas of the extended amygdala, which have been related to drug dependence for most drugs (see Chapter 3). Therefore, nicotine depends on dopamine for the behavioural effects that are most relevant for its reinforcing properties; this is likely to be the basis of the dependence-producing ability of tobacco. However, other neuronal systems related to substance dependence, such as opioid, glutamate, serotonin and glucocorticoid systems may also be modulated by nicotine (Dani & De Biasi, 2001; Kenny & Markou, 2001; Malin, 2001) and may be of importance to specific aspects of substance dependence.

Tolerance and withdrawal

Exposure to nicotine results in a high degree of tolerance, which appears to be mediated by several mechanisms, and which includes acute and long-term components (Swedberg, Henningfield & Goldberg, 1990; Perkins et al., 1993). Tolerance to some effects may be related to the upregulation of nicotine receptors in the central nervous system, but genetic factors also modulate the effects of nicotine including the development of tolerance (Collins & Marks, 1989). This may account for some individual differences in nicotine dependence (see Chapter 5).

Tolerance rapidly develops to the subjective effects of nicotine during the course of the day. Smokers generally consider that the first cigarette in the morning is more rewarding, which may be due to tolerance or to the relief from the withdrawal that develops overnight. Receptor desensitization (loss of sensitivity) may explain some of the behavioural effects of nicotine, acute and/or chronic tolerance, and relapse (Rosecrans & Karan, 1993).

Withdrawal from smoking may be accompanied by symptoms such as irritability, hostility, anxiety, dysphoric and depressed mood, decreased heart rate and increased appetite. The urge to smoke correlates with low blood nicotine levels (Russell, 1987), suggesting that smoking occurs to maintain a certain concentration of nicotine in the blood in order to avoid withdrawal symptoms. Thus, the continuity of tobacco use would be explained by both the positive and negative reinforcement of nicotine. Termination of prolonged nicotine administration to animals induces behaviours that suggest depression and increased anxiety, changes in trained behaviours, as well as weight gain. Reduction of locomotion, and decreased dopamine content and release in limbic structures, nucleus accumbens and striatum during nicotine withdrawal have been described in animal models, and may be correlated with behavioural changes due to nicotine withdrawal (Malin, 2001). Therefore, animal models for nicotine withdrawal have some external validity and are used in preclinical studies, mainly to describe possible future treatments for nicotine dependence.

The signs and symptoms of tobacco withdrawal, including effects on electrical activity of the brain, cognitive performance, anxiety, and response to stressful stimuli, can be largely mitigated by administration of pure nicotine in a variety of forms (e.g. gum, patch, nasal delivery) (Hughes, Higgins & Hatsukami, 1990; Heishman, Taylor & Henningfield, 1994; Pickworth, Heishman & Henningfield, 1995; Shiffman, Mason & Henningfield, 1998).

Humans report similar subjective effects from intravenous nicotine as from smoked tobacco (Henningfield, Miyasato & Jasinski, 1985; Jones, Garrett & Griffiths, 1999). Craving for tobacco is generally only partially relieved by the administration of pure forms of nicotine, since it can be elicited by factors that are not mediated by nicotine (e.g. the smell of smoke, the sight of other people smoking, and tobacco advertisements), through the process of conditioning and it can be reduced by constituents in tobacco smoke other than nicotine, such as "tar" (Butschky et al., 1995). These additional factors may have synergistic effects with nicotine in cigarettes to provide more effective relief from craving than nicotine delivered in cigarette smoke (Rose, Behm & Levin, 1993).

Pharmacological treatment of nicotine dependence

An improved understanding of dependence, and the identification and acceptance of nicotine as a dependence-producing drug, have been fundamental to the development of medications and behavioural treatments for nicotine dependence. There are currently many readily available treatments to help people reduce their smoking. Estimates are that over one million people have been successfully treated for nicotine dependence since the introduction of nicotine gum and the transdermal patch. All nicotine-replacement therapies are equally effective in helping people to quit smoking, and, combined with increased public service announcements in the media about the dangers of smoking, have produced a marked increase in successful quitting. However, treating dependence with medication alone is far less effective than when the medication is coupled with a behavioural treatment. In this case nicotine can prevent the physical withdrawal effects, while the individual attempts to deal with the craving and drug-seeking behaviour that have become habitual (see Chapter 3, section on behavioural therapies). The use of nicotine-based therapy is not intended for long-term use, but rather only at the beginning of treatment.

Although the major focus of pharmacological treatments of nicotine dependence has been nicotine-based, other treatments are being developed for the relief of symptoms of nicotine withdrawal. For example, the first non-nicotine prescription drug, the antidepressant bupropion, is currently used as a pharmacological treatment for nicotine dependence (Sutherland, 2002). Bupropion improves the abstinence rates of smokers, especially if combined with nicotine replacement therapy (O´Brien, 2001). Because depression is frequently associated with nicotine dependence – either by predisposing the individual to use tobacco, or on account of its development during nicotine dependence, or as a consequence of nicotine withdrawal – antidepressant agents have been tested for the treatment of nicotine dependence. This concept is explored more fully in Chapter 6 where comorbidity of substance use and mental illness are discussed.

Opioids

Introduction

Opiate drugs are compounds that are extracted from the poppy seed. These drugs opened the way to the discovery of the endogenous opioid system in the brain (Brownstein, 1993). The term "opioids" includes "opiates" as well as semisynthetic and synthetic compounds with similar properties. Evidence for the existence of opioid receptors was based on the observation that opiates (e.g. heroin and morphine) interact with specific binding sites in the brain. In 1976, the first evidence for the existence of multiple opioid receptors was reported (Martin et al., 1976) and pharmacological studies led to the classification of opioid binding sites into three receptor classes referred to as mu, delta and kappa receptors. Later, studies revealed that several subtypes of each receptor class exists (Pasternak, 1993).

The existence of opioid receptors suggested that these receptor sites might be the targets for opiate-like molecules that exist naturally in the brain. In 1975, two peptides that act at opiate receptors were discovered, Leu-enkephalin and Met-enkephalin (Hughes et al., 1975). Shortly after, other endogenous peptides were identified and more than 20 distinct opiate peptides are known today (Akil et al., 1997).

Behavioural effects

Intravenous injection of opioids produces a warm flushing of the skin and sensations described by users as a "rush"; however, the first experience with opiates can also be unpleasant, and can involve nausea and vomiting (Jaffe, 1990). Opioids have euphorogenic, analgesic, sedative, and respiratory depressant effects.

Numerous animal experiments using selective opioid compounds have shown that agonists of the mu receptor subtype, injected either peripherally or directly into the brain, have reinforcing properties. Delta agonists, as well as endogenous enkephalins, seem to produce reward, although to a lesser extent than mu agonists. Reinforcement by mu and delta agonists has been shown in several behavioural models, including drug self-administration, intracranial self-stimulation and conditioned place preference paradigms, and has been reviewed extensively (Van Ree, Gerrits & Vanderschuren, 1999). Pharmacological studies, therefore, have proposed that activation of both mu and delta receptors is reinforcing. It is also significant that the genetic inactivation of mu receptors abolished both the dependence-producing and analgesic effects of morphine, as well as actions of other clinically used opioid drugs. This demonstrated that mu receptors are critical for all the beneficial as well as detrimental effects of clinically relevant opiate drugs (Kieffer, 1999). Molecular studies, therefore, have highlighted mu receptors as the gate for opioid analgesia, tolerance and dependence.

Kappa receptors, however, appear to have an opposing effect on reward. The hypothesis of a mu/kappa control of mesolimbic dopaminergic neurons is best documented. It is important to note the observation that heroin is also self-administered in animals in the absence of these neurons, suggesting the existence of dopamine-independent mechanisms in opioid reinforcement (Leshner & Koob, 1999).

Mechanism of action

The three opioid receptors (mu, delta and kappa receptors) mediate activities of both exogenous opioids (drugs) and endogenous opioid peptides, and therefore represent the key players in the understanding of opioid-controlled behaviours. Opioid receptors belong to the superfamily of G protein-coupled receptors. Agonist binding to these receptors ultimately causes inhibition of neuronal activity.

Opioid receptors and peptides are strongly expressed in the central nervous system (Mansour et al., 1995; Mansour & Watson, 1993). In addition to its involvement in pain pathways, the opioid system is largely represented in brain areas involved in responses to psychoactive substances, such as the VTA and nucleus accumbens shell (Akil et al., 1997). Opioid peptides are involved in a wide variety of functions regulating stress responses, feeding, mood, learning, memory, and immune functions (for review, see Vaccarino & Kastin, 2001).

Tolerance and withdrawal

With repeated administration of opioid drugs, adaptive mechanisms change the functioning of opioid-sensitive neurons and neural networks. Tolerance develops, and higher doses of the drugs are required to gain the desired effect. Humans and experimental animals develop profound tolerance to opioids over periods of several weeks of escalating chronic administration. Tolerance involves distinct cellular and neural processes. Acute desensitization or tolerance of the opioid receptor develops in minutes during opioid use and abates in minutes to hours after exposure. There is also a long-term desensitization of the receptor that slowly develops and persists for hours to days after removal of opioid agonists. There are also counteradaptations to opioid effects of intracellular signalling mechanisms and in neuronal circuitry that contribute to tolerance. These processes have been recently reviewed (Williams, Christie & Manzoni, 2001).

Cessation of chronic opioid use is associated with an intensely dysphoric withdrawal syndrome, which may be a negative drive to reinstate substance use. The withdrawal is characterized by watering eyes, runny nose, yawning, sweating, restlessness, irritability, tremor, nausea, vomiting, diarrhoea, increased blood pressure and heart rate, chills, cramps and muscle aches, which can last 7–10 days (Jaffe, 1990). This was once thought to be sufficient to explain the persistence of opioid dependence (Collier, 1980). There is no doubt that the intensely dysphoric withdrawal syndrome plays an important role in maintaining episodes of opioid use, but opioid dependence, and relapse that occurs long after withdrawal cannot be explained solely on this basis (Koob & Bloom, 1988). Currently, long-term adaptations in neural systems are also thought to play an important role in dependence and relapse.

In conclusion, the data show complex and broad changes of the endogenous opioid system following repeated stimulation of mu receptors by opioids. The precise consequences of those changes remain unclear, but it is likely that the long-term dysregulation of the opioid system influences stress responses and drug-taking behaviour.

Neurobiological adaptations to prolonged use

Adaptations following chronic drug exposure extend well beyond reward circuits to other brain areas, notably those involved in learning and stress responses. Important regions are the amygdala, hippocampus and cerebral cortex, which are all connected to the nucleus accumbens. All these areas express opioid receptors and peptides, and the overall distribution of opioid peptide-expressing cells in neural circuits of dependence has been reviewed (Nestler, 2001; Koob & Nestler, 1997).

Repeated exposure to opioids induces drastic and perhaps irreversible modifications in the brain. Hallmarks of adaptations to chronic opioid use are tolerance, defined as a reduced sensitivity to the drug effects and generally referring to attenuation of analgesic efficacy. Drug craving and the physiological manifestations of drug withdrawal are also indications of long-term neuroadaptations. These phenomena are a consequence of sustained mu receptor stimulation by opiate drugs inducing neurochemical adaptations in opioid receptor-bearing neurons (Kieffer & Evans, 2002).

Pharmacological treatment of opioid dependence

Treatment of heroin dependence has been quite successful because of substitution therapy and methadone maintenance treatment in particular (see Box 4.1). Methadone is a synthetic opioid agonist that acts on the same receptors as opiate drugs, and therefore blocks the effects of heroin, eliminates withdrawal symptoms, and reduces craving. When properly used, methadone is non-sedating, non-intoxicating and does not interfere with regular activities. The medication is taken orally, and it suppresses opioid withdrawal for 24 hours. There is no cognitive blunting. Its most important feature is to relieve the craving associated with heroin dependence, thereby reducing relapse. Methadone maintenance treatment is safe, and very effective in helping people to stop taking heroin, especially when combined with behavioural therapies or counselling and other supportive services. Methadone maintenance treatment can also reduce the risk of contracting and transmitting HIV, tuberculosis and hepatitis (Krambeer et al., 2001).

BOX 4.1

Substitution therapy

Substitution therapy is defined as the administration under medical supervision of a prescribed psychoactive substance – pharmacologically related to the one producing dependence – to people with substance dependence, for achieving defined treatment aims (usually improved health and well-being). Substitution therapy is widely used in the management of opioid dependence and is often referred to as "opioid substitution treatment," "opioid replacement therapy", or "opioid pharmacotherapy". Agents suitable for substitution therapy of opioid dependence are those with some opioid properties, so that they have the capacity to prevent the emergence of withdrawal symptoms and reduce craving. At the same time they diminish the effects of heroin or other opioid drugs because they bind to opioid receptors in the brain. In general, it is desirable for opioid substitution drugs to have a longer duration of action than the drug they are replacing so as to delay the emergence of withdrawal and reduce the frequency of administration. As a result there is less disruption of normal life activities from the need to obtain and administer drugs, thereby facilitating rehabilitation efforts. Whereas non-prescribed opioids are usually injected or inhaled by drug users, these prescribed medicines are usually administered orally in the form of a solution or a tablet. Agents used in substitution therapy can also be prescribed in decreasing doses over short periods of time (usually less than one month) for detoxification purposes. Substitution maintenance treatment is associated with prescription of relatively stable doses of opioid agonists (e.g. methadone and buprenorphine) over a long period of time (usually more than 6 months). The mechanisms of action of opioid substitution maintenance therapy include prevention of disruption of molecular, cellular and physiological events and, in fact, normalization of those functions already disrupted by chronic use of usually short-acting opiates such as heroin. The context of delivery of substitution therapy has important implications for the quality of the interventions, both to maintain adequate control and to ensure responsible prescribing.

Since 1970, methadone maintenance treatment has grown substantially to become the dominant form of opioid substitution treatment globally. Because the treatment was initially controversial, it has been more rigorously evaluated than any other treatment for opioid dependence. The weight of evidence for benefits is substantial.

Source: WHO, 1998; Kreek, 2000.

A newer drug, Levo-alpha-acetyl-methadol (LAAM) resembles methadone: it is a synthetic opioid that can be used to treat heroin dependence, but it needs only to be taken three times per week, thus making it even easier for people to use this therapy.

Buprenorphine is another prescribed drug for management of opioid dependence that has the potential of improving access to drug treatment by bringing more people into treatment in primary health care settings (see Box 4.2). It has been widely used in France and is now being trialed in the USA.

BOX 4.2

Use of buprenorphine in treatment of opioid dependence

Whilst much of the work on substitution therapy has focused on methadone, several new synthetic oral opioids such as LAAM (L-alpha-acetyl-methadol), slow-release morphine and buprenorphine have been investigated as potential therapeutic agents in the treatment of opioid dependence. Buprenorphine in particular has been undergoing extensive clinical testing for treatment of opioid dependence and is likely to become the medication used in the management of opioid dependence not only in specialized clinics, but also in primary health care. Its pharmacological properties and resultant clinical characteristics – especially its relatively long duration of action and high safety profile – appear certain to ensure buprenorphine an important place in the overall treatment of opioid dependence.

Pharmacologically, buprenorphine is a partial agonist at the mu receptor and a weak antagonist at the kappa receptor. Because it binds tightly to, and dissociates slowly from these receptors, buprenorphine exhibits an agonist 'ceiling effect', most noticeably in its respiratory depression effect, which accords the medication a high degree of clinical safety. Its tight binding with slow dissociation from receptors also provides a blockade for the effects of subsequently-administered agonists, precipitates withdrawal in patients maintained on a sufficient dose of full agonist, and provides prolonged duration of action with poor reversibility by naloxone. Furthermore, buprenorphine's weak antagonist effect at the kappa receptor renders it devoid of psychotomimetic effects. Further research has demonstrated buprenorphine's limited levels of reinforcing efficacy in comparison to opioids, and established its ability to suppress heroin self-administration in opioid-dependent primates and humans.

The formulation containing both buprenorphine and the opioid antagonist naloxone has been recently introduced for maintenance therapy of opioid dependence. Adding naloxone to buprenorphine aims at reducing a risk of diversion and injecting use of prescribed buprenorphine. Over the past decade a series of controlled clinical trials, using such outcome measures as illicit opiate use, retention in treatment, craving and global rating of improvement, have substantiated buprenorphine's clinical safety and efficacy. When used in opioid substitution treatment for dependent pregnant women, it appears to be associated with a low incidence of neonatal withdrawal syndrome. Due to the above features, buprenorphine is a useful drug in the facilitation of withdrawal from opioids.

Sources: Barnett, Rodgers & Bloch, 2001; Fischer et al., 2000; Ling et al., 1998.

Heroin-assisted treatment of heroin dependence (see Box 4.3) has also been proposed.

Naloxone and naltrexone are medications that also block the effects of morphine, heroin and other opiates by acting as antagonists at the opioid receptors. They are especially useful in preventing relapse because they block

---

BOX 4.3

Heroin-assisted treatment of heroin dependence

Heroin prescription for treatment of opioid dependence, practised on a limited scale in the United Kingdom for many years, gained increased international interest in the early 1990s, with feasibility studies in Australia and a first national study of heroin-assisted treatment in Switzerland that started in 1994. This study led to the establishment of heroin-assisted treatment as one of the treatment options in Switzerland. The findings of the study showed that there were significant reductions in illicit drug use, improvement in health status and social integration (Uchtenhagen et al., 1999). Follow-up results at 18 months documented stability of improvements also after discharge from the programme (Rehm, 2001).

A review by a WHO expert group supported the main conclusions of the Swiss study, but also recommended further research in order to better identify the specific benefits of prescribed heroin (Ali et al., 1999). These recommendations have been respected in randomised controlled trials: one implemented in 1998-2001 in the Netherlands (van den Brink et al., 2002), one started in 2002 in Germany (Krausz, 2002). Other similar research projects are in preparation (Fischer et al., 2002). The shared objective of the trials is to test an additional therapeutic option for those heroin addicts for whom other treatments have failed and who are out of contact with the treatment system. An international network of scientists, engaged in the projects mentioned above, has emerged and organised three conferences for an exchange of methodological, therapeutic and practical problems and experience. The international debate on heroin-assisted treatment of opioid dependence, initially mainly political and controversial, tends to become more scientific and evidence-oriented (Bammer et al., 1999).

Sources: Ali et al., 1999; Bammer et al., 1999; Uctenhagen et al., 1999; Rehm et al., 2001; van den Brink et al., 2002; Krausz, 2002; Fischer et al. (2002).

---

all of the effects of opiates. The effects are relatively long-lasting, ranging from 1–3 days. This therapy begins after medically supervised detoxification, because naloxone and naltrexone do not protect against the effects of withdrawal, and can in fact precipitate withdrawal symptoms in dependent people. Naltrexone itself has no subjective effects or potential for the development of dependence. Patient noncompliance is a common problem. Therefore, a favourable treatment outcome requires that there also be a positive therapeutic relationship, effective counselling or therapy, and careful monitoring of medication compliance.

Cannabinoids

Introduction

Among all the cannabinoids contained in *Cannabis sativa*, delta-9-tetrahydrocannabinol (THC) is the major chemical with psychoactive effects and is metabolized to another active compound, 11-OH-delta-9-THC. Cannabinoids are generally inhaled by smoking, but may also be ingested. Peak intoxication through smoking is reached within 15–30 minutes and the effects last for 2–6 hours. Cannabinoids remain in the body for long periods and accumulate after repeated use. Cannabinoids may be found in the urine for 2–3 days after smoking a single cigarette and for up to 6 weeks after the last use in heavy users.

Several studies (e.g. Tramer et al. 2001) have demonstrated therapeutic effects of cannabinoids, e.g. in controlling nausea and vomiting in some cancer and AIDS patients. This has led to controversial discussion regarding the potential beneficial effects of cannabis itself in certain conditions (see Box 4.4).

Behavioural effects

The perception of time is slowed and there are feelings of relaxation and of sharpened sensory awareness. The perception of increased self-confidence and heightened creativity is not accompanied by better performance and there is impairment of short-term memory and of motor coordination. Analgesia, antiemetic and antiepileptic action, and increased appetite are

---

BOX 4.4

Therapeutic potential for cannabis

Therapeutic uses of D-9-tetrahydrocannabinol (THC) have led to discussions about the therapeutic potential of cannabis itself, although little research exists in this area and satisfactory clinical studies have not been conducted. In order to explore possible therapeutic uses of cannabis, several scientific issues need to be considered, including:

— the standardization of cannabis preparations required for some types of clinical and preclinical studies

— the difficulties inherent in the study of smoking as the mode of administration of a substance

— the need for a comparable placebo "cigarette" which would not be easily identified by experimental subjects and patients in controlled trials.

— the large number of patients which would be needed to study the comparative efficacy of smoking cannabis compared with other cannabinoids and other therapeutic agents.

— the possibility of using alternative delivery systems which could avoid smoking cannabis as well as the other components contained in its smokable form.In addition, the broader implications of such research on cannabis control policies would need to be carefully considered.

Source: WHO, 1997a.

central effects sometimes described to be of clinical relevance (O´Brien, 2001).

Cannabis derivatives produce clear subjective motivational responses in humans, leading to drug-seeking behaviour and repeated drug use. Indeed, cannabis derivatives are the most widely used illicit drugs in the world (Adams & Martin, 1996).

Animal studies have demonstrated that cannabinoids fulfil most of the common features attributed to substances with reinforcing properties (reviewed in Maldonado & Rodriguez de Fonseca, 2002). Thus, subjective effects have been demonstrated in animals by using a large range of doses of cannabinoids in the drug discrimination paradigm. The rewarding characteristics of these subjective effects have also been defined in animals by using the conditioned place preference and the intracranial self-stimulation paradigm. Animal studies have also revealed that cannabinoids interact with brain reward circuits and share with other psychoactive substances some biochemical features (e.g. changes in dopamine and opioid activity) that have been directly related to their reinforcing properties (Koob, 1992). These biochemical findings clearly support the dependence-producing ability of cannabinoids that has been reported in humans.

Mechanism of action

Cannabinoid receptors and their endogenous ligands together constitute what is now referred to as the 'endocannabinoid system'. Plant-derived cannabinoids or their synthetic analogues are classical cannabinoid receptor agonists (reviewed in Pertwee, 1999; Reggio & Traore, 2000; Khanolkar, Palmer & Makriyannis, 2000).

Cannabinoid compounds induce their pharmacological effects by activating two different receptors that have been identified and cloned: the CB-1 cannabinoid receptor, which is highly expressed in the central nervous system (Devane et al., 1988; Matsuda et al., 1990), and the CB-2 cannabinoid receptor, which is localized in the peripheral tissues mainly at the level of the immune system (Munro, Thomas & Abu-Shaar, 1993). THC and its analogues show good correlation between their affinity for these receptors and their effects, denoting that these receptors are the targets for these compounds. After the identification of the first cannabinoid receptor, the search for an endogenous ligand for this receptor was started. The discovery of the first endogenous cannabinoid (endocannabinoid) ligand took place in 1992 when the anandamide, arachidonoyl ethanolamide, was isolated from pig brain (Devane et al., 1992). A second type of endocannabinoid was discovered in 1995, also a derivative of arachidonic acid (Mechoulam et al., 1995; Sugiura et al., 1995). Recently, a third endocannabinoid ligand has been identified (Hanus et al., 2001). The identification of these endocannabinoid compounds and the development of potent and selective synthetic cannabinoid agonists, as well as selective cannabinoid antagonists has played a major role in the recent advances in cannabinoid pharmacology.

The endogenous ligands undergo depolarization-induced synthesis and release from neurons and are removed from the extracellular space by a carrier-mediated uptake process that is present in the membranes of neurons and astrocytes (Di Marzo et al., 1998; Maccarrone et al., 1998; Di Marzo, 1999; Piomelli et al., 1999; Hillard & Jarrahian, 2000). This is taken as evidence that these endogenous cannabinoids behave as transmitters in the brain.

Although cannabis is widely used, the mechanisms of its euphoriant and dependence-producing effects are largely unknown. There is a compelling body of evidence that delta-9-THC increases dopamine activity in the mesolimbic pathway projecting from the VTA to the nucleus accumbens, a key region in the development of dependence (see Chapter 3). In vivo studies have shown that delta-9-THC increases extracellular concentrations of dopamine in the nucleus accumbens (Chen et al., 1990). More recently, it has been shown by brain microdialysis that delta-9-THC increases extracellular dopamine concentration preferentially in the shell of the nucleus accumbens, similar to the action of many psychoactive substances (Tanda, Pontieri & Di Chiara, 1997). Systemic administration of delta 9-THC or synthetic cannabinoids also increases spontaneous firing of dopamine neurons within the VTA (French, 1997; Gessa et al., 1998).

The brain distribution of CB1 binding sites correlates with the effects of cannabinoids on memory, perception, motor control and anticonvulsant effects (Ameri, 1999). CB1 receptor agonists impair cognition and memory and alter motor function control. Thus, the cerebral cortex, hippocampus, lateral caudate-putamen, substantia nigra, pars reticulata, globus pallidus, entopeduncular nucleus and the molecular layer of the cerebellum are all populated with particularly high concentrations of CB1 receptors (Pertwee, 1997). Intermediate levels of binding are found in the nucleus accumbens. CB1 receptors are also found on pain pathways in the brain and spinal cord and at the peripheral terminals of primary sensory neurons (Pertwee, 2001) thus explaining the analgesic properties of cannabinoid receptor agonists. CB1 receptors are expressed on neurons of the heart, vas deferens, urinary bladder and small intestine (Pertwee, 1997).

The CB1 receptors located at nerve terminals (Pertwee, 1997; Ong & Mackie, 1999; Pertwee, 2001) suppress the neuronal release of transmitters that include acetylcholine, noradrenaline, dopamine, 5-hydroxy-tryptamine, GABA, glutamate and aspartate (Pertwee, 2001). CB2 receptors found in immune cells, with particularly high levels in B-cells and natural killer cells (Galiegue et al., 1995), are immunomodulatory (Molina-Holgado, Lledo & Guaza, 1997).

Tolerance and withdrawal

Tolerance rapidly develops to most effects of cannabis, cannabinoids, and related drugs acting at the CB1 cannabinoid receptor. The development of tolerance to antinociception, and to anticonvulsant and locomotor effects follow different time spans and occur to differing extents.

There is little evidence of withdrawal associated with cannabinoid use. In fact, withdrawal reactions after prolonged use of cannabinoids are rarely reported, probably because of the long half-life of cannabinoids, which prevents the emergence of withdrawal symptoms. Increased release of corticotrophin-releasing factor is a biochemical marker of stress that is increased during cannabinoid withdrawal (Rodriguez de Fonseca et al., 1997).

Neurobiological adaptations to prolonged use

Cannabis is sometimes regarded as an "innocuous" drug and the prevalence of lifetime and regular use has increased. However, people with schizophrenia who use cannabis are vulnerable to relapse and exacerbation of existing symptoms, while users report short-lived adverse effects, and regular use is related to the risk of dependence (Johns, 2001). Evidence linking cannabis to irreversible brain lesions and the induction of toxic encephalopathy in children is inconclusive.

It has been shown in several studies (as reviewed in Ameri, 1999) that long-term exposure to cannabis can produce long-lasting cognitive impairment, which may be due to residue drug in the brain, withdrawal reaction or direct neurotoxicity of cannabinoids, tar, carboxyhaemoglobin or benzopyrene. There is some evidence of impaired ability to focus attention and filter out irrelevant information, which increases with the number of years of use but is unrelated to frequency of use. The speed of information processing is delayed significantly with increasing frequency of use but is unaffected by duration of use. The results suggest that a chronic build-up of cannabinoids produces both short-term and long-term cognitive impairments (Solowij, Michie & Fox, 1995). In general, the data support a drug residue effect on attention, psychomotor tasks, and short-term memory during the 12–24 hour period immediately after cannabis use, but evidence is as yet insufficient to support or refute either a more prolonged drug residue effect, or a toxic effect on the central nervous system that persists even after drug residues have left the body (Pope, Gruber & Yurgelun-Todd, 1995).

A review of the preclinical literature suggests that both age during exposure and duration of exposure may be critical determinants of neurotoxicity. Cannabinoid administration for at least 3 months (8–10% of a rat's lifespan) was required to produce neurotoxic effects in peripubertal rodents, which would be comparable to about 3 years of exposure in rhesus monkeys and 7–10 years in humans. Studies of monkeys after having been exposed daily for up to 12 months have not consistently reported neurotoxicity, and the results of longer exposures have not yet been published (Scallet, 1991).

Cocaine (hydrochloride and crack)

Introduction

Cocaine is a powerful nervous system stimulant that can be taken intranasally, injected intravenously or smoked. The use of cocaine by many different cultures dates back for centuries. Cocaine is found in the leaves of *Erythroxylon coca*, trees that are indigenous to Bolivia and Peru.

Behavioural effects

Cocaine increases alertness, feelings of well-being and euphoria, energy and motor activity, feelings of competence and sexuality. Anxiety, paranoia and restlessness are also frequent. Athletic performance may be enhanced in sports where sustained attention and endurance is required. With excessive dosage, tremors, convulsions and increased body temperature are detected. Activation of the sympathetic nervous system occurs concomitantly with the behavioural effects. Tachycardia, hypertension, myocardial infarct and cerebrovascular haemorrhages may occur during cocaine overdose. As the effects of the drugs subside, the user feels dysphoric, tired, irritable and mildly depressed, which may lead to subsequent drug use to regain the previous experience (O´Brien, 2001).

There have been numerous papers reporting that cocaine can be self-administered by animals via the intravenous and oral routes (Caine & Koob 1994; Barros & Miczek, 1996; Rocha et al., 1998; Platt, Rowlett & Spealman, 2001). Cocaine's augmentative effect on intracranial self-stimulation requires activation of both D_1 and D_2 dopamine receptors (Kita et al., 1999). Conditioned place preference can be induced in rodents by administration of cocaine (Itzhak & Martin, 2002).

Mechanism of action

In the brain, cocaine acts as a monoamine transporter blocker, with similar affinities for dopamine, serotonin, and norepinephrine transporters (Ritz, Cone & Kuhar, 1990). Cocaine, and the dopamine transporter to which it binds, can be visualized in the human brain using positron emission tomography (PET) imaging (Fig. 4.2). The antagonism of the transporter proteins leaves more monoaminergic neurotransmitters available in the synaptic cleft to act upon presynaptic and postsynaptic receptors. It is widely accepted that the ability of cocaine to act as a reinforcer is due largely to its ability to block dopamine reuptake (Wise & Bozarth 1987; Woolverton & Johnson 1992; Sora et al., 2001). The reinforcing effects of psychostimulants are associated with increases in brain dopamine and D_2 receptor occupancy in humans as noted in PET studies (Volkow et al., 1999). However, both D_1 and D_2 receptors have been implicated in the reinforcing effects of cocaine. It has been demonstrated in animal studies that D_1 and D_2-like receptor

Fig. 4.2   Images of [(11)C] cocaine distribution in human brain at different time points after injection

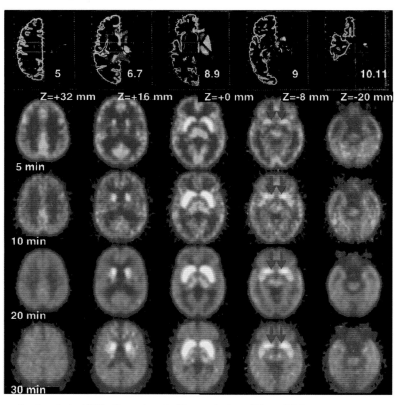

Source: Fowler et al., 2001. Reproduced with permission of the publisher.

antagonists attenuate cocaine self-administration (Caine & Koob 1994) while D_1 and D_2-like receptor agonists maintain cocaine self-administration (as reviewed in Platt, Rowlett & Spealman, 2001). Using PET to investigate the role of dopamine in the reinforcing effects of cocaine in humans it has been shown that the rate at which cocaine enters the brain and blocks the dopamine transporter is associated with the "high", and not merely with the presence of the drug in the brain (Volkow et al., 1999).

Despite the evidence pointing to a dopaminergic mechanism for cocaine reward, dopamine may not be the sole mediator of the reinforcing properties of cocaine, since dopamine transporter knock-out mice – mice that have had the dopamine transporter gene silenced so that the transporter is not expressed, (see Chapter 5) – continue to self-administer cocaine (Rocha et al., 1998). The serotonergic system may influence the reinforcing properties of cocaine, because cocaine also facilitates serotonin transmission in the nucleus accumbens (Andrews & Lucki, 2001).

Tolerance and withdrawal

In general, there appears to be little tolerance to the effects of cocaine, although there may be acute tolerance within a single session of repeated substance use (Brown, 1989).

Cocaine withdrawal does not result in the severe symptoms that characterize opioid withdrawal, but it does induce a "post-high down" (Brown, 1989), which can contribute to further cocaine use or use of another drug. During protracted withdrawal, the orbitofrontal cortex of people with cocaine dependence is hypoactive in proportion to the levels of dopamine D_2 receptors in the striatum. It is now proposed that the dependent state involves disruption of orbitofrontal cortex circuits related to compulsive repetitive behaviours (Volkow & Fowler, 2000).

Neurobiological adaptations to prolonged use

Cognitive deficits associated with chronic use of cocaine have been noted, and such deficits reflect changes to the underlying cortical, subcortical and neuromodulatory mechanisms that underpin cognition – and also interfere directly with rehabilitative programmes (Rogers & Robbins, 2001). Individuals who are dependent on cocaine have specific defects of executive functions, e.g. decision-making and judgement, and this behaviour is associated with dysfunction of specific prefrontal brain regions. PET studies suggest that stimulation of the dopaminergic system secondary to chronic use of cocaine activates a circuit that involves the orbitofrontal cortex, cingulate gyrus, thalamus and striatum. This circuit is abnormal in people with cocaine dependence and it is hypothesized that this abnormality contributes to the intense desire to use cocaine, resulting in the loss of control over the drive to take more cocaine (Volkow et al., 1996).

There appears to be strong evidence supporting the existence of a neurological syndrome following long-term use of cocaine. People with cocaine dependence exhibit impaired performance in tests of motor system functioning and have slower reaction times than non-dependent individuals. Evidence for EEG abnormalities among people recovering from cocaine dependence have also been found (Bauer, 1996).

Clinical and preclinical studies provide convincing evidence for persistent neurological and psychiatric impairments and possible neuronal degeneration associated with chronic use of cocaine or other stimulants. These impairments include multifocal and global cerebral ischaemia, cerebral haemorrhages, infarctions, optic neuropathy, cerebral atrophy, cognitive impairments, and mood and movement disorders. These may include a broad spectrum of deficits in cognition, motivation and insight, behavioural disinhibition, attention deficits, emotional instability, impulsiveness, aggressiveness, depression, anhedonia, and persistent movement disorders. The neuropsychiatric impairments accompanying stimulant use may contribute to the very high rate of relapse in individuals that can take place after years of abstinence.

Pharmacological treatment of cocaine dependence

Various approaches are being examined in the treatment of cocaine dependence. Because cocaine has potent effects on the dopamine transporter, medications that bind to the dopamine transporter have been tested. GBR 12909 is a selective and potent inhibitor of dopamine uptake that antagonizes the effects of cocaine on mesolimbic dopamine neurons in rats (Baumann et al., 1994), and blocks self-administration of cocaine in rhesus monkeys (Rothman & Glowa, 1995). Clinical trials of this drug are in the planning stage.

A novel strategy for treating cocaine dependence is the development of anti-cocaine antibodies, or immunotherapies to prevent cocaine from entering the brain. This approach differs significantly from traditional types of pharmacotherapies in that after cocaine is consumed, it is sequestered in the bloodstream by cocaine-specific antibodies that prevent its entry into the brain. One benefit from using a peripheral cocaine-blocking agent is that side effects typically associated with penetration of therapeutic drugs into the central nervous system are avoided.

The cocaine vaccine IPC-1010 has been tested in preclinical studies that were initiated by ImmuLogic Pharmaceutical Corporation in collaboration with Boston University and then continued under the name TA-CD in clinical studies conducted by Cantab Pharmaceuticals plc and Xenova Group plc in collaboration with Yale University, and support from The National Institute on Drug Abuse.

A series of studies assessed the preclinical effectiveness of anti-cocaine antibodies and the cocaine vaccine IPC-1010 on cocaine self-administration behaviour in rats. Active immunization with IPC-1010 significantly reduced both drug-seeking behaviour and the number of drug infusions earned compared to pre-immunization levels. Only rats having serum antibody levels greater than 0.05 mg/ml displayed attenuated drug-seeking behaviour and number of drug infusions across the range of doses examined. Active immunization with IPC-1010 with access to cocaine during immunization suggested that daily exposure to cocaine during the immunization period does not interfere with the ability of the immunotherapy to induce antibody formation and reduce cocaine self-administration behaviour. Studies also showed that immunization with IPC-1010 specifically decreased cocaine-seeking, and did not affect responding for another reward of food pellets.

In a phase I study, the safety and immunogenicity of TA-CD were evaluated in three groups of abstinent cocaine abusers (Kosten et al., 2002). Immunization with TA-CD induced cocaine-specific antibodies in the three groups of human subjects. The first clearly detectable anti-cocaine antibodies appeared on day 28 (14 days after the second immunization) which corresponded with the initial appearance of a decrease in cocaine self-administration behaviour in rats (Kantak et al., 2001). The antibody response was maximal after the third immunization and remained at this level for 4 months. As with rats, there was substantial variability between individuals in the magnitude of the antibody response. By one year after immunization, antibody levels in all three groups declined to baseline values. Adverse effects were minor and included small temperature elevations, mild pain and tenderness at the site of injection, and muscle twitch at the highest dose.

Phase II clinical trials with TA-CD are currently underway; however, press releases describing preliminary findings are available on the Internet. In the initial phase II study, an improved dosing regimen was initiated to boost anti-cocaine antibody levels. The immunotherapy produced high levels of antibodies against cocaine which approached levels produced in the rodent self-administration model.

In terms of clinical treatment with the cocaine immunotherapy, it is likely to work best with individuals who are highly motivated to quit using drugs altogether, since anti-cocaine antibodies are liable to have pharmacological specificity in addition to their behavioural specificity. The cocaine immunotherapy induces antibodies that are highly specific for recognizing cocaine and its active metabolite norcocaine and active derivative cocaethylene (Fox et al., 1996), and therefore they would not recognize structurally dissimilar stimulants.

It is clear from the present series of studies that the anti-cocaine actions of the cocaine immunotherapy emerge gradually over time once immunization begins. Therefore, the immunotherapy is not expected to immediately target craving for cocaine. Craving is significantly more common among inpatients than outpatients, but cocaine-abstinent individuals report less craving across outpatient treatment and follow-up compared to moderate and heavy cocaine users (Bordnick & Schmitz, 1998). On the basis of these considerations, it is hypothesized that treatment with the cocaine immunotherapy may eventually help ease craving and prevent relapse if it extinguishes cocaine use. Adjunct treatment with an anti-craving medication may help in this regard, particularly during the immunization process. How anti-cocaine antibodies interact with anti-craving medications deserves serious attention (e.g. Kuhar et al., 2001) as the development of these medications continues and the ability of the immunotherapy to block the reinforcing effects of cocaine in human clinical trials unfolds.

The ethical implications of this new type of therapy are considered in Chapter 7.

Amphetamines

Introduction

Amphetamines include Δ-amphetamine, L-amphetamine, ephedrine, methamphetamine, methylphenidate, and pemoline. Another member of this group is (-)cathinone, the active ingredient in freshly gathered leaves of the Khat shrub (*Catha edulis*), whose actions are very similar to that of amphetamine (Jaffe, 1990) (see Box 4.5). Amphetamines are used not only for the subjective "high" that they produce, but also to extend periods of wakefulness, as used by lorry drivers and students studying for exams. In addition, they are used as appetite suppressants, although this effect is short-lived. Medically, amphetamines are currently used only in the treatment of narcolepsy, and in treating the symptoms of attention deficit hyperactivity disorder (ADHD) in children. This condition is thought to be partly due to low cortical norepinephrine, which permits subcortical emotional systems to govern behaviour impulsively. When cortical arousal is facilitated with psychostimulants, children with ADHD are able to pay attention to the tasks they are engaged in (Panksepp, 1998) (see Box 4.6). Non-medical use of amphetamines and related stimulants is a growing problem worldwide (see Box 4.7).

Behavioural effects

Amphetamines are stimulants of the central nervous system that produce increased alertness, arousal, energy, motor and speech activity, increased self-confidence and ability to concentrate, an overall feeling of well-being and reduced hunger (Jacobs & Fehr, 1987; Hoffman & Lefkowitz, 1990). The short-term effects of low doses of amphetamine include restlessness, dizziness, insomnia, euphoria, mild confusion, tremor, and may induce panic or psychotic episodes. There is a general increase in alertness, energy and activity, and a reduction of fatigue and drowsiness. There may be heart palpitations, irregular heartbeat, increased respiration, dry mouth and suppression of appetite. With higher doses, these effects are intensified, leading to exhilaration and euphoria, rapid flow of ideas, feelings of increased mental and physical ability, excitation, agitation, fever and sweating. Paranoid thinking, confusion and hallucinations have been observed. Severe overdose may lead to high fever, convulsions, coma, cerebral haemorrhage and death (Jacobs & Fehr, 1987).

BOX 4.5

Khat

The leaves and buds of an East African plant, *Catha edulis*, which are chewed or brewed as a beverage. Used also in parts of the eastern Mediterranean and North Africa, khat is a stimulant with effects similar to those of amphetamine – the reason being that the main active ingredient in khat is cathinone, an amphetamine-like substance. Consumption of khat produces euphoria and increased alertness, although concentration and judgement are impaired. Heavy use can result in dependence and physical and mental problems resembling those produced by other stimulants.

Source: WHO, 1994.

BOX 4.6

Use of stimulant drugs to treat attention deficit hyperactivity disorder

Attention deficit hyperactivity disorder (ADHD) is characterized by hyperactivity, impulsivity and deficits in attention that are not appropriate for a child's developmental age. Psychostimulants, such as methylphenidate, are used in the treatment of ADHD. This use may seem paradoxical, however, it is believed that individuals with ADHD have low norepinephrine and dopamine activity and therefore have poor attention and difficulty in regulating behaviour based on external stimuli. The neurotransmitters norepinephrine and dopamine promote sensory and motor arousal. With too little cortical arousal, it is thought that subcortical emotional systems govern behaviour impulsively. When cortical arousal is facilitated with psychostimulants, the attention of children with ADHD improves and they are more able to concentrate on a task. Thus, with improved attention, individuals with ADHD can better regulate their own behaviour.

Source: Panksepp, 1998.

Amphetamine is a potent psychotomimetic, and can intensify symptoms or precipitate a psychotic episode in vulnerable individuals (Ujike, 2002). People who use amphetamine chronically often develop a psychosis very similar to schizophrenia (Robinson & Becker, 1986; Yui et al., 1999).

Amphetamine is readily self-administered by animals (Hoebel et al., 1983), shows robust place preference conditioning (Bardo, Valone & Bevins, 1999), discriminative stimulus effects (Bevins, Klebaur & Bardo, 1997), and brain stimulation reward effects (Phillips, Brooke & Fibiger, 1975; Glick, Weaver & Meibach, 1980).

Mechanism of action

The primary mechanism of action of amphetamine is to stimulate the release of dopamine from nerve terminals via the dopamine transporter. Thus, dopamine can be released independently of neuronal excitation. This contrasts with the effects of cocaine, which blocks the reuptake of monoamines in the nerve terminal, and thus only affects active neurons. Like cocaine, amphetamine also inhibits, to a certain extent, the reuptake of the catecholamines, thereby increasing their ability to activate receptors. Amphetamine may also directly activate catecholamine receptors, further contributing to monoaminergic activity.

Tolerance and withdrawal

Tolerance develops rapidly to many of the behavioural and physiological effects of amphetamines, such as suppression of appetite, insomnia, euphoria, and cardiovascular effects (Jacobs & Fehr, 1987). Interestingly, the effects of amphetamines on behaviour in children with ADHD and in people with narcolepsy do not show signs of tolerance. It is important to note that even though methamphetamine is used to treat ADHD in children, the therapeutic doses for ADHD and other disorders such as narcolepsy are much lower than the daily amounts taken for non-medical use.

Although tolerance develops to some aspects of psychostimulant use, sensitization, or an increase in the hyperactivity or stereotypy induced by amphetamine also occurs, even if the doses are spread out over days or weeks. Cross-sensitization with cocaine occurs, and is thought to be the result of increased dopamine in the striatum (Kalivas & Weber, 1988). Sensitization is thought to play a critical role in dependence (see Chapter 3).

Neurobiological adaptations to prolonged use

Long-term use of amphetamine may result in sleeping problems, anxiety, suppression of appetite, and high blood pressure. People who use amphetamine often take sedative/hypnotic drugs to counteract these effects, and thus the incidence of polydrug use is high (Jacobs & Fehr, 1987).

Amphetamine users sometimes ingest increasing quantities of amphetamine in "runs" that last 3–6 days. This continuous use has been modelled in animals, and changes in behaviour are observed consistent with hallucinatory-like effects. This pattern of use is neurotoxic and produces brain damage. Continuous infusion of low doses of amphetamine into rats produces a depletion of nigrostriatal dopamine, its precursors and metabolites, and receptors (Robinson & Becker 1986).

With long-term use of methamphetamine there is a decrease in dopamine D_2 receptor availability in the caudate and putamen, and a decrease in metabolic rate in the orbitofrontal cortex (Volkow et al., 2001a) (see Fig. 4.3), and loss of dopamine transporters that is associated with motor and cognitive impairment (Volkow et al., 2001b).

There are limited data available on the proportion of current amphetamine users who are dependent (see Box 4.7). A review of the medical literature indicates that some antidepressant drugs may decrease craving for amphetamines (Srisurapanont, Jarusuraisin & Kittirattanapaiboon, 2001). However, this may also be related to the comorbidity of psychostimulant dependence and depression (see Chapter 6).

Ecstasy

Introduction

Ecstasy or 3,4-methylenedioxymethamphetamine (MDMA) is a synthetic amphetamine, also known as XTC, E, Adam, MDM or "love drug" (Shaper, 1996). Ecstasy can be classified as a psychostimulant, belonging to the same group as cocaine and the amphetamines, since many of its acute effects are

Fig.4.3   Comparison of dopamine D2 receptor binding in the brains of a control subject and a person with methamphetamine dependence

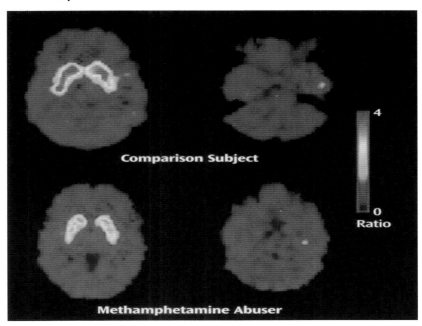

Source: Volkow et al., 2001a. Reproduced with permission from the publisher.

similar to these substances. Ecstasy is classifiable as a hallucinogen, due to the potential induction of hallucinations if used in extremely high doses (American Psychiatric Association, 1994; WHO, 2001). As the subjective effects of MDMA in humans are not the same as those produced by LSD and because the drug does not present similar structure or pharmacological activity to hallucinogens, the term "entactogens", meaning "entering in contact with yourself " (Nichols, 1986; Morgan, 2000) was proposed to define a new pharmacological class. As the understanding of the drug effects increases, its classification will be more accurate. Use of ecstasy has recently been associated with the global trend of dance parties (or "raves") and "techno" music (WHO, 2001).

Psychostimulant effects of MDMA are observed 20–60 minutes after oral ingestion of moderate doses (50–125 mg) of ecstasy and last from 2–4 hours (Grispoon & Bakalar, 1986). Peak plasma levels of ecstasy occur 2 hours after oral administration, and only residual levels are found 24 hours after the last dose (Verebey, Alrazi & Jafre, 1988; Cami et al., 1997). MDMA has a non-linear pharmacokinetic profile: consumption of elevated doses of the substance may produce disproportional elevation of plasma levels of ecstasy (Cami et al., 1997; de la Torre et al., 2000).

BOX 4.7

Growing epidemic of amphetamine-type stimulants (ATS) use

Amphetamine-type stimulants (ATS) refer to a group of drugs whose principal members include amphetamine and methamphetamine. However, a range of other substances also fall into this group, such as methcathinone, fenetylline, ephedrine, pseudoephedrine, methylphenidate and 3,4-methylenedioxymethamphetamine (MDMA) or 'Ecstasy' – an amphetamine-type derivative with hallucinogenic properties. The use of ATS is a global and growing phenomenon and in recent years, there has been a pronounced increase in the production and use of ATS worldwide.

Over the past decade, use of ATS has infiltrated its way into the mainstream culture in certain countries. Younger people in particular seem to possess a skewed sense of safety about these substances, believing rather erroneously that they are safe and benign. Meanwhile, ATS are posing a serious threat to the health, social and economic fabric of families, communities and countries. For many countries, the problem of ATS is relatively new, growing quickly and unlikely to go away. Geographically, its occurrence is spreading, but awareness of ATS is limited and responses are neither integrated nor consistent.

Recent data have shown a stabilization in ATS use in north America and western Europe, while the highest levels of abuse worldwide have emerged in East Asia and Oceania. According to a review conducted by UNDCP in 1996, there are about 20 countries in this region in which the abuse of ATS is more widespread than that of heroin and cocaine combined. In Japan, the Republic of Korea and the Philippines use of ATS is 5–7 times that of heroin and cocaine use.

Smoking, sniffing and inhaling are the most popular methods of ATS use, but ways to take the drug vary widely across the region. In countries such as Australia, where over 90% of those who report using ATS (mostly methamphetamine) inject, the drug represents a significant risk factor in the transmission of blood-borne viruses. The Philippines and Viet Nam are also reporting signs that injecting methamphetamine is increasing while in Thailand, the number of methamphetamine users now represents the majority of all new drug treatment cases. There are currently very limited data to indicate what proportion of current users are dependent. Researchers have pointed out that it is likely that dependence and chronic usage is associated with methamphetamine psychosis and related adverse consequences, and that because of the high rates of usage, levels of presentation of methamphetamine psychosis to mental health services are dramatically escalating.

In short, the present situation warrants immediate attention, with a major epidemic of methamphetamine use in Thailand that appears to be spreading across the entire Asia Pacific Region. Researchers have stressed an urgent need to map out this epidemic to assess the spread and scale of the problems, consequences and responses.

Sources: WHO, 1997b; Farrell et al., 2002; UNODCCP, 2002.

MDMA is widely distributed, easily crossing membranes and the blood-brain barrier. Its clearance depends partially on metabolism by the liver, between 3–7% is converted to the active substance methylenedioxyamphetamine (MDA), 28% is biotransformed to other metabolites, and around 65% is eliminated, unchanged, via the kidneys (Verebey, Alrazi & Jafre, 1988; Cami et al., 1997).

The half-life of ecstasy in plasma is 7.6 hours. This information is relevant when treating intoxication: 6–8 half-lives are necessary for complete elimination of ecstasy, giving a total time of around 48 hours for the drug to be completely eliminated. It can also be seen that at a plasma level of 8 mg/l – considered to be the level of severe intoxication – more than 24 hours would be necessary to decrease this to a plasma level lower than 1 mg/l, which produces less clinical effects. Therefore, 24 hours would be the estimated time of intensive care needed by intoxicated patients who had taken a few ecstasy capsules.

Behavioural effects

MDMA may produce subjective effects in humans that are similar to, but distinguishable from, those of the psychostimulants Δ-amphetamine and cocaine. Increased self-confidence, understanding and empathy together with enhanced sensation of proximity and intimacy with other people, and improvement of communication and relationship skills are described in uncontrolled studies. Euphoria and increased emotional and physical energy are presumed to occur with this psychostimulant (Downing, 1986; Nichols, 1986; WHO, 2001). Negative psychological effects of anxiety, paranoia, and depression can also occur (WHO, 2001).

Intravenous self-administration behaviour in primates (Beardsley, Balster & Harris, 1986) and in rats (Acquas et al., 2001) is maintained across a range of doses of ecstasy.

Mechanism of action

Similar to other amphetamines (McKenna & Peroutka, 1990), the effects of ecstasy may be related to several neurotransmitters including serotonin, dopamine, and norepinephrine (Downing, 1986; Nichols, 1986; Kalant, 2001; Montoya et al., 2002). However, serotonin plays the main role in mediating the effects of ecstasy (Shulgin, 1986; Mascaro et al, 1991; Marona-Lewicka et al., 1996; Kalant, 2001; Montoya et al., 2002). There is increased net serotonin release because MDMA binds to and blocks the serotonin transporter, thus blocking serotonin reuptake (Kalant, 2001). Eventually this leads to long-term depletion of serotonin and metabolite concentrations in the brain (WHO, 2001). MDMA also increases the release of dopamine (WHO, 2001).

Tolerance and withdrawal

Tolerance develops rapidly with use of ecstasy, and some individuals use progressively larger amounts of ecstasy to reinforce its psychoactive effect (McCann & Ricaurte, 1991; WHO, 2001). In some individuals, tolerance occurs to the pleasant psychoactive effects of ecstasy but not to the physical collateral effects, therefore any dose increase to augment the psychoactive effects may produce dysphoria (Grispoon & Bakalar, 1986). In this group of individuals, MDMA will not cause dependence, and thus the use of large amounts of ecstasy for long periods is rare (Peroutka, 1989). It is still necessary to define which are the social, genetic, cultural, environmental and hormonal factors involved in these long-term individual differences in the effects of ecstasy.

For 2–3 days following MDMA use, there may be residual effects associated with the acute withdrawal of the drug, including muscle stiffness and pain, headache, nausea, loss of appetite, blurred vision, dry mouth and insomnia (Kalant, 2001). Psychological effects may also be observed, most commonly depression, anxiety, fatigue, and difficulty in concentrating (Kalant, 2001). This is typical of the "crash" that is also seen following the use of amphetamines and cocaine.

Neurobiological adaptations to prolonged use

Neurotoxicity induced by MDMA is cumulative and is related to the dose and frequency of drug use (McKenna & Peroutka, 1990; Kalant, 2001). In animals, acute neurochemical effects are observed after doses of around 5–10 mg/kg of ecstasy and long-term effects occur after doses 4 times higher, or after frequent administration of smaller doses. A neurotoxic schedule of ecstasy reduces rat brain serotonin concentrations by 45%. Damage or neuroadaptation to the brain has been clearly demonstrated in both humans and in animal models, which show reduced serotonin concentrations, neurons, transporters and terminals (Kalant, 2001).

There are also long-term psychiatric and physical problems associated with MDMA use. Impairments of memory, decision-making and self-control are observed, as are paranoia, depression and panic attacks (Kalant, 2001; Montoya et al., 2002). There can also be major hepatic, cardiovascular and cerebral toxic effects (Kalant, 2001; Montoya et al., 2002). The long-term depletion of brain serotonin by ecstasy is also accompanied by impairment of body temperature control and behavioural responses (Shankaran & Gudelsky, 1999). The public health implications of these findings are apparent.

Volatile Solvents

Introduction

Several volatile chemicals (including gases such as nitric oxide, volatile solvents such as toluene, and aliphatic nitrites) produce effects on the central nervous system and are used mainly by children and adolescents due to their ready availability (see Box 4.8). The term inhalant applies to a diverse group of substances that can be found in products such as gasoline, nail-polish remover, paint stripper and adhesive glue (Weir, 2001). These compounds are intentionally sniffed either directly or from a solvent-soaked rag placed in the person's mouth or in a plastic bag. The volatile solvent compounds have few characteristics in common other than their toxicity and the behavioural effects they produce.

Behavioural effects

The intoxication induced by inhalation of solvent vapour produces some behavioural effects similar to those due to alcohol. Minutes after inhalation dizziness, disorientation and a short period of excitation with euphoria are observed, followed by a feeling of light-headedness and a longer period of depression of consciousness. In addition, marked changes in mental state are induced in people who misuse toluene and other solvents. Most users report elevation of mood and hallucinations. Potentially dangerous delusions such as believing one can fly or swim also occur, thoughts are likely to be slowed, time appears to pass more quickly, and tactile hallucinations are common (Evans & Raistrick, 1987). These behavioural effects are accompanied by visual disturbances, nystagmus, incoordination and unsteady gait, slurred speech, abdominal pain and flushing of the skin.

BOX 4.8

Use of volatile solvents

The term volatile solvent use describes the intentional inhalation of a variety of volatile substances (mostly organic solvents), for psychoactive effects. The term inhalants has come to encompass a group of psychoactive chemicals that are defined by the route of administration rather than by their effects on the central nervous system. Thus, such diverse substances as toluene, ether, and nitrites have been classified as inhalants because they are all taken in through the nose and mouth by inhalation.

Volatile solvent use (including glue sniffing, inhalant and solvent use) has now been reported in various parts of the world, mainly among adolescents, individuals living in remote communities and those whose occupations provide easy access to these substances. In certain countries volatile solvent use is associated with particular groups of young people such as street children and children from indigenous populations. Many products that can be used to achieve intoxication are readily available in the home and in a range of shops.

Sources: WHO, 1999; Brouette & Anton, 2001.

Animal studies have shown that, in common with classical depressant drugs, volatile solvents have biphasic effects on motor activity, disrupt psychomotor performance, have anticonvulsant effects, produce biphasic drug-like effects on rates of schedule-controlled operant behaviour, increase rates of punished responding, serve as reinforcers in self-administration studies and share discriminative stimulus effects with barbiturates and ethanol (Evans & Balster, 1991). Toluene is self-administered in primates (Weiss, Wood & Macys, 1979), and has biphasic effects on intracranial self-stimulation, increasing the frequency of self-stimulation at lower concentrations and decreasing it at higher concentrations. Several solvents contained in glue vapours, including toluene, induce conditioned place preference and activate the brain reward system in intracranial self-stimulation in rats, predicting the dependence-producing potential of volatile solvents (Yavich & Patkina, 1994; Yavich & Zvartau, 1994).

Mechanism of action

Little is known about the mechanism of action of the solvents, and they have received far less attention in research than other psychoactive substances. Most reviews consider the nature of the acute effects of volatile organic solvents by comparing their actions to those of classical depressant drugs such as the barbiturates, benzodiazepines and ethanol. Based on their physical effects it is assumed that solvents induce similar biochemical changes as ethanol and anaesthetics, and therefore the search for a GABAergic mechanism of action has been pursued. In mice, the discriminative stimulus effects of ethanol may be substituted for several volatile anaesthetics, toluene and other volatile solvents (Bowen & Balster, 1997). Acquisition of toluene discrimination by rats and mice, generalizes for GABAergic agents such as barbiturates and benzodiazepines, suggesting that toluene may have drug dependence potential of the CNS-depressant type (Knisely, Rees & Balster, 1990).

The commonly used solvents, including toluene, also affect ligand-gated ion channel activity. Toluene, similar to ethanol, reversibly enhances GABA(A) receptor-mediated synaptic currents. Therefore, the molecular sites of action of these compounds may overlap with those of ethanol and the volatile anaesthetics (Beckstead et al., 2000). Toluene has excitatory and inhibitory biphasic effects on neurotransmission that are related to GABAergic neurotransmission.

Dopamine in the nucleus accumbens is closely related to substance dependence for all psychoactive substances (Chapter 3). Acute inhalation of toluene by rats results in an increase in extracellular dopamine levels in the striatum (Stengard, Hoglund & Ungerstedt, 1994), and changes in neuronal firing of dopamine neurons of the VTA (Riegel & French, 1999). Therefore, this electrophysiological study suggests that mesolimbic dopamine neurotransmission can be changed by toluene exposure, pointing towards the same conclusion as the neurochemical studies.

Other evidence of dopamine involvement following toluene inhalation comes from studies on occupational toxicology. Subchronic inhalation exposure to concentrations of toluene likely to be found in occupational settings induces persistent changes in locomotor activity and the number of dopamine D_2 receptors in rat caudate (von Euler et al., 1993; Hillefors-Berglund, Liu & von Euler, 1995). Toluene-induced locomotor hyperactivity may be blocked by D_2 receptor antagonists (Riegel & French, 1999).

Tolerance and withdrawal

The acute neurobehavioural effects of volatile solvents, including anxiolysis and sedation, are those typically associated with central nervous system depressants, and these effects may lead to continued use, tolerance and withdrawal (Beckstead et al., 2000).

Tolerance may occur but it is considered difficult to estimate in humans. It seems to be established after 1–2 months of repetitive exposure to volatile solvents (American Psychiatric Association, 1994). Rats exposed to high environmental concentrations of toluene vapours for long periods of time, present tolerance to motor abnormalities (Himnan, 1984).

Withdrawal from volatile solvents in mice is characterized by increased susceptibility to convulsions and may be reversed or diminished by other solvent vapours, as well as by ethanol, midazolam and pentobarbital. These data support the hypothesis that the basis for volatile solvent use may be its ability to produce ethanol-like and depressant drug-like effects (Evans & Balster, 1991).

Neurobiological adaptations to prolonged use

Persistent changes in dopamine receptor binding and function have been found in rats exposed to low concentrations of toluene. In addition, acute inhalation exposure to toluene is accompanied by an increase in extracellular dopamine levels within the striatum (Stengard, Hoglund & Ungerstedt, 1994), while prolonged exposure does not significantly change extracellular dopamine levels in rat accumbens (Beyer et al., 2001).

Repeated exposure to toluene increased the acute motor-stimulant response to cocaine and potentiated and prolonged cocaine-induced increases in dopamine outflow in the nucleus accumbens, showing that repeated exposure to toluene enhances behavioural and neurochemical responses to subsequent cocaine administration in rats. This is evidence of the development of sensitization and cross-sensitization, which are key features in the development of dependence (see Chapter 3). These findings suggest that exposure to toluene alters neuronal function in an area known to be critically involved in substance dependence, by increasing sensitivity to other psychoactive substances and may, therefore, increase the probability of substance dependence (Beyer et al., 2001).

Organic solvent inhalation is the cause of several neuropathological changes that are associated with decreased cognitive functioning. Workers chronically exposed to mixtures of organic solvents in the environment at concentrations within or slightly exceeding the acceptable values, present with subtle cognitive deficits, detected through visual evoked potentials (Indulski et al., 1996). Chronic inhalation of primarily toluene-based solvents can produce a persistent paranoid psychosis, temporal lobe epilepsy and a decrease in IQ. These psychiatric and neurological sequelae of chronic solvent use are serious and potentially irreversible (Byrne et al., 1991). The degree to which these chronic neuropsychiatric effects modulate the persistent use of solvents or other substances needs clarification.

Hallucinogens

Introduction

The hallucinogens are a chemically diverse class, but are characterized by their ability to produce distortions in sensations, and to markedly alter mood and thought processes. They include substances from a wide variety of natural and synthetic sources, and are structurally dissimilar (Jacobs & Fehr, 1987). The name hallucinogen refers to hallucination-producing properties of these drugs. However, hallucinations are not the only effects caused by these drugs, and often occur only at very high doses. The hallucinations are most often visual, but can affect any of the senses, as well as the individual's perception of time, the world, and the self. The subjective effects vary greatly between individuals, and from one use to the next within the same person.

The hallucinogens are divided into classes based on structural similarity of the drugs. One class is related to lysergic acid diethylamide (LSD). These are the indolealkylamines, which are structurally similar to the neurotransmitter serotonin. This group includes LSA (d-lysergic acid amine, found in the seeds of several varieties of morning glory), psilocybin, and dimethyltryptamine (DMT). These latter three compounds are all naturally occurring.

The next group of hallucinogens consists of phenylethylamine drugs, of which mescaline, methylenedioxyamphetamine (MDA), and methylenedioxy-methamphetamine (MDMA) are the most popular members. MDMA, or ecstasy, is considered separately in this chapter due to its widespread use and current popularity. Paramethoxyamphetamine (PMA), dimethoxy-4-methylamphetamine (DOM) and trimethoxyamphetamine (TMA) are other members of this group. These drugs bear a close structural relationship with amphetamine.

Phencyclidine (PCP) and ketamine are dissociative anaesthetics that belong to the arylcycloalkylamine family of drugs, and act on glutamate receptors.

Finally, there is the atropinic family, which includes atropine, scopolamine and hyoscyamine. They are found naturally in many species of potato plants.

They are also found in *Atropa belladonna* (deadly nightshade), *Datura stramonium* (jimsonweed), and several related species throughout the world.

Cannabis is also classified as a hallucinogen, but is considered separately in this chapter.

Behavioural effects

These drugs produce increased heart rate and blood pressure, elevated body temperature, reduced appetite, nausea, vomiting, abdominal discomfort, rapid reflexes, motor incoordination and pupillary dilatation (Jacobs & Fehr, 1987).

The hallucinatory effects are related to dose, and distortions of any of the sensory modalities can occur. The melding of two sensory modalities is also possible (e.g. music being "seen"), and is called synaesthesia (Jacobs & Fehr, 1987). These drugs also affect thought processes and memory.

The intensity of the effects, and the emotional reaction to them, differ from person to person. Reactions can range from joy and euphoria to fear and panic. There can be a sense of deep insight, as well as psychotic episodes.

The effects of hallucinogens are quite similar between classes of drugs within this category, and range from excitation or depressant effects, analgesic and anaesthetic effects, depending on the dose taken and the situation. PCP and ketamine can produce hallucinations at very low doses.

Mechanism of action

LSD acts on the serotonin system, and is an autoreceptor agonist in the raphe nucleus. An autoreceptor is a receptor on a neuron for the transmitter that neuron releases. Activation of an autoreceptor acts as a negative feedback mechanism to turn down the firing of the neuron. This helps to regulate neuronal firing and to prevent overactivation of neurons. LSD also acts as a serotonin-2 agonist, or partial agonist (Jaffe, 1990). It is taken orally, and doses as low as 20–25 µg can produce effects.

PCP is a non-competitive antagonist at the N-methyl-D-aspartate (NMDA) receptor (Lodge & Johnson 1990). PCP-induced psychosis can last for weeks despite abstinence from substance use (Allen & Young 1978; Luisada 1978). Similarly to PCP, ketamine, a PCP analogue that is also a non-competitive NMDA receptor antagonist that exhibits higher selectivity than PCP for the NMDA receptor (Lodge & Johnson 1990), also induces psychotomimetic effects in healthy volunteers (Newcomer et al., 1999), and exacerbates symptoms in patients with schizophrenia (Lahti et al., 1995).

The atropinic class of hallucinogens are antagonists of muscarinic cholinergic receptors.

Tolerance and withdrawal

Tolerance develops rapidly to both the physical and psychological effects of the hallucinogens. The psychoactive effects will no longer occur after 3–4 days of repeated use, and will not recur unless a period of several days of abstinence occurs. There is no evidence of withdrawal occurring to any of the hallucinogens (Jacobs & Fehr, 1987).

Neurobiological adaptations to prolonged use

Few data are available on the long-term neurological effects of hallucinogens. "Flashbacks" may occur either shortly after using the drugs, or up to 5 years later (Jacob & Fehr, 1987). Flashbacks are spontaneous recurrences of experiences which occurred during a previous LSD episode. Other effects of long-term use include increased apathy, decreased interest, passivity, and failure to plan ahead, and there may also be disregard for social norms. However, it is difficult to ascribe these effects entirely to hallucinogens, as they are often used with other drugs as well. Finally, chronic use of hallucinogens can result in acute or long-term psychotic episodes.

Summary

It is evident that almost all psychoactive substances share the common property of increasing mesolimbic dopamine function. Not only psychostimulants such as cocaine (Kuczenski & Segal, 1992) and amphetamine (Carboni et al., 1989) but also narcotic analgesics (Di Chiara & Imperato, 1988b), nicotine (Imperato, Mulas & Di Chiara, 1986), ethanol (Imperato & Di Chiara, 1986) and phencyclidine (Carboni et al., 1989) stimulate dopamine transmission in the nucleus accumbens (Di Chiara & Imperato, 1988a), the main area of the ventral striatum. The implications of this with respect to dependence were discussed in Chapter 3.

The understanding of the acute and chronic effects of psychoactive substances on the brain has expanded greatly in recent years to begin to provide a substantial molecular and cellular fingerprint of the extensive changes in neuronal systems. The major realization has been that the use of psychoactive substances usurps the normal physiological mechanisms that mediate reward, learning and memory, and eventually results in remodelling of neuronal contacts and pathways, producing long-lasting, near-permanent changes. Furthering our understanding of the mechanisms involved still requires intensive research effort, and the availability of sophisticated molecular and biochemical tools should greatly facilitate this process.

Although psychoactive substances have these common effects, there is still considerable variability between drug classes in terms of primary physical and psychological effects, mechanisms of action, development of tolerance and withdrawal, and long-term effects (see Tables 4.1 and 4.2). Differences in the availability, cost, legality, marketing and cultural attitudes towards psychoactive substances and their use also affect which substances are used, and the development of dependence upon them. Thus, the study

Table 4.1 Summary of characteristics of selected psychoactive substances

Substance	Primary mechanism of action	Behavioural effects	Tolerance	Withdrawal	Effects of prolonged use
Ethanol	Increases activity of GABA-A receptors	Sedation Impaired memory Motor incoordination Anxiolysis	Metabolic tolerance occurs due to enzyme induction Behavioural tolerance develops through learning Tolerance also develops through changes to GABA-A receptor	Shaking, perspiration, weakness, agitation, headache, nausea, vomiting Seizures Delirium tremens	Altered brain function and morphology Cognitive impairments Decreased brain volume
Hypnotics and sedatives	Benzodiazepines: facilitate GABA's opening of GABA-A chloride channel Barbiturates: bind to a specific site on the GABA ionophore and increase chloride conductance	Sedation Anaesthesia Motor incoordination Cognitive impairments Memory impairment	Develops rapidly to most effects (except anticonvulsant) due to changes in GABA-A receptor	Anxiety, arousal, restlessness, insomnia, excitability, seizures	Memory impairment
Nicotine	Nicotinic cholinergic receptor agonist Increases sodium inflow through the channel, causing depolarization	Arousal, increased attention, concentration and memory; decreased anxiety and appetite; stimulant-like effects	Tolerance develops through metabolic factors, as well as receptor changes	Irritability, hostility, anxiety, dysphoria, depressed mood, decreased heart rate, increased appetite	Health effects due to smoking are well-documented. Difficult to dissociate effects of nicotine from other components of tobacco
Opioids	Mu and delta opioid receptor agonists	Euphoria, analgesia, sedation, respiratory depression	Short-term and long-term receptor desensitization Adaptations in intracellular signalling mechanisms	Watering eyes, runny nose, yawning, sweating, restlessness, chills, cramps, muscle aches	Long-term changes in opioid receptors and peptides Adaptations in reward, learning, stress responses

Table 4.1 Summary of characteristics of selected psychoactive substances (continued)

Substance	Primary mechanism of action	Behavioural effects	Tolerance	Withdrawal	Effects of prolonged use
Cannabinoids	CB1 receptor agonists	Relaxation, increased sensory awareness, decreased short-term memory, motor incoordination, analgesia, antiemetic and antiepileptic effects, increased appetite	Develops rapidly to most effects	Rare, perhaps due to long half-life of cannabinoids	Cognitive impairments, risk of relapse and exacerbation of mental illness
Cocaine	Monoamine (dopamine, norepinephrine, serotonin) transporter blocker (increases monoamines in synaptic cleft)	Increased alertness, energy, motor activity, feelings of competence; euphoria, anxiety, restlessness, paranoia	Perhaps short-term acute tolerance	Not much, except "post-high down"	Cognitive deficits, abnormalities on PET with orbitofrontal cortex Impaired motor function Decreased reaction times, EEG abnormalities, cerebral ischaemia, infarcts, haemorrhages
Amphetamines	Increased release of dopamine from nerve terminals via dopamine transporter Not dependent upon action potentials Inhibits monoamine oxidase (MAO)	Increased alertness, arousal, energy, motor activity, speech, self-confidence, concentration, feelings of well-being; decreased hunger, increased heart rate, increased respiration, euphoria	Develops rapidly to behavioural and physiological effects	Fatigue, increased appetite, irritability, emotional depression, anxiety	Sleep disturbances, anxiety, decreased appetite, increased blood pressure; decreased brain dopamine, precursors, metabolites and receptors
Ecstasy	Blocks serotonin reuptake	Increased self-confidence, empathy, understanding, sensations of intimacy, communication, euphoria, energy	May develop in some individuals	Nausea, muscle stiffness, headache, loss of appetite, blurred vision, dry mouth, insomnia, depression, anxiety, fatigue, difficulty concentrating	Neurotoxic to brain serotonin systems, leads to behavioural and physiological consequences

Table 4.1 Summary of characteristics of selected psychoactive substances (continued)

Substance	Primary mechanism of action	Behavioural effects	Tolerance	Withdrawal	Effects of prolonged use
Volatile solvents	Most likely GABA-A receptor mediated	Dizziness, disorientation, euphoria, light-headedness, increased mood, hallucinations, delusions, incoordination, visual disturbances, anxiolysis, sedation	Some tolerance develops (difficult to estimate)	Increased susceptibility to seizures	Changes in dopamine receptor binding and function; decreased cognitive function; psychiatric and neurological sequelae
Hallucinogens	Varies: LSD: serotonin autoreceptor agonist PCP: NMDA glutamate receptor antagonist Atropinics: muscarinic cholingergic receptor antagonists	Increased heart rate, blood pressure, body temperature; decreased appetite, nausea, vomiting, motor incoordination, papillary dilatation, hallucinations	Tolerance develops rapidly to physical and psychological effects	No evidence	Acute or chronic psychotic episodes, flashbacks or re-experiencing of drug effects long after drug use

Table 4.2 Features of major classes of psychoactive substances

Class	Examples	Most common behavioural effects
Stimulants	Amphetamine Cocaine Ecstasy Nicotine	Stimulation, arousal, increased energy, increased concentration, decreased appetite, increased heart rate, increased respiration, paranoia, panic
Depressants	Alcohol Sedatives/hypnotics Volatile solvents	Relaxation, disinhibition, motor impairments, memory and cognitive impairments, anxiolysis
Hallucinogens	Cannabinoids LSD Phencyclidine	Hallucinations, increased sensory awareness, motor and cognitive deficits
Opioids	Morphine Heroin	Euphoria, analgesia, sedation

of substance dependence must take these factors into account, while at the same time noting the similarities across drug classes. The next chapter examines genetic effects on substance use, both across and between substance groups. Chapter 6 discusses how substance use interacts with, precipitates, or may be a result of psychiatric illness. It is important to keep in mind that substance dependence is the result of not only the primary pharmacological properties of the psychoactive substance, but also the complex interplay of biological and environmental factors that surround its use.

References

Acquas E et al. (2001) Intravenous administration of ecstasy (3,4-methylenedioxymethamphetamine) enhances cortical and striatal acetylcholine release in vivo. *European Journal of Pharmacology*, **418**:207–211.

Adams IB, Martin BR (1996) Cannabis: pharmacology and toxicology in animals and humans. *Addiction*, **91**:1585–1614.

Ahijevych K (1999) Nicotine metabolism variability and nicotine addiction. *Nicotine and Tobacco Research*, **1**(Suppl.):S59–S62.

Akil H et al. (1997) Molecular and neuroanatomical properties of the endogenous opioid systems: implications for the treatment of opiate addiction. *Seminars in Neuroscience*, **9**:70–83.

Ali R et al. (1999) Report of the external panel on the evaluation of the Swiss scientific studies of medically prescribed narcotics to drug addicts. *Sucht*, **45**:160–170.

Allen RM, Young SJ (1978) Phencyclidine-induced psychosis. *American Journal of Psychiatry*, **135**:1081–1084.

Ameri A (1999) The effects of cannabinoids on the brain. *Progress in Neurobiology*, **58**:315–348.

American Psychiatric Association (1994) *Diagnostic and statistical manual of mental disorders,* 4th ed. Washington, DC, American Psychiatric Association.

Andrews CM, Lucki I (2001) Effects of cocaine on extracellular dopamine and serotonin levels in the nucleus accumbens. *Psychopharmacology* (Berlin), **155**:221–229.

Bammer G et al. (1999) The heroin prescribing debate: integrating science and politics. *Science*, **284**:1277–1278.

Bardo MT, Valone JM, Bevins RA (1999) Locomotion and conditioned place preference produced by acute intravenous amphetamine: role of dopamine receptors and individual differences in amphetamine self-administration. *Psychopharmacology*, **143**:39–46.

Barnard EA et al. (1998) International Union of Pharmacology. XV. Subtypes of gamma-aminobutyric acid-A receptors: classification on the basis of subunit structure and receptor function. *Pharmacological Reviews*, **50**:291–313.

Barnett PG, Rodgers JH, Bloch DA (2001) A meta-analysis comparing buprenorphine to methadone for treatment of opiate dependence. *Addiction*, **96**:683–690.

Barros HM, Miczek KA (1996) Withdrawal from oral cocaine in rats: ultrasonic vocalizations and tactile startle. *Psychopharmacology* (Berlin), 125:379–384.

Bauer LO (1996) Psychomotor and electroencephalographic sequelae of cocaine dependence. *NIDA Research Monograph*, **163**:66–93.

Baumann MH et al. (1994) GBR12909 attenuates cocaine-induced activation of mesolimbic dopamine neurons in the rat. *Journal of Pharmacology and Experimental Therapeutics*, **271**:1216–1222.

Beardsley PM, Balster RL, Harris LS (1986) Self-administration of methylenedioxymethamphetamine (MDMA) by rhesus monkeys. *Drug and Alcohol Dependence*, **18**:149–157.

Beckstead MJ et al. (2000) Glycine and gamma-aminobutyric acid(A) receptor function is enhanced by inhaled drugs of abuse. *Molecular Pharmacology*, **57**:1199–1205.

Benowitz NL et al. (2002) Slower metabolism and reduced intake of nicotine from cigarette smoking in Chinese-Americans. *Journal of the National Cancer Institute*, **94**:108–115.

Bevins RA, Klebaur JE, Bardo MT (1997) Individual differences in response to novelty, amphetamine-induced activity and drug discrimination in rats. *Behavioural Pharmacology*, **8**:113–123.

Beyer CE et al. (2001) Repeated exposure to inhaled toluene induces behavioural and neurochemical cross-sensitization to cocaine in rats. *Psychopharmacology*, **154**:198–204.

Bordnick PS, Schmitz JM (1998) Cocaine craving: an evaluation across treatment phases. *Journal of Substance Abuse*, **10**:9–17.

Bowen SE, Balster RL (1997) Desflurane, enflurane, isoflurane and ether produce ethanol-like discriminative stimulus effects in mice. *Pharmacology, Biochemistry and Behavior*, **57**:191–198.

Brouette T, Anton R (2001) Clinical review of inhalants. *American Journal of Addiction*, 10: 79–94.

Brown RM (1989) Pharmacology of cocaine abuse. In: *Cocaine, marijuana, and designer drugs: chemistry, pharmacology, and behavior*. Redda KK, Walker CA, Barnett G, eds. Boca Raton, FL, CRC Press.

Brownstein MJ (1993) A brief history of opiates, opioid peptides and opioid receptors. *Proceedings of the National Academy of Science of the United States of America*, **90**:5391–5393.

Butschky MF et al. (1995) Smoking without nicotine delivery decreases withdrawal in 12-hour abstinent smokers. *Pharmacology, Biochemistry and Behavior*, **50**:91–96.

Byrne A et al. (1991) Psychiatric and neurological effects of chronic solvent abuse. *Canadian Journal of Psychiatry*, **36**:735–738.

Caine SB, Koob GF (1994) Effects of dopamine D-1 and D-2 antagonists on cocaine self-administration under different schedules of reinforcement in the rat. *Journal of Pharmacology and Experimental Therapeutics*, **270**:209–218.

Cami J et al. (1997) Pharmacokinetics of ecstasy (MDMA) in healthy subjects. In: Congress of the European Association for Clinical Pharmacology and Therapeutics, 2nd - Berlin, Germany, 1997. *European Journal of Clinical Pharmacology*, 52:168.

Carboni E et al. (1989) Amphetamine, cocaine, phencyclidine and nomifensine increase extracellular dopamine concentrations preferentially in the nucleus accumbens of freely- moving rats. *Neuroscience*, **28**:653–661.

Carden SE, Coons EE (1990) Diazepam's impact on self-stimulation but not stimulation-escape suggests hedonic modulation. *Behavioral Neuroscience*, **104**:56–61.

Chen JP et al. (1990) Delta 9-tetrahydrocannabinol produces naloxone-blockable enhancement of presynaptic basal dopamine efflux in nucleus accumbens of conscious, freely-moving rats as measured by intracerebral microdialysis. *Psychopharmacology*, 102:156–162.

Clarke PBS, Pert A (1985) Autoradiographic evidence for nicotine receptors on nigrostriatal and mesolimbic dopaminergic projections. *Brain Research*, **348**:355.358.

Collier HO (1980) Cellular site of opiate dependence. *Nature*, **283**:625–629.

Collins AC, Marks MJ (1989) Chronic nicotine exposure and brain nicotinic receptors: influence of genetic factors. *Progress in Brain Research, 79:137-46.*

Corrigall WA (1999) Nicotine self-administration in animals as a dependence model. *Nicotine and Tobacco Research*, **1**:11–20.

Corringer PJ, Le Novere N, Changeux JP (2000) Nicotinic receptors at the amino acid level. *Annual Review of Pharmacology and Toxicology*, **40**:431–458.

Dani JÁ, De Biasi M (2001) Cellular mechanisms of nicotine addiction. *Pharmacology, Biochemistry and Behavior*, **70**:439–446.

Davis WM, Smith TE, Smith SG (1987) Intravenous and intragastric self-administration of chlordiazepoxide in the rat. *Alcohol and Drug Research*, **7**:511–516.

De la Torre R et al. (2000) Non-linear pharmacokinetics of MDMA ('ecstasy') in humans. *British Journal of Clinical Pharmacology*, **49**:104–109.

Devane WA et al. (1988) Determination and characterization of cannabinoid receptor in rat brain. *Molecular Pharmacology*, **34**:605–613.

Devane WA et al. (1992) Isolation and structure of a brain constituent that binds to the cannabinoid receptor. *Science*, **258**:1946–1949.

Di Chiara G (2000) Role of dopamine in the behavioural actions of nicotine related to addiction. *European Journal of Pharmacology*, **393**:295–314.

Di Chiara G, Imperato A (1988a) Drug abuse by humans preferentially increases synaptic dopamine concentrations in the mesolimbic system of freely-moving rats. *Proceedings of the National Academy of Science of the United States of America*, **94**:5274–5278.

Di Chiara G, Imperato A (1988b) Opposite effects of mu- and kappa-opiate agonists on dopamine release in the nucleus accumbens and in the dorsal caudate of freely-moving rats. *Journal of Pharmacology and Experimental Therapeutics*, **244**:1067–1080.

Di Marzo V (1999) Biosynthesis and inactivation of endocannabinoids: relevance to their proposed role as neuromodulators. *Life Sciences*, **65**:645–655.

Di Marzo V et al. (1998) Endocannabinoids: endogenous cannabinoid receptor ligands with neuromodulatory action. *Trends in Neuroscience*, **21**:521–528.

Downing J (1986) The psychological and physiological effects of MDMA on normal volunteers. *Journal of Psychoactive Drugs*, **18**:335–340.

Evans AC, Raistrick D (1987) Phenomenology of intoxication with toluene-based adhesives and butane gas. *British Journal of Psychiatry*, **150**:769–773.

Evans EB, Balster RL (1991) CNS depressant effects of volatile organic solvents. *Neuroscience and Biobehavioral Reviews*, **15**:233–241.

Fadda F, Rossetti ZL (1998) Chronic ethanol consumption: from neuroadaptation to neurodegeneration. *Progress in Neurobiology*, **56**:385–431.

Farrell M et al. (2002) Methamphetamine: drug use and psychoses becomes a major public health issue in the Asia-Pacific region. *Addiction*, **9**:771–772.

Feigenbaum JJ, Yanai J (1983) Evidence for the involvement of central dopaminergic receptors in the acute and chronic effects induced by barbiturates. *Neuropsychobiology*, **9**:83–87.

Fischer B et al. (2002) Heroin-assisted treatment as a response to the public health problem of opiate dependence in established market economies: an overview. *European Journal of Public Health*, **12**:228-34.

Fischer G et al. (2000) Treatment of opioid-dependent pregnant women with buprenorphine. *Addiction*, **95**:239–244.

Foulds J et al. (1997) Mood and physiological effects of subcutaneous nicotine in smokers and never-smokers. *Drug and Alcohol Dependence*, **44**:105–115.

Fowler JS et al. (2001) [(11)] Cocaine: PET studies of cocaine pharmacokinetics, dopamine transporter availability and dopamine transporter occupancy. *Nuclear Medicine and Biology*, **28**:561–572.

Fox BS et al. (1996) Efficacy of a therapeutic cocaine vaccine in rodent models. *Nature Medicine*, **2**:1129–1132.

French ED (1997) Delta 9-tetrahydrocannabinol excites rat VTA dopamine neurons through activation of cannabinoid CB1 but not opioid receptors. *Neuroscience Letters*, **226**:159–162.

Galiegue S et al. (1995) Expression of central and peripheral cannabinoid receptors in human immune tissues and leukocyte subpopulations. *European Journal of Biochemistry*, **232**:54–61.

Gessa GL et al. (1985) Low doses of ethanol activate dopaminergic neurons in the ventral tegmental area. *Brain Research*, 348:201–203.

Gessa GL et al. (1998) Cannabinoids activate mesolimbic dopamine neurons by an action on cannabinoid CB1 receptors. *European Journal of Pharmacology*, **341**:39–44.

Glick SD, Weaver LM, Meibach RC (1980) Lateralization of reward in rats: differences in reinforcing thresholds. *Science*, **207**:1093–1095.

Goldberg SR, Henningfield JE (1988) Reinforcing effects of nicotine in humans and experimental animals responding under intermittent schedules of IV drug injection. *Pharmacology, Biochemistry and Behavior*, **30**:227–234.

Goldberg SR et al. (1983) Control of behavior by intravenous nicotine injections in laboratory animals. *Pharmacology, Biochemistry and Behavior*, **19**:1011–1020.

Gomez TH, Roache JD, Meisch RA (2002) Orally delivered alprazolam, diazepam, and triazolam as reinforcers in rhesus monkeys. *Psychopharmacology* (Berlin), **161**:86–94.

Grahame NJ et al. (2001) Alcohol place preference conditioning in high- and low-alcohol preferring selected lines of mice. *Pharmacology, Biochemistry and Behavior*, **68**:805–814.

Griffiths RR, Weerts EM (1997) Benzodiazepine self-administration in humans and laboratory animals: implications for problems of long-term use and abuse. *Psychopharmacology* (Berlin), **134**:1–37.

Griffiths RR, Bigelow GE, Henningfield JE (1980) Similarities in animal and human drug-taking behavior. In: Mello NK, ed. *Advances in substance abuse*. Greenwich, CT, JAI Press:1–90.

Grispoon L, Bakalar J (1986) Can drugs be used to enhance the psychotherapeutic process? *American Journal of Psychotherapeutics*, **40**:393–404.

Grobin AC et al. (1998) The role of GABA(A) receptors in the acute and chronic effects of ethanol. *Psychopharmacology*, **139**:2–19.

Haefly WE (1978) Central action of benzodiazepines: general introduction. *British Journal of Psychiatry*, **133**:231–238.

Hanus L et al. (2001) 2-Arachidonyl glyceryl ether, an endogenous agonist of the cannabinoid CB1 receptor. *Proceedings of the National Academy of Science of the United States of America*, **98**:3662–3665.

Heishman SJ, Taylor RC, Henningfield JE (1994) Nicotine and smoking: a review of effects on human performance. *Experimental and Clinical Psychopharmacology*, 2:345–395.

Henningfield JE, Miyasato K, Jasinski DR (1985) Abuse liability and pharmacodynamic characteristics of intravenous and inhaled nicotine. *Journal of Pharmacology and Experimental Therapeutics*, **234**:1–12.

Henningfield JE, Keenan RM, Clarke PBS (1996) Nicotine. In: Schuster CR, Kuhar M, eds. *Pharmacological aspects of drug dependence*. Berlin, Springer-Verlag:272–314.

Hillard CJ, Jarrahian A (2000) The movement of *N*-arachidonoylethanolamine (anandamide) across cellular membranes. *Chemistry and Physics of Lipids*, **108**:123–134.

Hillefors-Berglund M, Liu Y, von Euler G (1995) Persistent, specific and dose-dependent effects of toluene exposure on dopamine D2 agonist binding in the rat caudate-putamen. *Toxicology*, **100**:185–194.

Himnan DJ (1984) Tolerance and reverse tolerance to toluene inhalation: effects on open-field behavior. *Pharmacology, Biochemistry and Behavior*, **21**:625–631.

Hodge CW et al. (2001) Allopregnanolone and pentobarbital infused into the nucleus accumbens substitute for the discriminative stimulus effects of ethanol. *Alcoholism: Clinical and Experimental Research*, 25:1441–1447.

Hoebel BG et al. (1983) Self-injection of amphetamine directly into the brain. *Psychopharmacology*, **81**:158–163.

Hoffman BB, Lefkowitz RJ (1990) Catecholamines and sympathomimetic drugs. In: Gilman AG et al., eds. *Goodman and Gilman's: The pharmacological basis of therapeutics*, 8th ed. New York, NY, Pergamon Press:187-220.

Holt RA, Bateson AN, Martin IL (1996) Chronic treatment with diazepam or abecarnil differently affects the expression of GABA(A) receptor subunit mRNAs in the rat cortex. *Neuropharmacology*, 35:1457–1463.

Hughes JR, Higgins ST, Hatsukami D (1990) Effects of abstinence from tobacco: a critical review. In: Kozlowski LT et al., eds. *Research advances in alcohol and drug problems*. New York, Plenum Publishing Corporation:317–398.

Hughes J et al. (1975) Identification of two related pentapeptides from the brain with potent opiate agonist activity. *Nature*, **258**:577–579.

Imperato A, Di Chiara G (1986) Preferential stimulation of dopamine release in the nucleus accumbens of freely-moving rats by ethanol. *Journal of Pharmacology and Experimental Therapeutics*, **239**:219–228.

Imperato A, Mulas A, Di Chiara G (1986) Nicotine preferentially stimulates dopamine release in the limbic system of freely moving rats. *European Journal of Pharmacology*, **132**:337–338.

Indulski JA et al. (1996) Neurological and neurophysiological examinations of workers occupationally exposed to organic solvent mixtures used in paint and varnish production. *International Journal of Occupational Medicine and Environmental Health*, **9**:235–244.

Itzhak Y, Martin JL (2002) Cocaine-induced conditioned place preference in mice: induction, extinction and reinstatement by related psychostimulants. *Neuropsychopharmacology*, 26:130–134.

Jacobs MR, Fehr KOB (1987) *Drugs and drug abuse: a reference text*, 2nd ed. Toronto, Addiction Research Foundation.

Jaffe JH (1990) Drug addiction and drug abuse. In: Gilman AG et al., eds. *Goodman and Gilman's pharmacological basis of therapeutics*, 8th ed. New York, NY, Pergamon Press:522–573.

Johns A (2001) Psychiatric effects of cannabis. *The British Journal of Psychiatry*, 178:116–122.

Jones HE, Garrett BE, Griffiths RR (1999) Subjective and physiological effects of intravenous nicotine and cocaine in cigarette smoking and cocaine abusers. *Journal of Pharmacology and Experimental Therapeutics*, 288:188–197.

Kalant H (1998) Research on tolerance: what can we learn from history? *Alcoholism: Clinical and Experimental Research*, 22:67–76.

Kalant H (2001) The pharmacology and toxicology of "ecstasy" (MDMA) and related drugs. *Canadian Medical Association Journal*, 165:917–928.

Kalivas PW, Weber B (1988) Amphetamine injection into the ventral mesencephalon sensitizes rats to peripheral amphetamine and cocaine. *Journal of Pharmacology and Experimental Therapeutics*, 245:1095–1102.

Kantak KM et al. (2001) Time course of changes in cocaine self-administration behavior during immunization with the cocaine vaccine IPC-1010. *Psychopharmacology*, 153:334–340.

Kenny PJ, Markou A (2001) Neurobiology of the nicotine withdrawal syndrome. *Pharmacology, Biochemistry and Behavior*, 70:531–549.

Khanolkar AD, Palmer SL, Makriyannis A (2000) Molecular probes for the cannabinoid receptors. *Chemistry and Physics of Lipids*, 108:37–52.

Kieffer BL (1999) Opioids: first lessons from knock-out mice. *Trends in Pharmacological Sciences*, 20:537–544.

Kieffer BL, Evans CJ (2002) Opioid tolerance: in search of the holy grail. *Cell*, 108:587–590.

Kita K et al. (1999) Effects of D1 and D2 dopamine receptor antagonists on cocaine-induced self-stimulation and locomotor activity in rats. *European Neuropsychopharmacology*, 9:1–7.

Knisely JS, Rees DC, Balster RL (1990) Discriminative stimulus properties of toluene in the rat. *Neurotoxicology and Teratology*, 12:129–133.

Koob GF (1992) Neural mechanisms of drug reinforcement. *Annals of the New York Academy of Sciences*, 28:171–191.

Koob GF (1995) Animal models of drug addiction. *Psychopharmacology: The Fourth Generation of Progress*, 66:759–772.

Koob GF and Bloom FE (1988) Cellular and molecular mechanisms of drug dependence. *Science*, 42:715–723.

Koob GF and Nestler EJ (1997) The neurobiology of drug addiction. *Journal of Neuropsychiatry and Clinical Neuroscience*, 9:482–497.

Kornetsky C et al. (1988) Brain stimulation reward: effects of ethanol. *Alcoholism: Clinical and Experimental Research*, 12:609–616.

Kosten TR et al. (2002) Human therapeutic cocaine vaccine: safety and immunogenicity. *Vaccine*, **20**:1196–1204.

Krambeer LL et al. (2001) Methadone therapy for opioid dependence. *American Family Physician*, **15**:2404–2410.

Kranzler HR (2000) Pharmacotherapy of alcoholism: gaps in knowledge and opportunities for research. *Alcohol and Alcoholism*, **35**:537–547.

Krausz M (2002) Modellprojekt: heroin als medicament [Model project: heroin as medication]. *Deutsches Ärzteblatt*, **99**:A26–A28.

Kreek MJ (2000) Methadone-related opioid agonist pharmacotherapy for heroin addiction: history, recent molecular and neurochemical research and future in mainstream medicine. *Annals of the New York Academy of Sciences*, **909**: 186-216.

Kuczenski R, Segal DS (1992) Differential effects of amphetamine and dopamine uptake blockers (cocaine, nomifensine) on caudate and accumbens dialysate dopamine and 3-methoxytyramine. *Journal of Pharmacology and Experimental Therapeutics*, **262**:1085–1094.

Kuhar MJ et al. (2001) Anticocaine catalytic antibodies have no affinity for RTI compounds: implications for treatment. *Synapse*, **41**:176–178.

Lahti AC et al. (1995) Ketamine activates psychosis and alters limbic blood flow in schizophrenia. *Neuroreport*, **6**:869–782.

Leshner AI, Koob GF (1999) Drugs of abuse and the brain. *Proceedings of the Association of American Physicians*, **111**:99–108.

Ling W et al. (1998) Buprenorphine maintenance treatment of opiate dependence: a multicenter, randomized clinical trial. *Addiction*, **93**:475–486.

Lodge D, Johnson KM (1990) Noncompetitive excitatory amino acid receptor antagonists. *Trends in Pharmacological Sciences*, **11**:81–86.

Luisada PV (1978) The phencyclidine psychosis: phenomenology and treatment. *NIDA Research Monograph*, **21**:241–253.

Lukas RJ et al. (1999) Current status of the nomenclature for nicotinic acetylcholine receptors and their subunits. *Pharmacological Reviews*, **51**:397–401.

McBride WJ (2002) Central nucleus of the amygdala and the effects of alcohol and alcohol-drinking behavior in rodents. *Pharmacology, Biochemistry and Behavior*, **71**:509–515.

McBride WJ, Li TK (1998) Animal models of alcoholism: neurobiology of high alcohol-drinking behavior in rodents. *Critical Reviews in Neurobiology*, **12**:339–369.

McCance-Katz EF, Kosten TR, Jatlow P (1998) Concurrent use of cocaine and alcohol is more potent and potentially more toxic than use of either alone: a multiple-dose study. *Biological Psychiatry*, **44**:250–259.

McCann U, Ricaurte G (1991) Lasting neuropsychiatric sequelae of methylenedioxymethamphetamine ("ecstasy") in recreational users. *Journal of Clinical Psychopharmacology*, **11**:302–305.

Maccarrone M et al. (1998) Anandamide hydrolysis by human cells in culture and brain. *Journal of Biological Chemistry*, **273**:32 332–32 339.

McKenna DJ, Peroutka SJ (1990) Neurochemistry and neurotoxicity of 3,4-methylenedioxymethamphetamine, MDMA ("ecstasy"). *Journal of Neurochemistry*, **54**:14–22.

Maldonado R, Rodriguez de Fonseca F (2002) Cannabinoid addiction: behavioural models and neural correlates. *Journal of Neuroscience*, **22**:3326–3331.

Malin DH (2001) Nicotine dependence studies with a laboratory model. *Pharmacology, Biochemistry and Behavior*, **70**:551–559.

Mansour A, Watson SJ (1993) Anatomical distribution of opioid receptors in mammalian: an overview. In: Hertz A, ed. *Opioids I*. Berlin, Springer-Verlag:79–105.

Mansour A et al. (1995) Opioid-receptor mRNA expression in the rat CNS: anatomical and functional implications. *Trends in Neuroscience*, **18**:22–29.

Marona-Lewicka D et al. (1996) Reinforcing effects of certain serotonin-releasing amphetamine derivates. *Pharmacology, Biochemistry and Behavior*, **53**:99–105.

Martin BR et al. (1976) ^{3}H-delta-9-tetrahydrocannabinol tissue and subcellular distribution in the central nervous system and tissue distribution in peripheral organs of tolerant and nontolerant dogs. *Journal of Pharmacology and Experimental Therapeutics*, **196**:128–144.

Mascaró BI et al. (1991) MDMA "extasis": revisión y puesta Al día. [MDMA "ecstasy": revision and updates]. *Revista Española de Drogodependencias*, **16**:91–101.

Mason BJ (2001) Treatment of alcohol-dependent outpatients with acamprosate: a clinical review. *Journal of Clinical Psychiatry*, **62**(Suppl.)20:S42–S48.

Matsuda LA et al. (1990) Structure of a cannabinoid receptor and functional expression of the cloned cDNA. *Nature*, **346**:561–564.

Mechoulam R et al. (1995) Identification of an endogenous 2-monoglyceride, present in canine gut, that binds to cannabinoid receptors. *Biochemical Pharmacology*, **50**:83–90.

Meisch RA (2001) Oral drug self-administration: an overview of laboratory animal studies. *Alcohol*, **24**:117–128.

Miyazawa A et al. (1999) Nicotinic acetylcholine receptor at 4.6 A resolution: transverse tunnels in the channel wall. *Journal of Molecular Biology*, **288**:765–786.

Molina-Holgado F, Lledo A, Guaza C (1997) Anandamide suppresses nitric oxide and TNF-alpha responses to Theiler's virus or endotoxin in astrocytes. *Neuroreport*, **8**:1929–1933.

Montoya AG et al. (2002) Long-term neuropsychiatric consequences of "ecstasy" (MDMA): a review. *Harvard Review of Psychiatry*, **10**:212–220.

Morgan MJ (2000) Ecstasy (MDMA): a review of its possible persistent psychological effects. *Psychopharmacology*, **152**:230–248.

Munro S, Thomas KL, Abu-Shaar M (1993) Molecular characterization of a peripheral receptor for cannabinoids. *Nature*, **365**:61–65.

Munzar P et al. (2001) High rates of midazolam self-administration in squirrel monkeys. *Behavioural Pharmacology*, **12**:257–265.

Naruse T, Asami T (1990) Cross-dependence on ethanol and pentobarbital in rats reinforced on diazepam. *Archives of International Pharmacodynamic Therapy*, **304**:147–162.

Nestler EJ (2001) Molecular basis of long-term plasticity underlying addiction. *Nature Reviews in Neuroscience*, **2**:119–128.

Newcomer JW et al. (1999) Ketamine-induced NMDA receptor hypofunction as a model of memory impairment and psychosis. *Neuropsychopharmacology*, **20**:106–118.

Nichols DE (1986) Differences between the mechanism of action of MDMA, MBDB, and the classic hallucinogens. Identification of a new therapeutic class: entactogens. *Journal of Psychoactive Drugs*, **18**:305–313.

Nutt DJ, Malizia AL (2001) New insights into the role of the GABA(A) benzodiazepine receptor in psychiatric disorder. *British Journal of Psychiatry*, **179**:390–396.

O´Brien CP (2001) Drug addiction and drug abuse. In: *Goodman and Gilman's*: *The pharmacological basis of therapeutics*, 10th ed. New York, McGraw Hill:621–667.

Ong WY, Mackie K (1999) A light and electron microscopic study of the CB1 cannabinoid receptor in primate brain. *Neuroscience*, **92**:1177–1191.

Panagis G et al. (2000) Effects of methyllycaconitine (MLA), an alpha-7 nicotinic receptor antagonist, on nicotine- and cocaine-induced potentiation of brain stimulation reward. *Psychopharmacology* (Berlin), **149**:388–396.

Panksepp J (1998) *Affective neuroscience: the foundations of human and animal emotions*. New York, NY, Oxford University Press.

Pasternak GW (1993) Pharmacological mechanisms of opioid analgesics. *Clinical Pharmacology*, **16**:1–18.

Paterson D, Nordberg A (2000) Neuronal nicotinic receptors in the human brain. *Progress in Neurobiology*, **61**:75–111.

Perkins KA et al. (1993) Chronic and acute tolerance to subjective effects of nicotine. *Pharmacology, Biochemistry and Behavior*, **45**:375–381.

Peroutka SJ (1989) "Ecstasy": a human neurotoxin? *Archives of General Psychiatry*, **46**:191.

Pertwee RG (1997) Pharmacology of cannabinoid CB1 and CB2 receptors. *Pharmacology and Therapeutics*, **74**:129–180.

Pertwee RG (1999) Pharmacology of cannabinoid receptor ligands. *Current Medicinal Chemistry*, **6**:635–664.

Pertwee RG (2001) Cannabinoid receptors and pain. *Progress in Neurobiology*, **63**:569–611.

Pfefferbaum A et al. (1998) A controlled study of cortical gray matter and ventricular changes in alcoholic men over a 5-year interval. *Archives of General Psychiatry*, **55**:905–912.

Phillips AG, Brooke SM, Fibiger HC (1975) Effects of amphetamine isomers and neuroleptics on self-stimulation from the nucleus accumbens and dorsal noradrenergic bundle. *Brain Research*, **1**:13–22.

Pickworth WB, Heishman SJ, Henningfield JE (1995) Relationships between EEG and performance during nicotine withdrawal and administration. *Brain Imaging of Nicotine and Tobacco Smoking.* Ann Arbor, MI, NPP Books:1–13.

Piomelli D et al. (1999) Structural determinants for recognition and translocation by the anandamide transporter. *Proceedings of the National Academy of Science of the United States of America*, **96**:5802–5807.

Platt DM, Rowlett JK, Spealman RD (2001) Discriminative stimulus effects of intravenous heroin and its metabolites in rhesus monkeys: opioid and dopaminergic mechanisms. *Journal of Pharmacology and Experimental Therapeutics*, **299**:760–767.

Pope HG Jr, Gruber AJ, Yurgelun-Todd D (1995) The residual neuropsychological effects of cannabis: the current status of research. *Drug and Alcohol Dependence*, **38**:25–34.

Reggio PH, Traore H (2000) Conformational requirements for endocannabinoid interaction with the cannabinoid receptors, the anandamide transporter and fatty acid amidohydrolase. *Chemistry and Physics of Lipids*, **108**:15–35.

Rehm J et al. (2001) Feasibility, safety, and efficacy of injectable heroin prescription for refractory opioid addicts: a follow-up study. *Lancet*, **358**:1417–1420.

Riegel AC, French ED (1999) An electrophysiological analysis of rat ventral tegmental dopamine neuronal activity during acute toluene exposure. *Pharmacology and Toxicology*, **85**:37–43.

Ritz MC, Cone EJ, Kuhar MJ (1990) Cocaine inhibition of ligand binding at dopamine, norepinephrine and serotonin transporters: a structure–activity study. *Life Sciences*, **46**:635–645.

Robinson TE, Becker JB (1986) Enduring changes in brain and behavior produced by chronic amphetamine administration: a review and evaluation of animal models of amphetamine psychosis. *Brain Research Reviews*, **11**:157–198.

Rocha BA et al. (1998) Cocaine self-administration in dopamine-transporter knockout mice. *Nature Neuroscience*, **1**:132–137.

Rodriguez de Fonseca F et al. (1997) Activation of corticotropin-releasing factor in the limbic system during cannabinoid withdrawal. *Science*, **276**:2050–2054.

Rogers RD, Robbins TW (2001) Investigating the neurocognitive deficits associated with chronic drug misuse. *Current Opinion in Neurobiology*, **11**:250–257.

Rose JE, Behm FM, Levin ED (1993) Role of nicotine dose and sensory cues in the regulation of smoke intake. *Pharmacology, Biochemistry and Behavior*, **44**:891–900.

Rosecrans JA, Karan LD (1993) Neurobehavioral mechanisms of nicotine action: role in the initiation and maintenance of tobacco dependence. *Journal of Substance Abuse Treatment*, **10**:161–170.

Rothman RB, Glowa JR (1995) A review of the effects of dopaminergic agents on humans, animals, and drug-seeking behavior, and its implications for medication development: focus on GBR12909. *Molecular Neurobiology*, **11**:1–19.

Royal College of Physicians (2000) *Nicotine addiction in Britain: a report of the Tobacco Advisory Group of the Royal College of Physicians.* London, Royal College of Physicians.

Russell MAH (1987) Nicotine intake and its regulation by smokers. In: Martin WR et al., eds. *Advances in behavioral biology. Vol 31. Tobacco smoking and nicotine.* New York, NY, Plenum Press:25–31.

Samson HH, Chappell A (2001) Muscimol injected into the medial prefrontal cortex of the rat alters ethanol self-administration. *Physiology and Behavior*, **74**:581–587.

Scallet AC (1991) Neurotoxicology of cannabis and THC: a review of chronic exposure studies in animals. *Pharmacology, Biochemistry and Behavior*, **40**:671–676.

Schilstrom B et al. (1998) Nicotine- and food-induced dopamine release in the nucleus accumbens of the rat: putative role of alpha-7 nicotinic receptors in the ventral tegmental area. *Neuroscience*, **85**:1005–1009.

Shankaran M, Gudelsky GA (1999) A neurotoxic regimen of MDMA suppresses behavioral, thermal and neurochemical responses to subsequent MDMA administration. *Psychopharmacology*, **147**:66–72.

Shaper AG (1996) Walking on the moon. *Lancet*, **347**:207–208.

Shiffman S, Mason KM, Henningfield JE (1998) Tobacco dependence treatments: review and prospectus. *Annual Review of Public Health*, **19**:335–358.

Shulgin AT (1986) The background and chemistry of MDMA. *Journal of Psychoactive Drugs*, **18**:291–304.

Solowij N, Michie PT, Fox AM (1995) Differential impairments of selective attention due to frequency and duration of cannabis use. *Biological Psychiatry*, **37**:731–739.

Sora I et al. (2001) Molecular mechanisms of cocaine reward: combined dopamine and serotonin transporter knockouts eliminate cocaine place preference. *Proceedings of the National Academy of Science of the United States of America*, **98**:5300–5305.

Soria R et al. (1996) Subjective and cardiovascular effects of intravenous nicotine in smokers and non-smokers. *Psychopharmacology* (Berlin), **128**:221–226.

Spyraki C, Kazandjian A, Varonos D (1985) Diazepam-induced place preference conditioning: appetitive and antiaversive properties. *Psychopharmacology* (Berlin), **87**:225–232.

Srisurapanont M, Jarusuraisin N, Kittirattanapaiboon P (2001) Treatment for amphetamine dependence and abuse. *Cochrane Database of Systematic Reviews*, **4**:CD003022.

Stengard K, Hoglund G, Ungerstedt U (1994) Extracellular dopamine levels within the striatum increase during inhalation exposure to toluene: a microdialysis study in awake, freely- moving rats. *Toxicology Letters*, **71**:245–255.

Streeton C, Whelan G (2001) Naltrexone: a relapse prevention maintenance treatment of alcohol dependence'– a meta-analysis of randomized controlled trials. *Alcohol and Alcoholism*, **36**:544–552.

Sugiura T et al. (1995) 2-Arachidonoylglycerol: a possible endogenous cannabinoid receptor ligand in the brain. *Biochemical and Biophysical Research Communications*, **215**:89–97.

Sutherland G (2002) Current approaches to the management of smoking cessation. *Drugs*, **62**(Suppl. 2):S53–S61.

Swedberg MDB, Henningfield JE, Goldberg SR (1990) Nicotine dependency: animal studies. In: Wonnacott S, Russell MAH, Stolerman IP, eds. *Nicotine psychopharmacology: molecular, cellular and behavioural aspects*. New York, Oxford University Press:38–76.

Szostak C, Finlay JM, Fibiger HC (1987) Intravenous self-administration of the short-acting benzodiazepine midazolam in the rat. *Neuropharmacology*, **26**:1673–1676.

Tanda G, Pontieri FE, Di Chiara G (1997) Cannabinoid and heroin activation of mesolimbic dopamine transmission by a common 1-opioid receptor mechanism. *Science*, **276**:2048–2050.

Taylor P (1996) Agents acting at the neuromuscular junction and autonomic ganglia. In: Hardman JG et al., eds. *Goodman and Gilman's pharmacological basis of therapeutics*, 9th ed. New York, NY, McGraw-Hill:177–197.

Tramer MR et al. (2001) Cannabinoids for control of chemotherapy induced nausea and vomiting: quantitative systematic review. *British Medical Journal*, **323**:16-21.

Tyndale RF, Sellers EM (2001) Variable CYP2A6-mediated nicotine metabolism alters smoking behavior and risk. *Drug Metabolism and Disposition*, **29**:548–552.

Uchtenhagen A et al. (1999) *Prescription of narcotics for heroin addicts: main results of the Swiss national cohort study*. Basel, Karger.

Ujike H (2002) Stimulant-induced psychosis and schizophrenia: the role of sensitization. *Current Psychiatry Reports*, **4**:177–184.

UNODCP (2002) Amphetamine-type stimulants threaten East Asia. *ODCCP Update*, March 2002:

United States Department of Health and Human Services (1988) *The health consequences of smoking: nicotine addiction. A report of the Surgeon General*. Washington, DC, US Government Printing Office.

Vaccarino AL, Kastin AJ (2001) Endogenous opiates: 2000. *Peptides*, **22**:2257–2328.

Van den Brink et al. (2002) *Medical co-prescription of heroin: two randomized controlled trials. Report to Government*. Utrecht, Central Committee on the Treatment of Heroin Addicts (available on the Internet at http://www.ccbh.nl).

Van Ree JM, Gerrits MA, Vanderschuren LJ (1999) Opioids, reward and addiction: an encounter of biology, psychology and medicine. *Pharmacological Reviews*, **51**:341–396.

Verebey K, Alrazi J, Jafre JH (1988) The complications of "ecstasy" (MDMA). *Journal of the American Medical Association*, **259**:1649–1650.

Vidal C (1996) Nicotinic receptors in the brain: molecular biology, function, and therapeutics. *Molecular Chemistry and Neuropathology*, **28**:3–11.

Vogel-Sprott M, Sdao-Jarvie K (1989) Learning alcohol tolerance: the contribution of response expectancies. *Psychopharmacology*, **98**:289–296.

Volkow ND, Fowler JS (2000) Addiction, a disease of compulsion and drive: involvement of the orbitofrontal cortex. *Cerebral Cortex*, **10**:318–325.

Volkow ND et al. (1996) Cocaine addiction: hypothesis derived from imaging studies with PET. *Journal of Addictive Diseases*, **15**:55–71.

Volkow ND et al. (1999) Reinforcing effects of psychostimulants in humans are associated with increases in brain dopamine and occupancy of D2 receptors. *Journal of Pharmacology and Experimental Therapeutics*, **291**:409–415.

Volkow ND et al. (2001a) Low level of brain dopamine D2 receptors in methamphetamine abusers: association with metabolism in the orbitofrontal cortex. *American Journal of Psychiatry*, **158**:2015–2021.

Volkow ND et al. (2001b) Association of dopamine transporter reduction with psychomotor impairment in methamphetamine abusers. *American Journal of Psychiatry*, **158**:377–382.

Von Euler G et al. (1993) Persistent effects of subchronic toluene exposure on spatial learning and memory, dopamine-mediated locomotor activity and dopamine D2 agonist binding in the rat. *Toxicology*, **77**:223–232.

Wang GJ et al. (2000) Regional brain metabolism during alcohol intoxication. *Alcoholism: Clinical and Experimental Research*, **24**:822–829.

Weir E (2001) Inhalant use and addiction in Canada. *Canadian Medical Association Journal*, **164**:397.

Weiss B, Wood RW, Macys DA (1979) Behavioral toxicology of carbon disulfide and toluene. *Environmental Health Perspectives*, **30**:39–45.

Wettstein JG, Gauthier B (1992) Discriminative stimulus effects of alprazolam and diazepam: generalization to benzodiazepines, antidepressants and buspirone. *Behavioural Pharmacology*, **3**:229–237.

WHO (1994) *Lexicon of alcohol and drug terms*. Geneva, World Health Organization.

WHO (1997a) *Cannabis: a health perspective and research agenda*. Geneva, World Health Organization (document WHO/MSA/PSA/97.4).

WHO (1997b) *Amphetamine-type stimulants: a report from the WHO Meeting on Amphetamines, MDMA and other Psychostimulants, Geneva, 12-15 November 1996*. Geneva, World Health Organization (document WHO/MSA/PSA/97.5).

WHO (1998) *Expert committee on drug dependence: thirtieth report*. Geneva, World Health Organization (WHO Technical Report Series, No. 873).

WHO (1999) Volatile solvents abuse: a global overview. *Geneva, World Health Organization (document WHO/HSC/SAB/99.7).*

WHO (2001) *Ecstasy: MDMA and other ring-substituted amphetamines*. Geneva, World Health Organization (document WHO/MSD/MSB/01.3).

Williams JT, Christie MJ, Manzoni O (2001) Cellular and synaptic adaptations mediating opioid dependence. *Physiological Reviews*, **81**:299–343.

Wise RA, Bozarth MA (1987) A psychomotor stimulant theory of addiction. *Psychological Reviews*, **94**:469–492.

Woolverton WL, Johnson KM (1992) Neurobiology of cocaine abuse. *Trends in Pharmacological Sciences*, **13**:193–200.

Yavich L, Zvartau E (1994) A comparison of the effects of individual organic solvents and their mixture on brain stimulation reward. *Pharmacology, Biochemistry and Behavior*, **48**:661–664.

Yavich L, Patkina N, Zvartau E (1994) Experimental estimation of addictive potential of a mixture of organic solvents. *European Neuropsychopharmacology*, **4**:111–118.

Yui K et al. (1999) Neurobiological basis of relapse prediction in stimulant-induced psychosis and schizophrenia: the role of sensitization. *Molecular Psychiatry*, **4**:512–523.

CHAPTER 5
Genetic Basis of Substance Dependence

Introduction

The aim of this chapter is to critically assess the evidence for a genetic contribution to the risk of developing psychoactive substance use and dependence in humans. While individual genetic differences contribute to the development of substance dependence, genetic factors are but one contributor to the complex interplay of physiological, social, cultural and personal factors that are involved. A list of commonly used genetic terms is provided in Box 5.1.

The classical (and popular) view of human genetics is one in which genetic mutation is the direct and usually only cause of a particular illness, for example, the single gene – or Mendelian – disorders such as Huntington's disease. Single gene diseases are caused by a specific mutated gene, and the mutation is both necessary and sufficient to cause the illness. Unlike single gene disorders, which are rare and might affect 1 in 10 000 people, complex disorders, such as substance dependence, are common in the population, often affecting 1 in 100 or more people. Complex disorders are clearly not caused by genes alone, but by the interaction between genes and the environment. Thus exposure to psychoactive substances could have a much greater effect on somebody who carries a genetic vulnerability to substance dependence, than on someone who does not.

Genetic vulnerability, or predisposition, to substance dependence is likely to be tied to several distinct genes (or multiple alleles), each producing a small effect, which might increase risk of developing substance dependence by 2–3 fold. Any one of the genes on its own will be insufficient to cause dependence, but several different genes may all contribute to the vulnerability. It is hypothesised that not everyone who carries a "risk gene" for substance use or dependence will become dependent, and likewise some of those who become dependent will not carry that particular genetic risk factor. It is the combination of the presence of several distinct genes or alleles which may be important, rather than a single gene. These genetic contributions to vulnerability seem likely to be distributed over several distinct regions (loci) on the chromosomes.

This chapter will address the genetics of substance use disorders in general, but will also specifically examine the data for opioid, alcohol and tobacco dependence, as these substances have received a substantial amount of

---

BOX 5.1

Commonly used genetic terms

Allele: One member of a pair of homologous genes in a diploid cell. An individual with identical alleles at a genetic locus is a homozygote; one with non-identical alleles is a heterozygote. In a case in which one allele leads to an observable gene product and the other has no phenotype, the functional allele is said to be dominant and the non-functional allele recessive.

Candidate genes: Genes with perceived relevance to the trait in question, which can be used to compare allele frequencies between affected and non-affected groups.

Gene: In genetics, a unit inferred from the pattern of inheritance; in molecular biology, defined narrowly as a section of DNA that is expressed as RNA or, more widely, as a coding sequence of DNA and associated regulatory sequences.

Gene locus: The specific place on a chromosome where a gene is located.

Heritability: The proportion of phenotypic variance that can be attributed to additive genetic variance.

Genotype: The genetic make-up of any organism.

Linkage: The more-frequent-than-random occurrence of two traits together due to the proximity of their corresponding genes on the same chromosome. The likelihood of a recombination event separating the two genes decreases with their increasing proximity on the chromosome.

Linkage studies: These studies use multiply-affected families to examine traits that are inherited together. The concept is based on the fact that genes that are located close to one another will be more likely to be inherited together from one parent than two genes located further apart.

Phenotype: The outward physical manifestation of the cell or individual due to actual expression of the alleles that are present.

Polygenic: A trait arising from more than one gene.

Polymorphism: The occurrence of something in several forms, e.g. the occurrence in a population of two or more alleles of a gene at a single genetic locus.

---

genetic research attention. However, one overwhelming finding from genetic studies of psychoactive substances is that the heritability (i.e. genetic contribution) of dependence for one substance correlates highly with dependence for other substances. Thus, there may be some common genetic components to substance dependence in general, as well as to dependence for specific psychoactive substances. There is also a high degree of association of substance dependence with mental illness (see Chapter 6). The most common types of genetic studies in humans and the types of information these studies provide are summarized below. Animal studies are also briefly presented.

Family, twin and adoption studies: estimations of heritability

Family, twin and adoption studies can be used to determine whether or not there is a genetic contribution to psychoactive substance use and dependence, but they do not provide evidence to determine which particular gene is involved. Twin and adoption studies also help to dissociate environmental factors from genetic factors.

Family studies examine the inheritance of traits through a family, in order to find out about patterns of inheritance and the relative risk of inheriting a disorder.

Twin studies are based on the fact that monozygotic (identical) twins share identical genetic material, while dizygotic (fraternal) twins share the same degree of genetic similarity as non-twin siblings. Presumably, twins raised together share very similar environments. If genetic effects are present, then monozygotic twins should be more alike, with respect to those effects, than dizygotic twins. This allows an estimation of the genetic contribution to psychoactive substance dependence. These types of studies provide evidence that variation in the vulnerability to substance dependence in populations is influenced by both individual genotypes and environmental differences (Heath et al., 1999a; Vanyukov & Tarter, 2000).

Adoption studies are capable of almost completely separating genetic and environmental influences on the variation in the vulnerability to a disorder (except contributions of antenatal and early postnatal environmental factors) (Heath et al., 1999a; Vanyukov & Tarter, 2000); in this way they complement the more traditional twin studies. Using adoption studies, environmental factors can be separated from genetic factors, since children adopted at birth are raised in an environment that is different from that of their genetic family. In this way, environmental factors such as socioeconomic status, learning about substance use, exposure to psychoactive drugs, etc., are randomized. For example, if a particular family shows a high level of substance dependence from generation to generation, it is difficult to know how much of this is attributable to shared genes, and how much is attributable to the shared environment. With adoption studies, the effect of the environment is factored out, and thus, it is easier to determine more clearly the contribution of genetics.

Identifying chromosomal locations of interest: linkage studies

Twin and adoption studies give an estimation of the proportion of variation in a trait that is due to genetics; however, they do not provide any information about which genes or chromosomes are involved. Linkage and association studies are used to identify regions of DNA that may be involved in the expression of a trait such as substance dependence. Linkage studies examine inheritance within related individuals, whereas association studies examine inheritance in unrelated individuals. The concept of linkage is based on the fact that genes located close to one another on a chromosome are more likely to be inherited together from one parent, than are two genes located further apart, due to the reassortment of genes that occurs during the process of recombination. The genes are said to be "linked" since there is a greater probability of the genes being inherited together. Linkage studies have been an important tool for the localization of chromosomal regions contributing to substance dependence; they support candidate gene studies and provide potential identities of unknown phenotype-related genes (Arinami, Ishiguro & Onaivi, 2000). The studies examine chromosomal locations that are inherited together in people who have the phenotype in question (e.g. who have nicotine dependence) in order to find areas of the chromosome important for the condition.

Candidate gene approach

The candidate gene approach requires the selection of genes that may have relevance to the phenotype in question. For example, it would be appropriate to investigate nicotinic receptor genes when examining the genetics of nicotine dependence. These studies examine candidate genes in people with or without dependence, to look for differences between these groups.

Animal studies

Many genetic studies on substance dependence employ animal models. Animal models have a great advantage in that the history of exposure to psychoactive substances and most other environmental factors can be controlled and manipulated allowing the use of powerful statistical analysis. In addition, genetic studies in animals allow for specific breeding studies that cannot be done with humans, and the results of these studies can be obtained in a relatively short period of time. Moreover, while early studies could only control the genetic make-up of experimental animals by in-breeding, modern transgenic and knockout methodology allows the genotype of these animals to be manipulated in a specified manner so that the role of specific genes in the behaviours of interest can be investigated.

Transgenic animals (usually mice) are created by injecting a foreign gene (transgene) into fertilized mouse eggs. The transgene integrates into the mouse chromosome in one or several copies in a random location. The eggs are then implanted into foster mothers. When the embryos develop to term, a proportion of them will have the transgene integrated into the mouse genome. The resulting transgenic founder animals are then bred to create transgenic lines of mice (Picciotto & Wickman, 1998; Bowers, 2000). The application of the transgenic approach depends on the understanding of mechanisms regulating gene expression in the mouse, which is currently relatively limited (Quinn, 1996; Spergel et al., 2001).

The gene knockout methodology allows the deletion of a gene – or a fragment of the gene – from the animal chromosomes. In this methodology a mutated copy of the gene of interest is introduced into cultured mouse embryonic stem cells. Through homologous recombination the mutated gene becomes integrated into the genome of the stem cell, and disrupts (or modifies, in the so-called knock-in technology) its function. Stem cells in which the gene is disrupted are injected into blastocysts, which are then implanted into foster mothers. Resulting mice have the gene disrupted in some but not all cells, and are further bred to create knockout lines of mice (Capecchi, 1994; Picciotto & Wickman, 1998).

Transgenic and knockout mice can serve as powerful research tools to observe the effects of gene modifications. However, results from transgenic and knockout studies need to be interpreted with caution for several reasons. The site of integration for the transgene into the mouse chromosome is random, and is as yet impossible to control. Therefore, some of the phenotypes observed in transgenic mice can be due to the functions of the transgene, but some can also be due to the disruption of the gene in which the transgene has been integrated. Creation of several transgenic lines is therefore necessary to verify that the observed phenotype is indeed due to the transgene (Bowers, 2000). The knockout technology does not have the problem of random transgene integration because the mutation in these mice is targeted to a specific gene. However, it has other problems, for example, the problem with background genotype (Crawley et al., 1997).

Both transgenic and knockout approaches are also faced with a problem of developmental compensation. That is, while the gene that is modified or over-expressed in the mutant animal could be important in the investigated phenotype, compensatory mechanisms could also occur during development (e.g. when a subunit of a receptor is knocked-out, another subunit could be over-expressed and compensate for the absence of the knocked-out subunit). If such compensation is occurring, the predicted change in the phenotype of the mutant mice will not occur. New methodologies, including inducible and brain region-specific transgenic and knockout approaches, are being developed, and should in future alleviate many such problems (Sauer, 1998; Le & Sauer, 2000).

Another approach used in animal studies is the quantitative trait loci (QTL) analysis. Substance dependence is considered to be a quantitative trait in which a combined action of multiple alleles leads to predisposition to dependence. This approach does not assume any prior knowledge of genes involved in substance-related disorders, and seeks to find them based on related phenotypes. QTL analysis is analogous to linkage studies in humans. As an example, inbred strains of mice that are genetically identical can be crossed with other inbred strains, and the absence or presence of a mapped sequence of DNA (marker) in each strain can be correlated with a quantitative measure of a phenotype (e.g. amount of psychoactive substance self-administered). Strong correlation of a phenotype with the presence of a genetic marker suggests that the genetic sequence in the proximity of this marker is involved in the regulation of this measure. Since the location of the marker sequence is mapped on mouse chromosomes, such analysis allows researchers to create genetic maps of loci important for the traits (Gora-Maslak et al., 1991; Grisel, 2000).

Genetics of tobacco dependence

Heritability of tobacco dependence

There is evidence of significant heritability of tobacco use among different populations, sexes and ages, as reported in a number of large-scale twin studies. Family and twin studies have demonstrated a genetic effect on "ever" smoking (or lifetime smoking, i.e. having smoked a cigarette at least once) (Cheng, Swan & Carmelli, 2000; McGue, Elkins & Iacono, 2000). A major genetic influence on the probability that an individual will become a smoker ("initiation") of about 60% has been observed, and continuation of the smoking habit once smoking has started ("persistence") of about 70% (Kaprio et al., 1982; Carmelli et al., 1992; Heath et al., 1995; Heath et al., 1999a; Koopmans et al., 1999; Sullivan & Kendler, 1999; Kendler, Thornton & Pedersen, 2000).

The initiation of smoking is separate from the development of nicotine dependence. One set of genetic factors was found to play a significant etiological role in both initiation and dependence, while another set of familial factors, probably in part genetic, solely influenced dependence (Kendler et al., 1999). In other words, genetic factors that contribute to variation in smoking initiation and dependence only partly overlap (Heath & Martin, 1993; Kendler et al., 1999; Madden et al., 1999; Sullivan & Kendler, 1999; Heath et al., 2002).

Other aspects of smoking, such as the age when the onset of smoking occurs, are also influenced by genetic effects in both sexes (Heath et al., 1999a; Koopmans et al., 1999). Once smoking is initiated, genetic factors determine to a large extent (86%) the quantity that is smoked (Kaprio et al., 1982; Koopmans et al., 1999). In addition some aspects of smoking, such as "never" smoking or intensity of smoking, showed a genetic contribution in males, which was not clear in females (Edwards et al., 1995). A study in adolescents demonstrated heritability estimates of over 80% for susceptibility to lifetime smoking and current use (Maes et al., 1999). Other aspects of smoking are also influenced by genetics, such as weight gain following cessation (Swan & Carmelli, 1995).

It is evident that there are different genetic contributions to different aspects of smoking behaviour, such as initiation, amount used, development of compulsive use, withdrawal symptoms, and development of tolerance. These factors individually contribute to the ICD-10 criteria for dependence

(Box 1.2). Thus, it can be seen that there are multiple genetic factors (as well as environmental factors such as availability and marketing) that contribute at different stages in the development of dependence.

Tobacco dependence and linkage studies

There is some evidence that smoking behaviour is associated with at least 14 different chromosomal locations (Bergen et al., 1999; Duggirala, Almasy & Blangero, 1999; Straub et al., 1999;). These studies suggest that the effect of any one gene on smoking behaviour is likely to be weak (Bergen et al., 1999; Arinami et al., 2000; Duggirala, Almasy & Blangero, 1999). One of the loci of interest is located on chromosome 5q near the locus for the dopamine D1 receptor, and this receptor has been associated with smoking (Comings et al., 1997; Duggirala, Almasy & Blangero, 1999).

Candidate genes for tobacco dependence

Nicotine is the primary compound in tobacco that establishes and maintains tobacco dependence (Henningfield, Miyasato & Jasinski, 1985). Smokers who are dependent on tobacco adjust their smoking to maintain their nicotine levels (Russell, 1987). Studies have been carried out to examine if genetic variation in the specific receptors for nicotine (Mihailescu & Drucker-Colin, 2000) as well as in pathways of nicotine elimination (Tyndale & Sellers, 2002) alter aspects of smoking behaviour.

Nicotinic receptors

Several types of evidence have suggested that a nicotinic receptor containing the β2-subunit is necessary for at least some of the reinforcing properties of nicotine (Mihailescu & Druker-Colin, 2000). However, no associations with changes in these receptors have been found (Silverman et al., 2000).

Recent studies of ethanol and tobacco use by humans suggest that common genes may influence the dependence on tobacco and ethanol. The results of one study of inbred mouse strains, selected on the basis of their response to ethanol, suggest that the α4 nicotinic receptor gene should be evaluated for its potential role in regulating ethanol and tobacco use in humans (Tritto et al., 2001).

Nicotine metabolism

Variation in the metabolic inactivation of nicotine is important because of the role of nicotine in producing tobacco dependence and regulating smoking patterns (Henningfield, Miyasato & Jasinski, 1985; Russel, 1987). Smoking is increased if the nicotine content in cigarettes is decreased or if nicotine excretion is increased, and smoking is decreased if nicotine is administered concurrently either intravenously or with a patch. The genes involved in nicotine metabolism may be important risk factors for smoking; the extent of variation is likely to be a major determinant of levels and accumulation of nicotine in the brain.

The metabolic enzyme CYP2A6 is genetically polymorphic (i.e. exists in more than one form). It is responsible for about 90% of the metabolic inactivation of nicotine to cotinine (Nakajima et al., 1996; Messina, Tyndale & Sellers, 1997). A significant impact of *CYP2A6* genetic variance has been found on the risk for tobacco dependence, age of starting smoking, the amount and patterns of cigarette smoking, duration of smoking, probability of quitting, and some aspects of risk of developing lung cancer (Miyamoto et al., 1999; Gu et al., 2000; Rao et al., 2000; Tyndale et al., 2002; Tyndale & Sellers, 2002). However, not all studies agree with these findings (Loriot et al., 2001; Tiihonen et al., 2000; Zhang et al., 2001).

Among Caucasian smokers those with genetically slow nicotine metabolism required fewer cigarettes per day, reflected in lower carbon monoxide levels, to maintain equal plasma nicotine levels, while those with the *CYP2A6* gene duplication (fast metabolizers) smoked more, and with greater intensity (Rao et al., 2000). In Caucasians, frequencies of genotypes with at least one decreased or inactive allele were higher in non-smokers than in smokers (Tyndale et al., 2002) indicating that slow nicotine inactivation modestly protects people from becoming smokers. It has also been shown that inhibiting CYP2A6 (mimicking the genetic defect) in smokers results in decreased smoking and rerouting of procarcinogens to other detoxifying pathways (Sellers, Kaplan & Tyndale, 2000; Sellers et al., 2002). Substantial variation in *CYP2A6* allele and genotype frequencies exists among ethnic groups (Oscarson et al., 1999; Tyndale et al., 2002). These data suggest that the *CYP2A6* genotype is likely to alter the risk for smoking and may alter the risk for smoking-related disease (Bartsch et al., 2000) among ethnic groups.

Genetics of alcohol dependence

Heritability of alcohol dependence

Heritability estimates of alcohol dependence depending on the diagnostic criteria used (e.g. DSM-IV, ICD-10; see Boxes 1.2 and 1.3) range from 52% to 63% (van den Bree et al., 1998a). It seems that some diagnostic systems are more sensitive in detecting genetic influences and may be more appropriate for studies attempting to find genes for alcohol dependence (van den Bree et al., 1998a).

Twin studies provide estimations of the heritability of predisposition to alcohol dependence of 51–65% in females and 48–73% in males (Carmelli et al., 1992; Kendler et al., 1994; Heath et al., 1997; Johnson et al., 1998; Han et al., 1999a; Prescott, Aggen & Kendler, 1999; Prescott & Kendler, 1999; Enoch

& Goldman, 2001). Heritability estimates were 66% in women and 42–75% in men for frequency of alcohol consumption (Heath et al., 1991; Heath & Martin, 1994) and 57% in women and 24–61% in men for average quantity consumed when drinking (Heath et al., 1991).

It is not clear if genetic risk is a major factor in the initiation of drinking or drinking during adolescence (Han et al., 1999a; Maes et al., 1999; Stallings et al., 1999). It may be that environmental effects explain most of the variation in initiation of drinking but genetic factors are more important in explaining the frequency of intoxication (Viken et al., 1999). Genetic factors contribute to the stability over time (68–80%) in frequency and in the quantity of alcohol consumed per drinking occasion (Kaprio et al., 1992; Carmelli et al., 1993).

Twin studies can also be used to examine other aspects of alcohol dependence. Estimated heritability of early alcohol use was significantly greater in boys (55%) than girls (11%) (Rose et al., 2001). Men (but not women) who are at increased genetic risk of alcohol dependence exhibited reduced sensitivity to alcohol (Heath et al., 1999b). The genetic risk for alcohol dependence was increased in those reporting a history of conduct disorder or major depression and in those with high neuroticism, social non-conformity, "tough-mindedness", novelty-seeking or (in women only) extraversion scores (Heath et al., 1997). Specific genes are also likely to influence the heritability for alcohol withdrawal syndrome (reviewed in Schuckit, 2000). In addition, genetic influences also alter treatment seeking (41%) for alcohol dependence, with shared environment explaining a further 40% of the variance (True et al., 1996).

These findings indicate further that there are genetic influences at many stages in the development of substance dependence, and indeed factors that influence treatment-seeking behaviour. The defining criteria of the phenotype in question can have major effects on the results of the study. Although it is clear that there is a genetic component to many aspects of alcohol drinking (e.g. initiation, frequency, quantity and response to alcohol), the relationship between genes and alcohol drinking behaviour is not a simple one.

Alcohol dependence and linkage studies

On chromosome 4q, one location identified was very close to the region of the alcohol dehydrogenase (ADH) genes (Long et al., 1998; Reich et al., 1998; Saccone et al., 2000); these genes have been associated with protective effects in Asians, as will be discussed later in this chapter (Reich et al., 1998). The finding of a linkage to 4q in a southwestern American Indian tribe and in Americans of European descent strongly supports a role for genes in this location in alcohol dependence. Linkage to chromosome 4p has also been seen near the β_1 GABA receptor gene (Long et al., 1998).

In a study of paired siblings (sib-pairs) in Finland, alcohol dependence showed weak evidence of linkage with a location on chromosome 6 and significant evidence of linkage to the serotonin receptor 1B G861C (see below); in a southwestern American Indian tribe, significant sib-pair linkage to chromosome 6 was also seen (Lappalainen et al., 1998). The strongest suggestions of linkage with susceptibility loci for alcohol dependence are on chromosomes 1 and 7, and more modest evidence for a locus on chromosome 2 (Reich et al., 1998). The best evidence for linkage has been seen on chromosome 11p (D11S1984), in close proximity to the dopamine receptor D4 (DRD4) and tyrosine hydroxylase (TH) genes (Long et al., 1998).

Candidate genes for alcohol dependence

Aldehyde dehydrogenase

Alcohol is metabolized to acetaldehyde, which in turn is metabolized to acetate before elimination from the body. The mitochondrial form of aldehyde dehydrogenase (ALDH2) is the enzyme primarily responsible for the metabolism of acetaldehyde to acetate (for reviews of ethanol metabolism and dependence see Agarwal (2001); Li (2000); Ramchandani et al. (2001). ALDH2 deficiency leads to an aversive response to alcohol due to elevated levels of acetaldehyde, resulting in increased hangover symptoms (Wall et al., 2000) and the alcohol flushing response, or alcohol sensitivity (Box 5.2) (Tanaka et al., 1997; Li, 2000). ALDH2 is found on chromosome 4p which has been linked to alcohol dependence in Asians and Europeans.

BOX 5.2

Alcohol flushing response or "alcohol sensitivity"

Some individuals show a cluster of symptoms following alcohol consumption, which have been related to elevated acetaldehyde levels. These elevations in acetaldehyde are due to alterations in ethanol metabolism, and can lead to the following symptoms:

– vasodilation, increased skin temperature, feeling of hotness, facial flushing

– increased heart rate and respiration

– decreased blood pressure

– bronchoconstriction

– nausea and headache

– euphoria or aversive reactions.

The neurotransmitters involved in this response are catecholamines, opioids, prostaglandins, histamine and bradykinin.

Source: Eriksson, 2001.

ALDH2*1 is a very active form found at high frequency among most ethnic populations, while the ALDH2*2 is inactive (or has very low activity) and is found at high frequency among Asians (e.g. Chinese, Japanese and Korean people). The ALDH2*2 has been demonstrated to be associated with substantial protection from alcohol in Japanese (Maezawa et al., 1995; Nakamura et al., 1996; Okamoto et al., 2001), Han Chinese (Chen et al., 1999), and Korean people (Lee et al., 2001). Genetic variation in ALDH2 in multiple ethnic groups alters the amount of ethanol consumed (Tanaka et al., 1997; Sun et al., 1999; Okamoto et al., 2001) and risk for binge drinking (Luczak et al., 2001). An association with liver disease was observed in some (Chao et al., 1997) but not all studies (Maruyama et al., 1999; Lee et al., 2001), and may be due to the effect on levels of consumption. Other variants of the ALDH2 are also under investigation.

Alcohol dehydrogenase

Alcohol dehydrogenase (ADH) metabolizes alcohol to acetaldehyde; it exists as a polygene family on chromosome 4p, which has been linked to alcohol dependence.

ADH2*2 allele frequency is lower in populations with alcohol dependence, indicating a protective role for ADH2*2 (Thomasson et al., 1994; Maezawa et al., 1995; Nakamura et al., 1996; Chen et al., 1999). For example, in aboriginal peoples of Taiwan (Thomasson et al., 1994) who have low frequencies of the protective allele ALDH2*2 (and thus would be more vulnerable), but who also have high frequencies of ADH2*2, (which is also protective), the protective effect of ADH2*2 is evident. This has also been seen in a Jewish population (Neumark et al., 1998; Shea et al., 2001). One study found that the ADH2 genotype had significant effects on both consumption and dependence in men, but not in women (Whitfield et al., 1998). ADH2 polymorphism was also associated with the risk of chronic alcohol-induced pancreatitis (Maruyama et al., 1999).

CYP2E1

Cytochrome P-450 2E1 (CYP2E1) is a hepatic enzyme that also metabolizes ethanol to acetaldehyde. In humans, the levels of hepatic CYP2E1 activity were found to vary by 15-fold. The 2E1 gene appears to be genetically polymorphic and rare 2E1 variant alleles are associated with altered ethanol metabolism (Watanabe, Hayashi & Kawajiri, 1994; Fairbrother et al., 1998; McCarver et al., 1998; Hu et al., 1999; Sun et al., 1999; Yoshihara et al., 2000a). Nicotine increases hepatic CYP2E1 in animal models, and smokers have higher CYP2E1 activity than non-smokers (Benowitz, Jacob & Saunders, 1999; Howard et al., 2001). Consistent with this, data from twin studies suggest that cigarette smoking may contribute to the development of tolerance to the effects of alcohol and a diminished sense of intoxication (Madden et al., 1995;

Madden, Heath & Martin, 1997), suggesting that smoking induces increased alcohol metabolism. While studies have not focused on whether genetic variation in *CYP2E1* alters the risk for smoking per se, an intriguing association between a *CYP2E1* polymorphism and levels of the nicotine metabolite cotinine suggests that CYP2E1, directly or indirectly, may alter smoking and/ or nicotine/cotinine metabolism (Yang et al., 2001). The determination of a role for genetic variation in *CYP2E1* in the risk for smoking is currently being investigated (Howard et al., 2002).

Chronic ethanol consumption results in the induction of CYP2E1, which is believed to play an important role in the pathogenesis of alcohol-induced liver disease and is responsible for the increased rates of ethanol metabolism observed in those consuming relatively high amounts of alcohol (Oneta et al., 2002). Genetic variants of *CYP2E1* can alter the relative inducibility, which may alter the impact on risk for alcohol dependence, or the resulting hepatic damage (Lucas et al., 1995; Ueno et al., 1996).

Genetics of opioid dependence

Heritability of opioid dependence

Heritability for opioid dependence is high, estimated at almost 70% (Tsuang et al., 2001). Twin studies consistently find higher concordance for opiate dependence in monozygotic than in dizygotic twins, indicating a significant genetic contribution (Lin et al., 1996; Tsuang et al., 1996;1999; 2001). Genetic risk for dependence can be divided into a common, or shared, vulnerability across different classes of drugs, and a genetic vulnerability to the specific drug in question. Opiate dependence has the lowest extent of common vulnerability to substance dependence, at 50%, indicating that there may be specific opiate-related neurochemical components to heroin dependence. It is clear from the above, that opiate use and dependence are at least in part influenced by genetic factors.

Opioid dependence and linkage studies

There have been no family-based genetic linkage studies of opioid dependence in humans.

Candidate genes for opioid dependence

The candidate gene approach requires the selection of genes with perceived relevance to the trait in question. In the case of opioids this is easy, as the receptor pharmacology is well understood and there are consequently good candidate genes from the endogenous opioid system. Data from genetic epidemiology tell us that the highest genetic contribution to opioid dependence is from unique genetic effects – i.e. those not connected with dependence on other drugs – pointing to components of the endogenous opioid system as good candidate genes. All three known receptors (mu, delta, and kappa), and genes coding for opioid ligands have been screened for genetic variation (Mayer & Hollt, 2001).

Mu opioid receptor

The mu opioid receptor subtype is the primary target of morphine and the mediator of the reinforcement and reward effect of opioids, which makes the mu opioid receptor gene the outstanding candidate for genetic vulnerability. The data however, have not consistently associated this gene with opioid dependence. Sequencing of the mu opioid receptor gene identified five single nucleotide polymorphisms (single base pair changes in nucleotide sequence) in the gene (Bond et al., 1998). However this polymorphism was not associated with heroin dependence in a sample of heroin-dependent individuals from China (Li et al., 1997) or Germany (Franke et al., 2001). However a study among Hong Kong Chinese people found a significant association (Szeto et al., 2001). Persons expressing a mu opioid receptor variant have altered hypothalamic–pituitary–adrenal axis function and altered responses to other physiological processes regulated through activation of the mu opioid receptor (Wand et al., 2002). Natural sequence variations in the mu opioid receptor gene have little influence on ligand binding or receptor down-regulation but could modify receptor density and signalling (Befort et al., 2001).

Kappa opioid receptor

The kappa opioid receptor has also been examined and positive association was seen in one study (Mayer et al., 1997), but was not replicated in a second (Franke et al., 1999). Seven allelic variants in the kappa-1 opioid receptor gene have been discovered, (LaForge et al., 2000; Mayer & Hollt, 2001), but there is no evidence that any are functional.

Dopamine D4 receptor

The dopamine D4 receptor (DRD4) has also shown evidence for association with opioid dependence (Kotler et al., 1997; Li et al., 1997; Vandenbergh et al., 2000) although this is not supported in another study (Franke et al., 2000).

Prodynorphin

Prodynorphin has also been examined (Zimprich et al., 2000). However, prodynorphin allelic distributions were not significantly different in people with heroin dependence and controls.

CYP2D6

Opioid metabolizing enzymes are also strong candidate genes for involvement in susceptibility. The most significant finding in opioid dependence is the association found between oral codeine dependence and the metabolizing enzyme CYP2D6 (Tyndale, Droll & Sellers, 1997). Many opioids (e.g. codeine, oxycodone and hydrocodone) are metabolized by CYP2D6 to metabolites of increased activity, principally morphine. It is estimated that 4–10% of Caucasians lack CYP2D6 activity due to inheritance of two non-functional alleles. Tyndale, Droll & Sellers (1997) found that of a group of people with dependence on oral opiates, there were no poor metabolizers of CYP2D6 (Fisher's exact test, $p <$ or $= 0.05$). This is in contrast with 4% of people in the non-dependent group being poor metabolizers of CYP2D6, suggesting that the CYP2D6 variant genotype offers protection against oral opioid dependence. However, this finding remains controversial (Mikus et al., 1998).

Genetics of the combined risk of dependence on tobacco, alcohol, opioids and other psychoactive substances

Heritability of substance dependence

Genetic risk influences the predisposition to use and to the development of dependence on alcohol, tobacco and opioids individually. However, there is also a genetic contribution to use of, and dependence on, a combination of alcohol, tobacco and other substances (Carmelli et al., 1992; Reed et al., 1994; Swan, Carmelli & Cardon, 1996, 1997; Daeppen et al., 2000; Hopfer, Stallings & Hewitt, 2001; Tsuang et al., 2001).

The classic adoption studies of Cadoret have been instrumental in defining the importance of genetic factors in substance abuse (Cadoret et al., 1986, 1995). These studies demonstrated that substance abuse was significantly greater in adoptees whose biological parents were dependent on alcohol or other psychoactive substances, or who had a personality disorder. This led to a model in which two genetic factors and an independent, environmental factor from the adoptive family increase the risk of substance abuse.

The co-occurrence of lifetime tobacco and alcohol dependence has a substantial genetic correlation suggesting a common genetic vulnerability (True et al., 1999). Environmental features have a large influence on the initiation of alcohol and tobacco use in adolescents, whereas alcohol and tobacco use in slightly older young adults was more influenced by genetic risk factors (Koopmans, van Doornen & Boomsma, 1997). People who smoke are also at greater risk for severe alcohol dependence (Daeppen et al., 2000). Significant genetic correlations exist between problem drinking and ever smoking or using at least one half-pack (10 cigarettes) per day (Hopfer, Stallings & Hewitt, 2001). The shared genetic influence on alcohol use and smoking in women is clearest for those subjects with the highest severity of alcohol use (Hopfer, Stallings & Hewitt, 2001).

Smoking has been shown to be a significant risk factor for promoting the progression of alcohol dependence (Bucholz, Heath & Madden, 2000). This effect may occur by diminishing the effects of alcohol, because nicotine can increase the activity of the alcohol-metabolizing enzyme CYP2E1 (Madden et al., 1995). However, alcohol dependence is associated with more serious nicotine withdrawal (Madden et al., 1997). This indicates that tobacco and alcohol dependence share a considerable proportion of genes (Carmelli et al., 1990; Hettema, Corey & Kendler, 1999; Vanyukov & Tarter, 2000). This common genetic influence may partially explain the clinical and epidemiological observations that people who are dependent on alcohol are also often dependent on tobacco.

Family studies show strong familial aggregation of substance dependence (Meller et al., 1988; Mirin et al., 1991; Kendler, Davis & Kessler, 1997; Bierut et al., 1998; Merikangas et al., 1998). One estimate is that there is an eight-fold increased risk of substance dependence amongst relatives of dependent people compared to controls, which applied to a wide range of substances including opioids, cannabis, sedatives and cocaine (Bierut et al., 1998; Merikangas et al., 1998).

A major population-based twin study has been used to examine the role of genes in the familial transmission of substance dependence (Kendler & Prescott, 1998). This large-scale study showed that genetic factors substantially influence vulnerability to substance dependence. Family environment is also important, but family environment predominantly influences initiation, whereas genetic factors have a stronger influence on heavy use and dependence (van den Bree et al., 1998b; Kendler 2001). These studies place heritability estimates for substance dependence at between 50% and 80%.

Few studies specifically address the interrelationship or overlap of heritability between opioid dependence and alcohol dependence. There is evidence of both common and specific additive factors transmitted in families (Beirut et al., 1998). Overall the evidence suggests that independent causative factors mainly operate for alcohol and opioid dependence, although there may be some common genetic factors related to dependence in general.

Linkage studies of substance dependence

The well-established links between alcohol dependence and smoking have been recently reviewed (Narahashi et al., 2001). Approximately one-third of the loci that showed evidence for linkage to smoking behaviour also showed evidence for linkage to alcohol dependence (Bergen et al., 1999). Strong evidence for linkage to chromosome 15 was observed in a family study involving people with alcohol dependence and heavy smokers (Merette et al., 1999). Of note, linkage with alcohol was found on chromosome 19q12-13, which may be due to linkage with smoking and the polymorphic CYP2A6 enzyme (19q13.2) which can inactivate nicotine (Messina, Tyndale & Sellers, 1997).

Candidate genes involved in substance dependence

Candidate gene studies examine alleles that might reasonably be thought to be involved in a disorder. Currently the best candidate allelic variants fulfil at least two criteria: the variant has been shown to alter function, and the variant has a good likelihood of being biologically relevant (Stoltenberg & Burmeister, 2000).

There are two main types of genes that have been associated with drug dependence; those that are likely to be specific to the particular dependence [e.g. nicotinic receptors and smoking, ethanol metabolism and alcohol dependence (Grant et al., 1999)] and those that may play a common role in either all or a subset of dependencies. Genetic alterations in various combinations of the genes for neurotransmitters and receptors (i.e. serotonin, norepinephrine, GABA, glutamate and opioid) that modify dopamine neuron function may put individuals at risk for dependence (Comings & Blum, 2000; Quattrocki, Baird & Yurgelun-Todd, 2000). Like other behavioural disorders, substance dependence is polygenically (i.e. many genes) inherited and each gene is likely to account for only a small percentage of the variance. In each subsequent section, gene candidates that may affect dependence more generally will follow the candidate genes specific to tobacco, alcohol and opioid dependence.

GABAergic systems

Inhibition of GABAergic systems in the substantia nigra fine-tunes the amount of dopamine released at the nucleus accumbens, an important site for the effects of all psychoactive substances (see Chapters 3 and 4). $GABA_A$ receptor blockers reduce some ethanol-induced behaviours, such as motor impairment and sedation. The role of this receptor in alcohol dependence is further supported by effective alleviation of alcohol withdrawal symptoms by $GABA_A$ agonists (Parsian & Cloninger, 1997). In addition, one of the clusters of $GABA_A$ receptors is located on chromosome 4, at a locus which is thought to feature prominently in alcohol dependence. Thus the GABAergic system may alter risk for smoking and alcohol dependence (Loh & Ball, 2000).

Nicotine can stimulate the firing rate of dopamine neurons in the ventral tegmental area (VTA), but GABAergic neurons may also be an important target for the effects of nicotine on the central nervous system.

$GABA_A$ receptor $\alpha 1$. No association has been found with any type of substance dependence (Parsian & Cloninger, 1997).

$GABA_A$ receptor $\alpha 3$. An association was found for alcohol dependence, but not with its subtypes (Parsian & Cloninger, 1997).

$GABA_A$ receptor $\alpha 6$. There is some evidence for the involvement of this receptor subunit in alcohol dependence, in both animal and human studies. A locus for acute effects of alcohol is located on mouse chromosome 11 and encodes the GABA$_A$ receptor $\gamma2$, $\alpha1$, $\alpha6$, and $\beta2$ subunits, suggesting a role for these subunits in response to alcohol (Hood & Buck, 2000). A GABA$_A$ receptor variant a6 subunit segregates in a rat line which voluntarily avoids alcohol consumption, providing support for a possible role for variants of this receptor subtype to alter genetic predisposition to alcohol preference (Saba et al., 2001). Different variants of the $\alpha6$ subunit are associated with lower alcohol response (Iwata, Virkkunen & Goldman, 2000), alcohol dependence (Loh et al., 2000) and with Korsakoff's psychosis (Loh et al., 1999).

GABA$_A$ receptor $\beta1$. GABA$_A$ receptor $\beta1$ gene variants were associated with alcohol dependence (Parsian & Zhang, 1999).

GABA$_A$ receptor $\beta2$. GABA$_A$ receptor $\beta2$ variants were tested and found not to associate with alcohol dependence or alcohol withdrawal (Sander et al., 1999a). The BanI RFLP at the GABA$_A$ $\beta2$ receptor subunit gene associated with both alcohol dependence and Korsakoff's psychosis (Loh et al., 1999).

GABA$_A$ receptor $\beta3$. An association of GABA$_A$ receptor $\beta3$ variants was found with severe alcohol dependence (Noble et al., 1998a).

GABA$_A$ receptor $\gamma2$. Functionally relevant variation in GABA$_A$ $\gamma2$, or a closely linked gene, is correlated genetically with some behavioural responses to alcohol in certain strains of mice (Hood & Buck, 2000). No association in humans has been found (Hsu et al., 1998; Sander et al., 1999a), except in the presence of antisocial personality disorder (see Box 6.1) (Loh et al, 2000).

GABA$_B$ receptor R1. Data suggest that GABA$_B$ R1 variants do not contribute a substantial effect to the genetic variance of alcohol dependence (Sander et al., 1999b). Nevertheless, possible evidence of potential allelic associations emphasize the need for further studies to test more defined phenotype–genotype relationships.

Dopamine system

Because of its importance in brain reward circuits, the mesolimbic dopaminergic system has been implicated in the reinforcing effects of many substances including nicotine and ethanol (Uhl et al., 1998; Merlo Pich, Chiamulera & Carboni, 1999; Comings & Blum, 2000) (see also Chapter 3). Accordingly, polymorphisms of genes in the dopaminergic system are plausible functional candidate genes for tobacco and alcohol dependence. Studies over the past decade have shown that alleles of the dopamine receptor system are associated with alcohol and tobacco dependence, dependence on other psychoactive substances, novelty-seeking, obesity, compulsive gambling and several personality traits. This is an example of genetic variation in a system (e.g. dopamine), which may alter a number of behaviours including alcohol and tobacco dependence.

Dopamine D1 receptor. As mentioned previously, smoking behaviour (as defined by the number of cigarettes per day for one year) has been linked to a genetic location on chromosome 5q (D5S1354) (Duggirala, Almasy & Blangero, 1999) that is near the dopamine receptor D1 (DRD1) locus. An association was made between a polymorphism, and smoking, alcohol use, illicit drug use, compulsive shopping, compulsive eating and gambling (Comings et al., 1997), although not all studies confirm a role for DRD1 in alcohol use (Hietala et al., 1997; Sander et al., 1995). These results suggest a role for genetic variants of the DRD1 gene in some dependence-related behaviours, and further, suggest an interaction of genetic variants of the DRD1 and DRD2 genes (Comings et al., 1997).

Dopamine D2 receptor. Variants of the dopamine receptor D2 (DRD2) gene have been associated with dependence on alcohol, nicotine, cocaine and opioids, and with novelty-seeking, obesity and gambling, but the results have not been consistent (Noble, 2000; Noble et al., 1998b). It is hypothesized that the DRD2 gene is involved in reinforcement (see Chapter 3).

Among non-Hispanic Caucasians who smoked at least one pack of cigarettes per day, had unsuccessfully attempted to stop smoking, and were not dependent on alcohol or other drugs, the DRD2 A1 allele was more prevalent than in controls (Comings et al., 1996), although this is not observed in all studies (Singleton et al., 1998). There was a significant, inverse relationship between the prevalence of the DRD2 A1 allele and the age of onset of smoking and the maximum duration of time since the smokers had quit smoking on their own (Comings et al., 1996). These results support the concept that the DRD2 gene is one of a multifactorial set of risk factors associated with smoking (Comings et al., 1996).

In summary, DRD2 may not alter risk for alcohol dependence, but alcohol-dependent patients with the DRD2 A1 allele may have greater severity of their disorder across a range of problem drinking indices (Connor et al., 2002).

There are a few examples where the DRD2 genetic variation has been examined in conjunction with other genes. Variants of both the DRD2 and GABA$_A$ receptor subunit β3 genes have been associated with risk for alcohol dependence; however, the risk for alcohol dependence is more robust when these variants are combined than when they are considered separately (Noble et al., 1998a). Similarly, DRD2 variant and ADH2 have been shown to have a stronger association with risk for alcohol dependence when combined than when alone (Amad et al., 2000).

Dopamine D3 receptor. The DRD3 receptor is found at high levels in the nucleus accumbens, a region involved in drug reward and dependence (see Chapter 3). A variant of the DRD3 gene has been shown in some studies to alter function. The role of this variant in tobacco smoking has not been studied, but it has been shown to alter use of some other substances and psychiatric disorders. Studies of DRD3 and alcohol dependence demonstrated no significant association (Parsian et al., 1997; Henderson et al., 2000).

Dopamine D4 receptor. A variant of the DRD4 gene has been identified and is thought to play a role in nicotine dependence. When exposed to smoking cues before smoking either high-nicotine cigarettes or control cigarettes, individuals with the DRD4 variant allele had greater craving, more arousal, less positive affect, and more attention to the smoking cues than did those without the variant allele (Hutchison et al., 2002a). These preliminary results suggest that the rewarding effects of smoking and the beneficial effects of nicotine replacement therapy may depend, in part, on genetic factors involved in dopamine transmission.

An association study on the DRD4 gene showed that African-Americans who had at least one variant allele had a higher risk of smoking, a shorter time to the first cigarette in the morning, and an earlier age at smoking initiation (Shields et al., 1998). After smoking cessation counselling, none of the smokers with the variant allele were abstinent at 2 months, compared with 35% of the smokers who were homozygous for the non-variant genotype. The analysis of Caucasians did not suggest a similar risk.

Some studies have shown an association between alcohol dependence and DRD4 receptor variation (George et al., 1993; Hutchison et al., 2002b), while others have not (Parsian et al., 1997; Ishiguro et al., 2000; Albanese et al., 2001).

It is interesting that the DRD4 variation increased the risk for alcohol dependence in individuals with protective *ALDH2*2* variants, indicating the overriding of the protective effects of *ALDH2*2* by the DRD4 variant (Muramatsu et al., 1996).

Dopamine D5 receptor. Several functional polymorphisms in DRD5 have been identified (Cravchik & Gejman, 1999); however, for smoking initiation, there was no significant association with the four DRD5 markers studied. While these data are not consistent with a strong role for DRD5 in the etiology of smoking behaviours, one study suggested the involvement of the locus in the variation of risk of substance use and antisocial behaviour (Vanyukov et al., 2000), indicating that further studies may be warranted.

Dopamine transporter. A polymorphism of the dopamine transporter has been identified which can alter rates of transcription (production of messenger RNA, mRNA) (Michelhaugh et al., 2001) and which is associated with altered levels of the dopamine transporter protein in the brain (Heinz et al., 2000), suggesting that the polymorphism results in functional differences. However, no association with substance dependence has been found.

Dopamine beta hydroxylase. Smokers with a particular dopamine beta hydroxylase (DBH) genotype smoked fewer cigarettes when compared to those without the genotype (McKinney et al., 2000). Heavy smokers (>20 cigarettes per day) had a higher frequency of the DBH variant allele when compared to light smokers (McKinney et al., 2000).

Monoamine Oxidase A. Central dopaminergic reward pathways give rise to dependence and are activated by nicotine and alcohol indicating that allelic variants in genes involved in dopamine metabolism may be important in dependence. Monoamine oxidase (MAO) is involved in the metabolism of neurotransmitters including dopamine, serotonin and norepinephrine. There are two distinct forms of MAO: MAO-A and MAO-B; both are encoded in genes on the X chromosome.

MAO activity is reduced by smoking (Checkoway et al., 1998). One study found that smokers with a certain MAO-A genotype smoked more cigarettes than those without that genotype (McKinney et al., 2000).

Low platelet MAO activity has been associated with alcohol dependence, making genetic variation in these genes of interest. Variations in the MAO-A and MAO-B genes differ between people with alcohol dependence and controls (Parsian et al., 1995). A variant of the MAO-A gene is associated with both a risk for alcohol dependence and lower age of onset of substance dependence in males (Vanyukov et al., 1995).

Significant associations of alcohol dependence with MAO-A alleles were found among the Han Chinese people, but not among aboriginal Taiwanese groups (Hsu et al., 1996). A functional polymorphism in the MAO-A allele was identified and the frequency was increased in males with antisocial personality disorder and alcohol dependence, but not in those with alcohol dependence alone or in controls (Samochowiec et al., 1999; Schmidt et al., 2000).

Catechol-O-methyltransferase. Catechol-O-methyltransferase (COMT) inactivates catecholamines and catechol drugs. A common genetic polymorphism in humans is associated with a 3–4 fold variation in COMT enzyme activity (Lachman et al., 1996). Since ethanol and nicotine use are associated with rapid release of dopamine in limbic areas, it is conceivable that subjects who inherit low activity alleles would inactivate dopamine more slowly, thereby altering their vulnerability to the development of dependence. A functional polymorphism resulting in increased enzyme activity has been associated with alcohol dependence and polysubstance use (Vandenbergh et al., 1997; Horowitz et al, 2000). No association was found between this COMT polymorphism and smoking initiation, smoking persistence and smoking cessation (David et al., 2002).

Men with a specific COMT genotype (30% of all subjects) reported 27% higher weekly alcohol consumption compared with the two other genotype groups (Kauhanen et al., 2000). The results indicate that COMT polymorphism may contribute to the amount of alcohol intake, not only in people with alcohol dependence, but also in a general male population. Visual and auditory disturbances among people with alcohol dependence in withdrawal symptoms were significantly different among COMT genotypes (Nakamura et al., 2001), suggesting that COMT activity could partially affect the appearance of delirium tremens in these individuals.

Tyrosine Hydroxylase. Tyrosine hydroxylase (TH) is the rate-limiting enzyme in the biosynthesis of catecholamines. Nicotine has been shown to regulate TH, and mice with more TH are less sensitive to nicotine. No association was found between a TH genetic polymorphism and cigarette smoking (Lerman et al., 1997).

Results to date suggest that no major influence on alcohol dependence is exerted through genes associated with the TH variants (Geijer et al., 1997; Ishiguro et al., 1998; Albanese et al., 2001).

Serotonergic systems

Genes in the serotonin system are plausible candidates for association with smoking or alcohol dependence because of the role of serotonin in mood regulation, impulse control, appetite and aggression (Veenstra-VanderWeele et al., 2000). Nicotine can increase serotonin release suggesting that some aspects of smoking might be altered by variation in the serotonergic system (e.g. variable mood disturbances during withdrawal resulting in altered cessation rates). In addition, a number of serotonin reuptake inhibitors are being examined for their utility in smoking cessation and in preventing weight gain associated with smoking cessation. Alterations in the serotonergic neurotransmission have been frequently described for patients suffering from alcohol dependence, anxiety disorders and narcolepsy, thus the serotonergic system provides additional candidate genes for genetic variation in alcohol dependence and smoking.

Serotonin receptors. While functional polymorphisms have been identified in serotonin receptors and associated with relevant personality dimensions (e.g. harm-avoidance, reward dependence), there are no reports of associations between serotonin receptors and smoking behaviour. In the studies of serotonin receptor variants and alcohol dependence there are some positive and many negative findings (Yoshihara et al., 2000b). A clearer phenotype, including personality variables, may be required before a better picture of the role of serotonin receptors in the genetic risk for alcohol-related behaviours can be elucidated.

Serotonin Receptor 1B. The 5HT1B receptor gene variant (G861C) has not been associated with alcohol dependence (Gorwood et al., 2002; Kranzler et al., 2002), either alone or with a comorbid antisocial diagnosis (Kranzler et al.,

2002). However for people with alcohol dependence with inactive ALDH2, but not for those with active ALDH2, there was an association with the 5HT1B receptor variant (G861GC), suggesting its involvement in the development of some type of alcohol dependence (Hasegawa et al., 2002).

Serotonin Receptor 2A. Data suggest that there may be a relatively small genetic variability in the HTR2A receptor gene involved in the development of alcohol dependence (Nakamura et al., 1999; Hwu & Chen, 2000; Preuss et al., 2001; Hasegawa et al., 2002).

Serotonin Receptor 2C. There is no evidence of HTR2C allele association with alcohol dependence (Lappalainen et al., 1999; Schuckit et al., 1999; Fehr et al., 2000; Parsian & Cloninger, 2001).

Serotonin Receptor 5. There was no evidence of HTR 5 allele differences in a Finnish study of people with alcohol dependence and controls (Iwata et al., 1998).

Serotonin Receptor 7. The HTR 7 L279 variant was not significantly associated with alcohol dependence or impulsivity, however it may be a predisposing allele in a subgroup of people with alcohol dependence and multiple behavioural problems (Pesonen et al., 1998).

Tryptophan Hydroxylase. Genetic variation in tryptophan hydroxylase (TPH) could significantly alter serotonergic neurotransmission and thus alter the risk for dependence.

No association of TPH alleles with smoking status has been found (Lerman et al., 2001), however, individuals with a specific genotype start smoking at an earlier age (Lerman et al, 2001). In addition, another study found an association with smoking initiation but not with progression to nicotine dependence (Sullivan et al., 2001). These data suggest that variation in the production of serotonin may be involved in the etiology of smoking initiation.

A higher frequency of the TPH A allele was found in Japanese people with alcohol dependence and histories of drinking-related antisocial behaviours (Ishiguro et al., 1999) and in Finnish people with alcohol dependence who were also criminal offenders (Nielsen et al., 1998). However, no association was found between the TPH A allele and alcohol dependence without personality disorders (Han et al., 1999b; Ishiguro et al., 1999; Fehr et al., 2001).

Serotonin transporter. The serotonin transporter (5-HTT) gene (*SLC6A4*) is a plausible candidate gene for smoking and predisposition to alcohol dependence because of its association with psychological traits relevant to smoking and drinking behaviour. A specific polymorphism of this gene has been associated with numerous psychiatric disorders (e.g. depression, anxiety disorders, bipolar disorders and schizophrenia).

Other systems of interest

Cholecystokinin. The neuropeptide cholecystokinin (CCK) plays an important role in the functioning of the central nervous system via an interaction with dopamine and other neurotransmitters. The interaction of CCK with the dopaminergic system has been implicated in the behaviours associated with psychoactive drugs (Vaccarino, 1994; Crawley & Corwin, 1994).

Acute and chronic exposure to nicotine results in weight loss that is associated with an increase in CCK in the hypothalamus; CCK antagonists ameliorate symptoms of nicotine withdrawal, consistent with a role of the CCK gene as a risk factor for smoking (Comings et al., 2001)

Opioid receptors. Both ethanol and opioids activate the mesolimbic dopamine reward system, and genetic differences in the sensitivity of the endogenous opioid system to alcohol may be an important factor in determining the risk for the development of alcohol dependence or excessive alcohol consumption (Gianoulakis, 2001). No consistent associations have been identified.

Glutamate transporter. Glutamate-mediated excitatory pathways play an important role in the pathogenesis of alcohol dependence. The astroglial glutamate transporter EAAT2 confers vulnerability to alcohol dependence; however, no association of a polymorphism with alcohol dependence, or with alcohol dependence with severe physiological withdrawal symptoms, or alcohol dependence with antisocial behaviour, was observed (Sander et al., 2000).

Confounding issues in linkage and candidate gene studies

Environment

Twin and family studies indicate a significant genetic risk for alcohol and tobacco dependence and a substantial role for environmental factors (Stoltenberg & Burmeister, 2000; Crabbe, 2002). It is important to remember the latter source of variation in risk and to look for ways to integrate studies of genetic and environmental influence (see later in this chapter). This difficult task was reviewed for a series of complex disorders (Kiberstis & Roberts, 2002). However, recent developments in genetics raise the possibility of sorting out the complex interactions between genotype and environment that determine the development of the individual behavioural phenotype. This is clearly a direction that needs much attention.

Genetic heterogeneity

In addition to genetic and diagnostic heterogeneity, it is anticipated that increased risk for many complex disorders such as substance dependence, requires multiple genetic variants in combination (Stoltenberg & Burmeister,

2000; Crabbe, 2002). Many psychiatric disorders are likely to be caused by multiple genes that interact with each other (Cooper, 2001). This suggests that having one predisposing allele does not imply high risk; in fact, the majority of carriers are not expected to express the disorder (Stoltenberg & Burmeister, 2000). Issues of genetic heterogeneity create complexity for linkage studies, as well as for studies that examine only one gene, or allelic variant at a time (Wahlsten, 1999).

Phenotype

At least some genetic defects appear to predispose populations to forms of dependence that do not fall into the neatly defined categories in DSM-IV or ICD-10 (Boxes 1.2 and 1.3). This is certainly the case for tobacco dependence where other ways of determining dependence have been proposed and used (e.g. Fagerstrom & Schneider, 1989; Heatherton et al., 1991). Likewise, it was found that different symptoms of alcohol dependence yielded heritability estimates ranging from 3% to 53% (Slutske et al., 1999), and the same has been observed with alternative diagnostic tools for alcohol dependence (van den Bree et al., 1998a). These findings indicate the need to clearly define the phenotype of interest. In other words, clearly defining the endpoint (e.g. relative risk for drinking over 8 drinks per day, alcohol withdrawal, relative risk for initiation of smoking, initial tolerance) may improve the ability to identify specific genes involved.

Comorbidity

Many psychiatric disorders co-occur with substance dependence (see Chapter 6). Comorbidity among disorders will be understood only with increased knowledge of the underlying neurobiology of the disorders. Behavioural genetic approaches will allow investigators to directly test causes of each disorder as well as the comorbidity, and to estimate the size of the effect of each contributing factor.

Methodological issues

Candidate gene studies have often found conflicting results. The reasons for differences in findings include:

— inconsistencies in the definitions of "smokers" (i.e. ever vs. never, former, >100 cigarettes in lifetime, dependence) and "smoking behaviour" (i.e. initiation, maintenance, quitting, cessation, relapse);

— issues concerning functionless polymorphisms, methodology (e.g. erroneous genotyping techniques) and statistical power;

— ethnic ancestry.

Differences in definitions of "smokers", "drinkers" and "ethnic ancestry" are likely to contribute substantially to the differing outcomes of studies. Another issue is that "attractive" candidate genes will be studied in many laboratories, and there is often a bias towards reporting positive findings.

A further issue is the practice of examining one gene and sometimes one allele at a time. While this is simpler and requires smaller sample sizes, examples exist which indicate that only when two or more genetically variable genes (e.g. ALDH2 and ALD) are examined together, will meaningful results be found. Another limitation of the candidate gene approach is the amount of knowledge of the biology of the disorder being studied. This issue further supports integrating research approaches, using chromosomal locations identified by linkage or QTL studies, as well as candidate genes identified in model systems such as *Drosophila*, to identify other potential candidate genes. To understand the genetic contributions to smoking and drinking behaviours, many aspects of the behaviour need to be assessed, as different genes may affect the various behaviours differentially. Large studies of multiple gene variants and clearly-defined phenotypes will lead to clearer understanding of the specific genes and mechanisms involved.

Future directions

The genetic approaches and findings outlined in this chapter provide an indication of the promise that genetic research offers. These genetic data can be, and have been, used to improve our understanding of the etiology of substance dependence and variation in risk between individuals. Once genes are identified which alter the predisposition to dependence, a major challenge will be to understand how the functions of these genes interact with the environmental influences on dependence (Swan, 1999). Analysis of specific genes will allow a rational exploration of biochemical underpinnings of the actions of nicotine, alcohol and other substances, and makes possible a link between behavioural change, genetic predisposition and biochemical action. Such genes, and the proteins they encode, will become primary targets for creating novel diagnostic tools as well as the basis of novel behavioural and pharmacological treatments.

Genetic information may be useful for identifying individuals at increased risk for substance dependence (and thus for refining prevention approaches), and for predicting the health consequences of substance dependence (e.g. hepatic toxicity). By gaining a better understanding of genes that are involved in initiation, maintenance and cessation of substance dependence, novel pharmacological and behavioural treatment approaches may be created (Swan, 1999; Sellers & Tyndale, 2000; Marteau & Lerman, 2001; Johnstone, York & Walton, 2002). This research field also offers great potential for using a person's genetic information to personalize treatment approaches (i.e. choosing the appropriate treatment, drug and dose) and for minimizing adverse reactions. Again, it is important to emphasize that a certain genetic make-up does not necessarily mean that a person will develop dependence, but it may provide useful information for treatment and prevention approaches.

In summary, the improved understanding of genetic influences on substance dependence promises to increase our understanding of dependence-producing processes, and should provide novel prevention and treatment approaches.

Social and cultural aspects

It should be emphasized that complex genetic risk factors and protective factors for dependence operate within a biological, social and cultural milieu, which affects the outcome for each individual person. The following section briefly highlights some of the relevant social and cultural factors.

Risk factors and protective factors for dependence: an overview

Research on risk factors for dependence involves comparisons of people with and without dependence, and longitudinal studies with subjects who become dependent or avoid dependence. There are both environmental risk factors (e.g. social class, mobility, social change, peer culture, educational style and occupational risk groups) and individual risk factors (e.g. genetic disposition, child abuse, personality disorders) (Uchtenhagen, 2000a,b). Cultural norms, attitudes and views about substance use (e.g. social acceptability, tolerance, stigma) and local, national or regional policies on illicit drugs, tobacco and alcohol may also be considered as environmental risk factors.

Risk factors for problem drug use include family disruption and dependence problems in the family, poor performance at school, social deprivation, young age of onset of substance use, and depression and suicidal behaviour during adolescence (Lloyd, 1998).

While risk factors emphasize negative influences and the importance of prevention, protective factors stress positive alternatives and the necessity of health promotion. Protective factors can have an independent main effect or act as intervening variables between risk factors and behavioural outcome.

Individuals draw upon environmental or personal resources that may enable them to cope better with stress and health-related challenges (Antonovsky, 1987). This concept in social psychology is mirrored in sociology in the theory of social capital. Social capital is the sum of the resources that an individual or a group has access to through social, family or institutional relationships (Klingemann et al., 2001).

Environmental resources include economic situation, social support, social integration, learning models and temporal factors (Schmid, 2000). With respect to temporal factors, age at onset of substance use is important as well as events in life that can be characterized by a higher vulnerability to substance use, such as experimenting with drugs when entering adolescence, compensating for stress factors when entering the professional adult world, and facing retirement between the ages of 55 and 65 years (see Vogt, 2000a,b).

There is some empirical evidence that social inequality and class differences are related to risky use of both licit and illicit psychoactive substances. For example, the decline in smoking in some countries has been more rapid in men and women from higher socioeconomic classes, and drinking shows an inverse relationship with occupational status (Marmot, 1997). As regards illicit substances, ecological studies have shown that the poverty status of communities is a powerful predictor of fatal drug overdoses of cocaine and opioids in developed countries. For example, in a study in an urban community in New York, 69 % of the variance in fatal drug overdoses was explained by poverty status (Marzuk et al., 1997).

Poverty also is associated with problems of nutrition and a wide array of negative contextual conditions: malnourished individuals are especially vulnerable to adverse effects of consumption of licit and illicit substances (Charness, 1999). General health status and nutritional state play an important role: for example diabetes, hypertension and hepatitis C virus increase vulnerability to alcohol (Regev & Jeffers, 1999; Weathermon & Crabb, 1999. More specifically, health-related knowledge about alcohol use and anti-drinking attitudes lowered the odds of drinking (Epstein et al., 1995).

Personal resources include coping skills, self-efficacy, risk perception, optimism, health-related behaviour, ability to resist social pressure and general health behaviour. These resources will interact with and possibly be enhanced by community programmes that can fulfil the needs of people to resort less frequently to substance use, and that provide a healthy environment in which the individual feels less pressured to use licit and illicit substances.

Summary

Family, twin and adoption studies provide strong evidence for a significant, but not exclusive, genetic contribution to the development of substance use and dependence. Environmental factors, and individual specific experiences, are also of major importance. Family and adoption studies that have focused on general risk for substance use show that substance dependence is a familial trait, which can be attributed to either shared environment or shared genes. Twin studies consistently show higher monozygotic than dizygotic concordance for substance dependence, indicating a genetic effect.

The significant and complex genetic contributions to substance dependence continue to motivate efforts to identify allelic variants that contribute to dependence vulnerability, even if each allelic variant contributes only a modest fraction to the whole problem. Genotypes at loci containing vulnerability alleles could provide improved approaches to treating vulnerable individuals and thus maximize the use of resources for prevention and treatment. Individual and societal suffering could be relieved by better understanding the complex human processes of dependence through careful application of complex genetic approaches.

The two main approaches to estimate genetic and environmental components of phenotypic variance are twin and adoption studies. Twin studies strongly indicate the presence of genetic risk factors for multiple aspects of smoking and alcohol dependence, including initiation, continuation, amount consumed and cessation. Moreover a plethora of studies indicate considerable commonality between tobacco and alcohol dependence, making the identification of both common and substance-unique genetic influences crucial and challenging. In addition to estimating genetic liability, these studies provide further information about environmental contributions, identifying that which is shared (i.e. that which both twins have in common and which contributes to their similarity) and that which is non-shared (contributing to the relative dissimilarity) (Heath, Madden & Martin, 1998; Vanyukov & Tarter, 2000; Jacob et al., 2001).

Table 5.1 Summary of heritability of dependence on selected substances

Substance	Heritability estimates (%)	Linkage	Candidate genes
Nicotine	60–80	Chromosome 5q near D1 receptor loci	CYP2A6 Dopamine D4 receptor Dopamine Beta hydroxylase
Alcohol	52–63	Loci on chromosomes 4q, 6, 1, 7, 2, 11p, 10q	ALDH2 ADH CYP2E1 $GABA_A$ α6, β1, β3, γ2 Dopamine D4 receptor COMT (catechol-O methyltransferase) Serotonin 2A receptor
Opioids	70	None identified	CYP2D6
Combined risk for substance dependence in general	50–80	Loci on chromosome 15, 19q12-13	Dopamine D1 receptor Dopamine D2 receptor Dopamine D4 receptor Monoamine oxidase A

References

Agarwal DP (2001) Genetic polymorphisms of alcohol metabolizing enzymes. *Pathology and Biology* (Paris), **49**:703–709.

Albanese V et al. (2001) Quantitative effects on gene silencing by allelic variation at a tetranucleotide microsatellite. *Human Molecular Genetics*, **10**:1785–1792.

Amad S et al. (2000) Association of D2 dopamine receptor and alcohol dehydrogenase 2 genes with Polynesian alcoholics. *European Psychiatry*, **15**:97–102.

Antonovsky A (1987) *Unraveling the mystery of health: how people manage stress and stay well.* San Francisco, CA, Jossey-Bass.

Arinami T, Ishiguro H, Onaivi ES (2000) Polymorphisms in genes involved in neurotransmission in relation to smoking. *European Journal of Pharmacology*, **410**:215–226.

Bartsch H et al. (2000) Genetic polymorphism of CYP genes, alone or in combination, as a risk modifier of tobacco-related cancers. *Cancer Epidemiology Biomarkers Preview*, **9**:3–28.

Befort K et al. (2001) A single nucleotide polymorphic mutation in the human [micro] -opioid receptor severely impairs receptor signalling. *The Journal of Biological Chemistry*, **276**:3130–3137.

Benowitz NL, Jacob III P, Saunders S (1999) Carbon monoxide, cigarette smoke and CYP2E1 activity [abstract]. *Clinical Pharmacology and Therapeutics*, **63**:154.

Bergen AW et al. (1999) A genome-wide search for loci contributing to smoking and alcohol dependence. *Genetic Epidemiology*, **17**(Suppl.1):S55–S60.

Bierut LJ et al. (1998) Familial transmission of substance dependence: alcohol, marijuana, cocaine, and habitual smoking: a report from the Collaborative Study on the Genetics of Alcoholism. *Archives of General Psychiatry*, **55**:982–988.

Bond C et al. (1998) Single nucleotide polymorphism in the human mu-opioid receptor gene alters beta-endorphin binding and activity: possible implications for opiate addiction. *Proceedings of the National Academy of Science of the United States of America*, **95**:9608–9613.

Bowers BJ (2000) Applications of transgenic and knockout mice in alcohol research. *Alcohol Research and Health*, **24**:175–184.

Bucholz KK, Heath AC, Madden PA (2000) Transitions in drinking in adolescent females: evidence from the Missouri adolescent female twin study. *Alcoholism: Clinical and Experimental Research*, **24**:914–923.

Cadoret RJ et al. (1986) An adoption study of genetic and environmental factors in drug abuse. *Archives of General Psychiatry*, **43**:1131–1136.

Cadoret RJ et al. (1995) Adoption study demonstrating two genetic pathways to drug abuse. *Archives of General Psychiatry*, **52**:42–52.

Capecchi MR (1994) Targeted gene replacement. *Scientific American*, **270**:52–59.

Carmelli D, Heath AC, Robinette D (1993) Genetic analysis of drinking behavior in World War II veteran twins. *Genetic Epidemiology*, **10**:201–213.

Carmelli D et al. (1990) Heritability of substance use in the NAS-NRC Twin Registry. *Acta Geneticae Medicae et Gemellologiae* (Roma), **39**:918.

Carmelli D et al. (1992) Genetic influence on smoking: a study of male twins. *New England Journal of Medicine*, **327**:829–833.

Chao YC et al. (1997) Alcoholism and alcoholic organ damage and genetic polymorphisms of alcohol metabolizing enzymes in Chinese patients. *Hepatology*, **25**:112–117.

Charness ME (1999) Intracranial voyeurism: revealing the mammillary bodies in alcoholism. *Alcoholism: Clinical and Experimental Research*, **23**:1941–1944.

Checkoway H (1998) A genetic polymorphism of MAO-B modifies the association of cigarette smoking and Parkinson's disease. *Neurology*, **50**:1458–1461.

Chen CC et al. (1999) Interaction between the functional polymorphisms of the alcohol-metabolism genes in protection against alcoholism. *American Journal of Human Genetics*, **65**:795–807.

Cheng LS, Swan GE, Carmelli D (2000) A genetic analysis of smoking behavior in family members of older adult males. *Addiction*, **95**:427–435.

Comings DE, Blum K (2000) Reward deficiency syndrome: genetic aspects of behavioral disorders. *Progress in Brain Research*, **126**:325–341.

Comings DE et al. (1996) The dopamine D2 receptor (DRD2) gene: a genetic risk factor in smoking. *Pharmacogenetics*, **6**:73–79.

Comings DE et al. (1997) Studies of the potential role of the dopamine D1 receptor gene in addictive behaviors. *Molecular Psychiatry*, **2**:44–56.

Comings DE et al. (2001) Cholecystokinin (CCK) gene as a possible risk factor for smoking: a replication in two independent samples. *Molecular Genetics and Metabolism*, **73**:349–353.

Connor JP et al. (2002) D2 dopamine receptor (DRD2) polymorphism is associated with severity of alcohol dependence. *European Psychiatry*, **17**:17–23.

Cooper B (2001) Nature, nurture and mental disorder: old concepts in the new millennium. *British Journal of Psychiatry*, **178**(Suppl. 40):S91–S101.

Crabbe JC (2002) Genetic contributions to addiction. *Annual Review of Psychology*, **53**:435–462.

Cravchik A, Gejman PV (1999) Functional analysis of the human D5 dopamine receptor missense and nonsense variants: differences in dopamine binding affinities. *Pharmacogenetics*, **9**:199–206.

Crawley JN, Corwin RL (1994) Biological actions of cholecystokinin. *Peptides*, **15**:731–755.

Crawley JN et al. (1997) Behavioral phenotypes of inbred mouse strains: implications and recommendations for molecular studies. *Psychopharmacology* (Berlin), **132**:107–124.

Daeppen JB et al. (2000) Clinical correlates of cigarette smoking and nicotine dependence in alcohol-dependent men and women: the Collaborative Study Group on the Genetics of Alcoholism. *Alcohol and Alcoholism*, **35**:171–175.

David SP et al. (2002) No association between functional catechol *O*-methyl transferase 1947A>G polymorphism and smoking initiation, persistent smoking or smoking cessation. *Pharmacogenetics*, **12**:265–268.

Duggirala R, Almasy L, Blangero J (1999) Smoking behavior is under the influence of a major quantitative trait locus on human chromosome 5q. *Genetic Epidemiology*, **17** Suppl 1:S139–S144.

Edwards KL, Austin MA, Jarvik GP (1995) Evidence for genetic influences on smoking in adult women twins. *Clinical Genetics*, **47**:236–244.

Enoch MA, Goldman D (2001) The genetics of alcoholism and alcohol abuse. *Current Psychiatry Reports*, 3:144–151.

Epstein JA et al. (1995) The role of social factors and individual characteristics in promoting alcohol use among inner-city minority youths. *Journal of Studies on Alcohol*, **56**:39–46.

Eriksson CJP (2001) The role of acetaldehyde in the actions of alcohol: update 2000. *Alcoholism: Clinical and Experimental Research*, **25** (Suppl):S15–S32.

Fagerstrom KO, Schneider NG (1989) Measuring nicotine dependence: a review of the Fagerstrom Tolerance Questionnaire. *Journal of Behavioral Medicine*, **12**:159–182.

Fairbrother KS et al. (1998) Detection and characterization of novel polymorphisms in the CYP2E1 gene. *Pharmacogenetics*, **8**:543–552.

Fehr C et al. (2000) Sex differences in allelic frequencies of the 5-HT2C Cys23Ser polymorphism in psychiatric patients and healthy volunteers: findings from an association study. *Psychiatric Genetics*, **10**:59–65.

Fehr C et al. (2001) Serotonergic polymorphisms in patients suffering from alcoholism, anxiety disorders and narcolepsy. *Progress in Neuropsychopharmacology and Biological Psychiatry*, **25**:965–982.

Franke P et al. (1999) Human delta-opioid receptor gene and susceptibility to heroin and alcohol dependence. *American Journal of Medical Genetics*, **88**:462–464.

Franke P et al. (2000) DRD4 exon III VNTR polymorphism-susceptibility factor for heroin dependence: results of a case-control and a family-based association approach. *Molecular Psychiatry*, **5**:101–104.

Franke P et al. (2001) Nonreplication of association between mu-opioid receptor gene (OPRM1) A118G polymorphism and substance dependence. *American Journal of Medical Genetics*, **105**:114–119.

Geijer T et al. (1997) Tyrosine hydroxylase and dopamine D4 receptor allelic distribution in Scandinavian chronic alcoholics. *Alcoholism: Clinical and Experimental Research*, **21**:35–39.

George SR et al. (1993) Polymorphisms of the D4 dopamine receptor alleles in chronic alcoholism. *Biochemical and Biophysical Research Communications*, **196**:107–114.

Gianoulakis C (2001) Influence of the endogenous opioid system on high alcohol consumption and genetic predisposition to alcoholism. *Journal of Psychiatry and Neuroscience*, **26**:304–318.

Gora-Maslak G et al. (1991) Use of recombinant inbred strains to identify quantitative trait loci in psychopharmacology. *Psychopharmacology* (Berlin), **104**:413–424.

Gorwood P et al. (2002) Reappraisal of the serotonin 5-HT(1B) receptor gene in alcoholism: of mice and men. *Brain Research Bulletin*, **57**:103–107.

Grant JD et al. (1999) An assessment of the genetic relationship between alcohol metabolism and alcoholism risk in Australian twins of European ancestry. *Behavior Genetics*, **29**:463–472.

Grisel JE (2000) Quantitative trait locus analysis. *Alcohol Research and Health*, **24**:169–174.

Gu DF et al. (2000) The use of long PCR to confirm three common alleles at the CYP2A6 locus and the relationship between genotype and smoking habit. *Annals of Human Genetics*, **64**:383–390.

Han C, McGue MK, Iacono WG (1999a) Lifetime tobacco, alcohol and other substance use in adolescent Minnesota twins: univariate and multivariate behavioral genetic analyses. *Addiction*, **94**:981–993.

Han L et al. (1999b) No coding variant of the tryptophan hydroxylase gene detected in seasonal affective disorder, obsessive–compulsive disorder, anorexia nervosa, and alcoholism. *Biological Psychiatry*, **45**:615–619.

Hasegawa Y et al. (2002) Association of a polymorphism of the serotonin 1B receptor gene and alcohol dependence with inactive aldehyde dehydrogenase-2. *Journal of Neural Transmission*, **109**:513–521.

Heath AC, Martin NG (1993) Genetic models for the natural history of smoking: evidence for a genetic influence on smoking persistence. *Addictive Behaviors*, **18**:19–34.

Heath AC, Martin NG (1994) Genetic influences on alcohol consumption patterns and problem drinking: results from the Australian NH & MRC twin panel follow-up survey. *Annals of the New York Academy of Sciences*, **708**:72–85.

Heath AC, Madden PA, Martin NG (1998) Statistical methods in genetic research on smoking. *Statistical Methods in Medical Research*, **7**:165–186.

Heath AC et al. (1991) The inheritance of alcohol consumption patterns in a general population twin sample. II. Determinants of consumption frequency and quantity consumed. *Journal of Studies on Alcohol*, **52**:425–433.

Heath AC et al. (1995) Personality and the inheritance of smoking behavior: a genetic perspective. *Behavior Genetics*, **25**:103–117.

Heath AC et al. (1997) Genetic and environmental contributions to alcohol dependence risk in a national twin sample: consistency of findings in women and men. *Psychological Medicine*, **27**:1381–1396.

Heath AC et al. (1999a) Genetic and social determinants of initiation and age at onset of smoking in Australian twins. *Behavior Genetics*, **29**:395–407.

Heath AC et al. (1999b) Genetic differences in alcohol sensitivity and the inheritance of alcoholism risk. *Psychological Medicine*, **29**:1069–1081.

Heath AC et al. (2002) Estimating two-stage models for genetic influences on alcohol, tobacco or drug use initiation and dependence vulnerability in twin and family data. *Twin Research*, **5**:113–124.

Heatherton TF et al. (1991) The Fagerstrom Test for Nicotine Dependence: a revision of the Fagerstrom Tolerance Questionnaire. *British Journal of Addiction*, **86**:1119–1127.

Heinz A et al. (2000) Genotype influences in vivo dopamine transporter availability in human striatum. *Neuropsychopharmacology*, **22**:133–139.

Henderson AS et al. (2000) COMT and DRD3 polymorphisms, environmental exposures, and personality traits related to common mental disorders. *American Journal of Medical Genetics*, **96**:102–107.

Henningfield JE, Miyasato K, Jasinski DR (1985) Abuse liability and pharmacodynamic characteristics of intravenous and inhaled nicotine. *Journal of Pharmacology and Experimental Therapeutics*, **234**:1–12.

Hettema JM, Corey LA, Kendler KS (1999) A multivariate genetic analysis of the use of tobacco, alcohol, and caffeine in a population based sample of male and female twins. *Drug and Alcohol Dependence*, **57**:69–78.

Hietala J et al. (1997) Allelic association between D2 but not D1 dopamine receptor gene and alcoholism in Finland. *Psychiatric Genetics*, **7**:19–25.

Hood HM, Buck KJ (2000) Allelic variation in the GABA A receptor gamma2 subunit is associated with genetic susceptibility to ethanol-induced motor incoordination and hypothermia, conditioned taste aversion, and withdrawal in BXD/Ty recombinant inbred mice. *Alcoholism: Clinical and Experimental Research*, **24**:1327–1334.

Hopfer CJ, Stallings MC, Hewitt JK (2001) Common genetic and environmental vulnerability for alcohol and tobacco use in a volunteer sample of older female twins. *Journal of Studies on Alcohol*, **62**:717–723.

Horowitz R et al. (2000) Confirmation of an excess of the high enzyme activity COMT val allele in heroin addicts in a family-based haplotype relative risk study. *American Journal of Medical Genetics*, **96**:599–603.

Howard LA, Sellers EM, Tyndale RF (2002) The role of pharmacogenetically-variable cytochrome P450 enzymes in drug dependence. *Pharmacogenomics*, **3**:185–199.

Howard LA et al. (2001) Low doses of nicotine and ethanol induce CYP2E1 and chlorzoxazone metabolism in rat liver. *Journal of Pharmacology and Experimental Therapeutics*, **299**:542–550.

Hsu YP et al. (1996) Association of monoamine oxidase A alleles with alcoholism among male Chinese in Taiwan. *American Journal of Psychiatry*, **153**:1209–1211.

Hsu YP et al. (1998) Search for mutations near the alternatively spliced 8-amino acid exon in the GABA A receptor gamma2 subunit gene and lack of allelic association with alcoholism among four aboriginal groups and Han Chinese in Taiwan. *Brain Research. Molecular Brain Research*, **56**:284–286.

Hu Y et al. (1999) Structural and functional characterization of the 5'-flanking region of the rat and human cytochrome P450 2E1 genes: identification of a polymorphic repeat in the human gene. *Biochemical and Biophysical Research Communications*, **263**:286–293.

Hutchison KE et al. (2002a) The DRD4 VNTR polymorphism influences reactivity to smoking cues. *Journal of Abnormal Psychology*, **111**:134–143.

Hutchison KE et al. (2002b) The DRD4 VNTR polymorphism moderates craving after alcohol consumption. *Health Psychology*, **21**:139–146.

Hwu HG, Chen CH (2000) Association of 5HT2A receptor gene polymorphism and alcohol abuse with behavior problems. *American Journal of Medical Genetics*, **96**:797–800.

Ishiguro H et al. (1998) Systematic search for variations in the tyrosine hydroxylase gene and their associations with schizophrenia, affective disorders, and alcoholism. *American Journal of Medical Genetics*, **81**:388–396.

Ishiguro H et al. (1999) The 5' region of the tryptophan hydroxylase gene: mutation search and association study with alcoholism. *Journal of Neural Transmission*, **106**:1017–1025.

Ishiguro H et al. (2000) Association study between genetic polymorphisms in the 14-3-3 eta chain and dopamine D4 receptor genes and alcoholism. *Alcoholism: Clinical and Experimental Research*, **24**:343–347.

Iwata N, Virkkunen M, Goldman D (2000) Identification of a naturally occurring Pro385-Ser385 substitution in the GABA(A) receptor alpha6 subunit gene in alcoholics and healthy volunteers. *Molecular Psychiatry*, **5**:316–319.

Iwata N et al. (1998) Identification of a naturally occurring Pro15-Ser15 substitution in the serotonin 5A receptor gene in alcoholics and healthy volunteers. *Molecular Brain Research*, **58**:217–220.

Jacob T et al. (2001) An integrative approach for studying the etiology of alcoholism and other addictions. *Twin Research*, **4**:103–118.

Johnson EO et al. (1998) Extension of a typology of alcohol dependence based on relative genetic and environmental loading. *Alcoholism: Clinical and Experimental Research*, **22**:1421–1429.

Johnstone EC, York EE, Walton RT (2002) Genetic testing: the future of smoking cessation therapy? *Expert Reviews in Molecular Diagnosis*, **2**:60–68.

Kaprio J et al. (1982) Cigarette smoking and alcohol use in Finland and Sweden: a cross-national twin study. *International Journal of Epidemiology*, **11**:378–386.

Kaprio J et al. (1992) Consistency and change in patterns of social drinking: a 6-year follow-up of the Finnish twin cohort. *Alcoholism: Clinical and Experimental Research*, **16**:234–240.

Kauhanen J et al. (2000) Association between the functional polymorphism of catechol-*O*-methyltransferase gene and alcohol consumption among social drinkers. *Alcoholism: Clinical and Experimental Research*, **24**:135–139.

Kendler KS (2001) Twin studies in psychiatric disorders. *Archives of General Psychiatry*, **58**:1005–1014.

Kendler KS, Prescott CA (1998) Cocaine use, abuse and dependence in a population-based sample of female twins. *British Journal of Psychiatry*, **173**:345–350.

Kendler KS, Davis CG, Kessler RC (1997) The familial aggregation of common psychiatric and substance use disorders in the National Comorbidity Survey: a family history study. *British Journal of Psychiatry*, **170**:541–548.

Kendler KS, Thornton LM, Pedersen NL (2000) Tobacco consumption in Swedish twins reared apart and reared together. *Archives of General Psychiatry*, **57**:886–892.

Kendler KS et al. (1994) A twin-family study of alcoholism in women. *American Journal of Psychiatry*, **151**:707–715.

Kendler KS et al. (1999) A population-based twin study in women of smoking initiation and nicotine dependence. *Psychological Medicine*, **29**:299–308.

Kiberstis P, Roberts L (2002) It's not just the genes. *Science*, **296**:685.

Klingemann H et al. (2001) *Promoting self-change from problem substance use. Practical implications for policy, prevention and treatment.* Dordrecht, Kluwer Academic Publishers.

Koopmans JR, van Doornen LJ, Boomsma DI (1997) Association between alcohol use and smoking in adolescent and young adult twins: a bivariate genetic analysis. *Alcoholism: Clinical and Experimental Research*, 21:537–546.

Koopmans JR et al. (1999) The genetics of smoking initiation and quantity smoked in Dutch adolescent and young adult twins. *Behavior Genetics*, 29:383–393.

Kotler M et al. (1997) Excess dopamine D4 receptor (D4DR) exon III seven repeat allele in opioid-dependent subjects. *Molecular Psychiatry*, 2:251–254.

Kranzler HR, Hernandez-Avila CA, Gelernter J (2002) Polymorphism of the 5-HT1B receptor gene (HTR1B): strong within-locus linkage disequilibrium without association to antisocial substance dependence. *Neuropsychopharmacology*, 26:115–122.

Lachman HM et al. (1996) Human catechol-*O*-methyltransferase pharmacogenetics: description of a functional polymorphism and its potential application to neuropsychiatric disorders. *Pharmacogenetics*, 6:243–250.

LaForge KS, Yuferov V, Kreek MJ (2000) Opioid receptor and peptide gene polymorphisms: potential implications for addictions. *European Journal of Pharmacology,* 410:249-268.

Lappalainen J et al. (1998) Linkage of antisocial alcoholism to the serotonin 5-HT1B receptor gene in two populations. *Archives of General Psychiatry*, 55:989–994.

Lappalainen J et al. (1999) HTR2C Cys23Ser polymorphism in relation to CSF monoamine metabolite concentrations and DSM-III-R psychiatric diagnoses. *Biological Psychiatry*, 46:821–826.

Le Y, Sauer B (2000) Conditional gene knockout using cre recombinase. *Methods in Molecular Biology*, 136:477–485.

Lee HC et al. (2001) Association between polymorphisms of ethanol-metabolizing enzymes and susceptibility to alcoholic cirrhosis in a Korean male population. *Journal of Korean Medical Science*, 16:745–750.

Lerman C et al. (1997) Lack of association of tyrosine hydroxylase genetic polymorphism with cigarette smoking. *Pharmacogenetics*, 7:521–524.

Lerman C et al. (2001) Tryptophan hydroxylase gene variant and smoking behavior. *American Journal of Medical Genetics*, 105:518–520.

Li TK (2000) Pharmacogenetics of responses to alcohol and genes that influence alcohol drinking. *Journal of Studies on Alcohol*, 61:5–12.

Li TK et al. (1997) Association analysis of the dopamine D4 gene exon III VNTR and heroin abuse in Chinese subjects. *Molecular Psychiatry*, 2:413–416.

Lin N et al. (1996) The influence of familial and non-familial factors on the association between major depression and substance abuse/dependence in 1874 monozygotic male twin pairs. *Drug and Alcohol Dependence*, 43:49–55.

Lloyd C (1998) Risk factors for problem drug use: identifying vulnerable groups. *Drugs Education, Prevention and Policy*, 5:217–232.

Loh EW, Ball D (2000) Role of the GABA(A)beta2, GABA(A)alpha6, GABA(A)alpha1 and GABA(A)gamma2 receptor subunit genes cluster in drug responses and the development of alcohol dependence. *Neurochemistry International*, 37:413–423.

Loh EW et al. (1999) Association between variants at the GABA(A)beta2, GABA(A)alpha6 and GABA(A)gamma2 gene cluster and alcohol dependence in a Scottish population. *Molecular Psychiatry*, **4**:539–544.

Loh EW et al. (2000) Association analysis of the GABA(A) receptor subunit genes cluster on 5q33-34 and alcohol dependence in a Japanese population. *Molecular Psychiatry*, **5**:301–307.

Long JC et al. (1998) Evidence for genetic linkage to alcohol dependence on chromosomes 4 and 11 from an autosome-wide scan in an American Indian population. *American Journal of Medical Genetics*, **81**:216–221.

Loriot MA et al. (2001) Genetic polymorphisms of cytochrome P450 2A6 in a case-control study on lung cancer in a French population. *Pharmacogenetics*, **11**:39–44.

Lucas D et al. (1995) Cytochrome P450 2E1 genotype and chlorzoxazone metabolism in healthy and alcoholic Caucasian subjects. *Pharmacogenetics*, **5**:298–304.

Luczak SE et al. (2001) Binge drinking in Chinese, Korean, and White college students: genetic and ethnic group differences. *Psychology of Addictive Behaviors*, **15**:306–309.

McCarver DG (1998) A genetic polymorphism in the regulatory sequences of human CYP2E1: association with increased chlorzoxazone hydroxylation in the presence of obesity and ethanol intake. *Toxicology and Applied Pharmacology*, **152**:276–281.

McGue M, Elkins I, Iacono WG (2000) Genetic and environmental influences on adolescent substance use and abuse. *American Journal of Medical Genetics*, **96**:671–677.

McKinney EF et al. (2000) Association between polymorphisms in dopamine metabolic enzymes and tobacco consumption in smokers. *Pharmacogenetics*, **10**:483–491.

Madden PA, Heath AC, Martin NG (1997) Smoking and intoxication after alcohol challenge in women and men: genetic influences. *Alcoholism: Clinical and Experimental Research*, **21**:1732–1741.

Madden PA et al. (1995) Alcohol sensitivity and smoking history in men and women. *Alcoholism: Clinical and Experimental Research*, **19**:1111–1120.

Madden PA et al. (1997) Nicotine withdrawal in women. *Addiction*, **92**:889–902.

Madden PA et al. (1999) The genetics of smoking persistence in men and women: a multicultural study. *Behavior Genetics*, **29**:423–431.

Maes HH et al. (1999) Tobacco, alcohol and drug use in eight- to sixteen-year-old twins: the Virginia Twin Study of Adolescent Behavioral Development. *Journal of Studies on Alcohol*, **60**:293–305.

Maezawa Y et al. (1995) Alcohol-metabolizing enzyme polymorphisms and alcoholism in Japan. *Alcoholism: Clinical and Experimental Research*, **19**:951–954.

Marmot M (1997) Inequality, deprivation and alcohol use. *Addiction*, **92**(Suppl. 1):S13–S20.

Marteau TM, Lerman C (2001) Genetic risk and behavioural change. *British Medical Journal*, **322**:1056–1059.

Maruyama K et al. (1999) Genotypes of alcohol-metabolizing enzymes in relation to alcoholic chronic pancreatitis in Japan. *Alcoholism: Clinical and Experimental Research*, **23**(Suppl 4):S85–S91.

Marzuk PM et al. (1997) Poverty and fatal accidental drug overdoses of cocaine and opiates in New York City: an ecological study. *American Journal of Drug and Alcohol Abuse*, **23**:221–228.

Mayer P, Hollt V (2001) Allelic and somatic variations in the endogenous opioid system of humans. *Pharmacology and Therapeutics*, **91**:167–177.

Mayer P et al. (1997) Association between a delta-opioid receptor gene polymorphism and heroin dependence in man. *Neuroreport*, **8**:2547–2550.

Meller WH et al. (1988) Specific familial transmission in substance abuse. *The International Journal of the Addictions*, **23**:1029–1039.

Merette C et al. (1999) Evidence of linkage in subtypes of alcoholism. *Genetic Epidemiology*, **17**(Suppl. 1):S253–S258.

Merikangas KR et al. (1998) Familial transmission of substance use disorders. *Archives of General Psychiatry*, **55**:973–979.

Merlo Pich E, Chiamulera C, Carboni L (1999) Molecular mechanisms of the positive reinforcing effect of nicotine. *Behavioral Pharmacology*, **10**:587–596.

Messina ES, Tyndale RF, Sellers EM (1997) A major role for CYP2A6 in nicotine C-oxidation by human liver microsomes. *Journal of Pharmacology and Experimental Therapeutics*, **282**:1608–1614.

Michelhaugh SK et al. (2001) The dopamine transporter gene (SLC6A3) variable number of tandem repeats domain enhances transcription in dopamine neurons. *Journal of Neurochemistry*, **79**:1033–1038.

Mihailescu S, Drucker-Colin R (2000) Nicotine, brain nicotinic receptors, and neuropsychiatric disorders. *Archives of Medical Research*, **31**:131–144.

Mikus G et al. (1998) Relevance of deficient CYP2D6 in opiate dependence. *Pharmacogenetics*, **8**:565–568.

Mirin SM et al. (1991) Psychopathology in drug abusers and their families. *Comprehensive Psychiatry*, **32**:36–51.

Miyamoto M et al. (1999) CYP2A6 gene deletion reduces susceptibility to lung cancer. *Biochemical and Biophysical Research Communications*, **261**:658–660.

Muramatsu T et al. (1996) Association between alcoholism and the dopamine D4 receptor gene. *Journal of Medical Genetics*, **33**:113–115.

Nakajima M et al. (1996) Role of human cytochrome P4502A6 in C-oxidation of nicotine. *Drug Metabolism and Disposition*, **24**:1212–1217.

Nakamura A et al. (2001) Association between catechol-*O*-methyltransferase (COMT) polymorphism and severe alcoholic withdrawal symptoms in male Japanese alcoholics. *Addiction Biology*, **6**:233–238.

Nakamura K et al. (1996) Characteristics of Japanese alcoholics with the atypical aldehyde dehydrogenase 2*2. I. A comparison of the genotypes of ALDH2, ADH2,

ADH3, and cytochrome P-4502E1 between alcoholics and nonalcoholics. *Alcoholism: Clinical and Experimental Research*, **20**:52–55.

Nakamura T et al. (1999) Association of a polymorphism of the 5HT2A receptor gene promoter region with alcohol dependence. *Molecular Psychiatry*, 4:85–88.

Narahashi T et al. (2001) Mechanisms of alcohol-nicotine interactions: alcoholics versus smokers. *Alcoholism: Clinical and Experimental Research*, **25**(Suppl. ISBRA):S152–S156.

Neumark YD et al. (1998) Association of the ADH2*2 allele with reduced ethanol consumption in Jewish men in Israel: a pilot study.'*Journal of Studies on Alcohol*, **59**:133–139.

Nielsen DA et al. (1998) A tryptophan hydroxylase gene marker for suicidality and alcoholism. *Archives of General Psychiatry*, **55**:593–602.

Noble EP (2000) Addiction and its reward process through polymorphisms of the D2 dopamine receptor gene: a review. *European Psychiatry*, **15**:79–89.

Noble EP et al. (1998a) D2 dopamine receptor and GABA(A) receptor beta3 subunit genes and alcoholism. *Psychiatry Research*, **81**:133–147.

Noble EP et al. (1998b) D2 and D4 dopamine receptor polymorphisms and personality. *American Journal of Medical Genetics*, **81**:257–267.

Okamoto K et al. (2001) Effect of ALDH2 and CYP2E1 gene polymorphisms on drinking behavior and alcoholic liver disease in Japanese male workers. *Alcoholism: Clinical and Experimental Research*, **25**(Suppl.):S19–S23.

Oneta CM et al. (2002) Dynamics of cytochrome P4502E1 activity in man: induction by ethanol and disappearance during withdrawal phase. *Journal of Hepatology*, **36**:47–52.

Oscarson M et al. (1999) Characterization and PCR-based detection of a CYP2A6 gene deletion found at a high frequency in a Chinese population. *FEBS Letters*, **448**:105–110.

Parsian A, Cloninger CR (1997) Human GABA(A) receptor alpha1 and alpha3 subunits genes and alcoholism. *Alcoholism: Clinical and Experimental Research*, **21**:430–433.

Parsian A, Zhang ZH (1999) Human chromosomes 11p15 and 4p12 and alcohol dependence: possible association with the GABRB1 gene. *American Journal of Medical Genetics*, **88**:533–538.

Parsian A, Cloninger CR (2001) Serotonergic pathway genes and subtypes of alcoholism: association studies. *Psychiatric Genetics*, **11**:89–94.

Parsian A et al. (1995) Monoamine oxidases and alcoholism. I. Studies in unrelated alcoholics and normal controls. *American Journal of Medical Genetics*, **60**:409–416.

Parsian A et al. (1997) No association between polymorphisms in the human dopamine D3 and D4 receptors genes and alcoholism. *American Journal of Medical Genetics*, **74**:281–285.

Pesonen U et al. (1998) Mutation screening of the 5-hydroxytryptamine7 receptor gene among Finnish alcoholics and controls. *Psychiatry Research*, **77**:139–145.

Picciotto MR, Wickman K (1998) Using knockout and transgenic mice to study neurophysiology and behavior. *Physiology Reviews*, **78**:1131–1163.

Prescott CA, Kendler KS (1999) Genetic and environmental contributions to alcohol abuse and dependence in a population-based sample of male twins. *American Journal of Psychiatry*, **156**:34–40.

Prescott CA, Aggen SH, Kendler KS (1999) Sex differences in the sources of genetic liability to alcohol abuse and dependence in a population-based sample of US twins. *Alcoholism: Clinical and Experimental Research*, **23**:1136–1144.

Preuss UW et al. (2001) Impulsive traits and 5-HT2A receptor promoter polymorphism in alcohol dependents: possible association but no influence of personality disorders. *Neuropsychobiology*, **43**:186-191.

Quattrocki E, Baird A, Yurgelun-Todd D (2000) Biological aspects of the link between smoking and depression. *Harvard Review of Psychiatry*, **8**:99–110.

Quinn JP (1996) Neuronal-specific gene expression — the interaction of both positive and negative transcriptional regulators. *Progress in Neurobiology*, **50**:363–379.

Ramchandani VA, Bosron WF, Li TK (2001) Research advances in ethanol metabolism. *Pathology and Biology* (Paris), **49**:676–682.

Rao Y et al. (2000) Duplications and defects in the CYP2A6 gene: identification, genotyping, and in vivo effects on smoking. *Molecular Pharmacology*, **58**:747–755.

Reed T et al. (1994) Correlations of alcohol consumption with related covariates and heritability estimates in older adult males over a 14- to 18-year period: the NHLBI Twin Study. *Alcoholism: Clinical and Experimental Research*, **18**:702–710.

Regev A, Jeffers L (1999) Hepatitis C and alcohol. *Alcoholism: Clinical and Experimental Research*, **23**:1543–1551.

Reich T et al. (1998) Genome-wide search for genes affecting the risk for alcohol dependence. *American Journal of Medical Genetics*, **81**:207–215.

Rose RJ et al. (2001) Drinking or abstaining at age 14? A genetic epidemiological study. *Alcoholism: Clinical and Experimental Research*, **25**:1594–1604.

Russell MAH (1987) Nicotine intake and its regulation by smokers. In: Martin WR et al., eds. *Advances in behavioral biology. Vol. XX. Tobacco, smoking and nicotine.* New York, NY, Plenum Press:25–50.

Saba L et al. (2001) The R100Q mutation of the GABA(A) alpha(6) receptor subunit may contribute to voluntary aversion to ethanol in the sNP rat line. *Molecular Brain Research*, **87**:263–270.

Saccone et al. (2000) A genome screen of maximum number of drinks as an alcoholism phenotype. *American Journal of Medical Genetics*, **96**:632-637.

Samochowiec J et al. (1999) Association of a regulatory polymorphism in the promoter region of the monoamine oxidase A gene with antisocial alcoholism. *Psychiatry Research*, **86**:67–72.

Sander T et al. (1995) Dopamine D1, D2 and D3 receptor genes in alcohol dependence. *Psychiatric Genetics*, **5**:171–176.

Sander T et al. (1999a) Association analysis of sequence variants of GABA(A) alpha6, beta2, and gamma2 gene cluster and alcohol dependence.'*Alcoholism: Clinical and Experimental Research*, **23**:427–431.

Sander T et al. (1999b) Association analysis of exonic variants of the gene encoding the GABA(B) receptor and alcohol dependence. *Psychiatric Genetics*, 9:69–73.

Sander T et al. (2000) Genetic variation of the glutamate transporter EAAT2 gene and vulnerability to alcohol dependence. *Psychiatric Genetics*, 10:103–107.

Sauer B (1998) Inducible gene targeting in mice using the Cre/lox system. *Methods*, 14:381–392.

Schuckit MA (2000) Genetics of the risk for alcoholism. *American Journal of the Addictions*, 9:103–112.

Schuckit MA et al. (1999) Selective genotyping for the role of 5-HT2A, 5-HT2C, and GABA alpha6 receptors and the serotonin transporter in the level of response to alcohol: a pilot study. *Biological Psychiatry*, 45:647–651.

Schmid H (2000) Protektive faktoren. [Protective factors.] In: Uchtenhagen A, Zieglgänsberger W, eds. *Suchtmedizin: konzepte, strategien und therapeutsches management.* [*Addiction medicine: concepts, strategies and therapeutic management.*] Munich, Urban & Fischer Verlag:226–234.

Schmidt LG et al. (2000) Different allele distribution of a regulatory MAOA gene promoter polymorphism in antisocial and anxious–depressive alcoholics. *Journal of Neural Transmission*, 107:681–689.

Sellers EM, Tyndale RF (2000) Mimicking gene defects to treat drug dependence. *Annals of the New York Academy of Sciences*, 909:233–246.

Sellers EM, Kaplan HL, Tyndale RF (2000) Inhibition of cytochrome P4502A6 increases nicotine's oral bioavailability and decreases smoking. *Clinical Pharmacology and Therapeutics*, 68:35–43.

Sellers EM et al. (2002, in press) Inhibiting CYP2A6 decreases smoking and increases the detoxification of the procarcinogen 4-(methylnitrosamino)-(3-pyridyl)-1-butanone (NNK). *Nicotine and Tobacco Research* (in press).

Shea SH et al. (2001) ADH2 and alcohol-related phenotypes in Ashkenazic Jewish American college students. *Behavior Genetics*, 31:231–239.

Shields PG et al. (1998) Dopamine D4 receptors and the risk of cigarette smoking in African- Americans and Caucasians. *Cancer Epidemiology and Biomarkers Preview*, 7:453–458.

Silverman MA et al. (2000) Haplotypes of four novel single nucleotide polymorphisms in the nicotinic acetylcholine receptor beta2 subunit (CHRNB2) gene show no association with smoking initiation or nicotine dependence. *American Journal of Medical Genetics*, 96:646–653.

Singleton AB et al. (1998) Lack of association between the dopamine D2 receptor gene allele DRD2*A1 and cigarette smoking in a United Kingdom population. *Pharmacogenetics*, 8:125–128.

Slutske WS et al. (1999) The heritability of alcoholism symptoms: "indicators of genetic and environmental influence in alcohol-dependent individuals" revisited. *Alcoholism: Clinical and Experimental Research*, 23:759–769.

Spergel DJ et al. (2001) Using reporter genes to label selected neuronal populations in transgenic mice for gene promoter, anatomical, and physiological studies. *Progress in Neurobiology*, 63:673–686.

Stallings MC et al. (1999) A twin study of drinking and smoking onset and latencies from first use to regular use. *Behavior Genetics*, **29**:409–421.

Stoltenberg SF, Burmeister M (2000) Recent progress in psychiatric genetics — some hope but no hype. *Human Molecular Genetics*, **9**:927–935.

Straub RE et al. (1999) Susceptibility genes for nicotine dependence: a genome scan and follow up in an independent sample suggest that regions on chromosomes 2, 4, 10, 16, 17 and 18 merit further study. *Molecular Psychiatry*, **4**:129–144.

Sullivan PF, Kendler KS (1999) The genetic epidemiology of smoking. *Nicotine and Tobacco Research*, **1**(Suppl. 2):S51–S57; S69–S70.

Sullivan PF et al. (2001) Association of the tryptophan hydroxylase gene with smoking initiation but not progression to nicotine dependence. *American Journal of Medical Genetics*, **105**:479–484.

Sun F et al. (1999) Association of genetic polymorphisms of alcohol-metabolizing enzymes with excessive alcohol consumption in Japanese men. *Human Genetics*, **105**:295–300.

Swan GE (1999) Implications of genetic epidemiology for the prevention of tobacco use. *Nicotine and Tobacco Research*, **1**(Suppl. 1):S49–S56.

Swan GE, Carmelli D (1995) Characteristics associated with excessive weight gain after smoking cessation in men. *American Journal of Public Health*, **85**:73–77.

Swan GE, Carmelli D, Cardon LR (1996) The consumption of tobacco, alcohol, and coffee in Caucasian male twins: a multivariate genetic analysis. *Journal of Substance Abuse*, **8**:19–31.

Swan GE, Carmelli D, Cardon LR (1997) Heavy consumption of cigarettes, alcohol and coffee in male twins. *Journal of Studies on Alcohol*, **58**:182–190.

Szeto CY et al. (2001) Association between mu-opioid receptor gene polymorphisms and Chinese heroin addicts. *Neuroreport*, **12**:1103–1106.

Tanaka F et al. (1997) Polymorphism of alcohol-metabolizing genes affects drinking behavior and alcoholic liver disease in Japanese men. *Alcoholism: Clinical and Experimental Research*, **21**:596–601.

Thomasson HR et al. (1994) Low frequency of the ADH2*2 allele among Atayal natives of Taiwan with alcohol use disorders. *Alcoholism: Clinical and Experimental Research*, **18**:640–643.

Tiihonen J et al. (2000) CYP2A6 genotype and smoking. *Molecular Psychiatry*, **5**:347–348.

Tritto T et al. (2001) Potential regulation of nicotine and ethanol actions by alpha4-containing nicotinic receptors. *Alcohol*, **24**:69–78.

True WR et al. (1996) Models of treatment seeking for alcoholism: the role of genes and environment. *Alcoholism: Clinical and Experimental Research*, **20**:1577–1581.

True WR et al. (1999) Common genetic vulnerability for nicotine and alcohol dependence in men. *Archives of General Psychiatry*, **56**:655–661.

Tsuang MT et al. (1996) Genetic influences on DSM-III-R drug abuse and dependence: a study of 3,372 twin pairs. *American Journal of Medical Genetics*, **67**:473–477.

Tsuang MT et al. (1999) Genetic and environmental influences on transitions in drug use. *Behavior Genetics*, **29**:473–479.

Tsuang MT et al. (2001) The Harvard Twin Study of Substance Abuse: what we have learned. *Harvard Review of Psychiatry*, **9**:267–279.

Tyndale RF, Sellers EM (2002) Genetic variation in CYP2A6-mediated nicotine metabolism alters smoking behavior. *Therapeutic Drug Monitoring*, **24**:163–171.

Tyndale RF, Droll KP, Sellers EM (1997) Genetically deficient CYP2D6 metabolism provides protection against oral opiate dependence. *Pharmacogenetics*, **7**:375–379.

Tyndale RF et al. (2002) CYP2A6 lower activity genotypes are associated with decreased risk for smoking and varying frequency among ethnic groups. In: *Microsomes and drug oxidations*. Sapporo, Japan: International Symposium on Microsomes and Drug Oxidations:150.

Uchtenhagen A (2000a) Determinanten für drogenkonsum und –abhängigkeit. [Determinants of drug use and addiction.] In: Uchtenhagen A, Zieglgänsberger W, eds. *Suchtmedizin: konzepte, strategien und therapeutsches management. [Addiction medicine: concepts, strategies and therapeutic management.]* Munich, Urban & Fischer Verlag:193–195.

Uchtenhagen A (2000b) Risikofaktoren und schutzfaktoren: eine übersicht. [Risk and protective factors: an overview.] In: Uchtenhagen A, Zieglgänsberger W, eds. *Suchtmedizin: konzepte, strategien und therapeutsches management. [Addiction medicine: concepts, strategies and therapeutic management.]* Munich, Urban & Fischer Verlag:195–198.

Ueno Y et al. (1996) Effect of the cytochrome P450IIE1 genotype on ethanol elimination rate in alcoholics and control subjects. *Alcoholism: Clinical and Experimental Research*, **20**(Suppl. 1):A17–A21.

Uhl GR et al. (1998) Dopaminergic genes and substance abuse. *Advances in Pharmacology*, **42**:1024–1032.

Vaccarino FJ (1994) Nucleus accumbens dopamine-CCK interactions in psycho-stimulant reward and related behaviors. *Neuroscience and Biobehavioral Reviews*, **18**:207–214.

Vandenbergh DJ et al. (1997) High-activity catechol-*O*-methyltransferase allele is more prevalent in polysubstance abusers. *American Journal of Medical Genetics*, **74**:439–442.

Vandenbergh DJ et al. (2000) Long forms of the dopamine receptor (DRD4) gene VNTR are more prevalent in substance abusers: no interaction with functional alleles of the catechol-*o*-methyltransferase (COMT) gene. *American Journal of Medical Genetics*, **96**:678–683.

van den Bree MB, Svikis DS, Pickens RW (1998a) Genetic influences in antisocial personality and drug use disorders. *Drug and Alcohol Dependence*, **49**:177–187.

van den Bree MB et al. (1998b) Genetic analysis of diagnostic systems of alcoholism in males. *Biological Psychiatry*, **43**:139–145.

Vanyukov MM, Tarter RE (2000) Genetic studies of substance abuse. *Drug and Alcohol Dependence*, **59**:101–123.

Vanyukov MM et al. (1995) Preliminary evidence for an association of a dinucleo-tide repeat polymorphism at the MAOA gene with early onset alcoholism/substance abuse. *American Journal of Medical Genetics*, **60**:122–126.

Vanyukov MM et al. (2000) Antisociality, substance dependence, and the DRD5 gene: a preliminary study. *American Journal of Medical Genetics*, **96**:654–658.

Veenstra-van der Weele J, Anderson GM, Cook EH Jr (2000) Pharmacogenetics and the serotonin system: initial studies and future directions. *European Journal of Pharmacology*, **410**:165–181.

Viken RJ et al. (1999) Longitudinal analyses of the determinants of drinking and of drinking to intoxication in adolescent twins. *Behavior Genetics*, **29**:455–461.

Vogt I (2000a) Risikoperioden im lebenszyklus. [Risk periods in the life cycle.] In: Uchtenhagen A, Zieglgänsberger W, eds. *Suchtmedizin: konzepte, strategien und therapeutsches management. [Addiction medicine: concepts, strategies and therapeutic management.]* Munich, Urban & Fischer Verlag:212–215.

Vogt I (2000b) Geschlechtsspezifische gefährdungen. [Gender specific dangers.] In: Uchtenhagen A, Zieglgänsberger W, eds. *Suchtmedizin: konzepte, strategien und therapeutsches management. [Addiction medicine: concepts, strategies and therapeutic management.]* Munich, Urban & Fischer Verlag:215–219.

Wall TL et al. (2000) Hangover symptoms in Asian Americans with variations in the aldehyde dehydrogenase (ALDH2) gene. *Journal of Studies on Alcohol*, **61**:13–17.

Wahlsten D (1999) Single-gene influences on brain and behavior. *Annual Review of Psychology*, **50**:599–624.

Wand GS et al. (2002) The mu-opioid receptor gene polymorphism (A118G) alters HPA axis activation induced by opioid receptor blockade. *Neuropsycho-pharmacology*, **26**:106–114.

Watanabe J, Hayashi S, Kawajiri K (1994) Different regulation and expression of the human CYP2E1 gene due to the RsaI polymorphism in the 5'-flanking region. *Journal of Biochemistry* (Tokyo), **116**:321–326.

Weathermon R, Crabb D (1999) Alcohol and medication interactions. *Alcohol Health and Research World*, **23**:40–54.

Whitfield JB et al. (1998) ADH genotypes and alcohol use and dependence in Europeans. *Alcoholism: Clinical and Experimental Research*, **22**:1463–1469.

Yang M et al. (2001) Individual differences in urinary cotinine levels in Japanese smokers: relation to genetic polymorphism of drug-metabolizing enzymes. *Cancer Epidemiology and Biomarkers Preview*, **10**:589–593.

Yoshihara E et al. (2000a) The effects of the ALDH2*1/2, CYP2E1 C1/C2 and C/D genotypes on blood ethanol elimination. *Drug and Chemical Toxicology*, **23**:371–379.

Yoshihara E et al. (2000b) The human serotonin receptor gene (HTR2) MspI polymorphism in Japanese schizophrenic and alcoholic patients. *Neuro-psychobiology*, **41**:124–126.

Zhang X et al. (2001) Lack of association between smoking and CYP2A6 gene polymorphisms in a Japanese population. *Nihon Arukoru Yakubutsu Igakkai Zasshi*, **36**:486–490.

Zimprich A et al. (2000) An allelic variation in the human prodynorphin gene promoter alters stimulus-induced expression. *Journal of Neurochemistry*, **74**:472–477.

CHAPTER 6

Concurrent Disorders

Introduction

Over the past decade, there has been increasing awareness that there is a high degree of comorbidity (co-occurrence in the same individual) between various psychiatric disorders. That is, individuals with a history of one psychiatric disorder are much more likely than would be expected by chance to have a history of another psychiatric disorder (Robins & Regier, 1991; Kessler et al., 1994). Most relevant to this report are data indicating that there is high comorbidity between any mental disorder and substance dependence. Specifically, these data indicate that:

- Lifetime prevalence of alcohol disorder is 22.3% for individuals with any mental disorder compared to 14% for the general population, and that the odds of having an alcohol disorder if a person also has any mental disorder are 2.3 times higher than if there is no mental disorder (Regier et al., 1990).

- Among people with substance (except alcohol) use disorders, 53% also suffer from at least one other mental disorder, with an odds ratio of 4.5 when compared to people without substance (other than alcohol) disorders (Regier et al., 1990).

- Higher percentages of people with mental illness, particularly those with schizophrenia, smoke tobacco than in the general population and among people without mental illness. Depending on the particular mental illness, it has been reported that 26–88% of psychiatric patients smoke compared to 20–30% of the general population (Glassman et al., 1990; Breslau, 1995; Hughes et al., 1986).

Despite the fact that the majority of studies were undertaken in a few developed countries and the degree of comorbidity in many cultures is vastly unknown, this high degree of comorbidity between mental disorders and substance use disorders strongly suggests that these disorders are linked because of shared neurobiological and behavioural abnormalities. Although most scientists and clinicians would agree with this suggestion, it remains unclear as to what the causal factors are. That is, does mental illness lead to substance dependence, or does substance dependence lead to mental illness, or are both mental illness and substance dependence independent symptomatic manifestations of the same underlying neuropathologies? These are topics of considerable recent interest and research at both the clinical and preclinical levels.

The purpose of this chapter is to present several hypotheses that may explain the high degree of comorbidity between mental illness and substance dependence. Emphasis will be placed on the comorbidity of schizophrenia and depression with illicit drug dependence, tobacco smoking and alcohol use, with particular reference to dependence on psychostimulants and tobacco. Schizophrenia and depression were selected on the basis of high societal and economic costs of these two disorders (Rupp & Keith, 1993; Mauskopf et al., 1999; Meltzer, 1999; Wong & Licinio, 2001), and on the fact that they appear to be highly associated with substance use disorders. Generally, research findings over the past decade will be highlighted, although older findings will also be referred to where relevant. Finally, directions for future clinical and preclinical research will be discussed, as well as considerations for treatment and prevention of substance use disorders.

It is also important to recognize that the effects of many psychoactive substances can produce psychiatric-like syndromes. For example, as discussed in Chapter 4, amphetamines and cocaine can induce psychotic-like symptoms, and some drugs can produce hallucinations, which are an aspect of some psychoses. Furthermore, psychoactive substances alter mood states, producing either euphoria and feelings of well-being, or inducing depression, especially during substance withdrawal. Psychoactive substances can alter cognitive functioning, which is also a core feature of many mental illnesses. These factors all suggest common neurobiological mechanisms to both mental illnesses and substance dependence.

Research into the comorbidity of mental illness with substance dependence will provide new insights into both disorders, and may provide improved treatment and prevention strategies for both disorders independently, and when they co-occur. Research in developing countries, among the general population, and among people seeking or receiving treatment is also of extreme importance for better understanding the relationship between biological and environmental factors related to comorbidity.

Hypotheses that may explain the observed comorbidity

As discussed above, the high comorbidity between any mental illness and substance dependence in humans in certain populations (Rounsaville et al., 1982; Robins et al., 1984; Rounsaville et al., 1987; Robins & Regier, 1991; Rounsaville et al., 1991; Kessler et al., 1994; Kosten, Markou & Koob, 1998) is likely to reflect similarities in the neurobiology of these psychiatric disorders.

Four neurobiological hypotheses can be postulated to explain this comorbidity.

1. Psychoactive substance use disorders and other mental illnesses are different symptomatic expressions of the same pre-existing neurobiological abnormalities.
2. Repeated substance administration leads – through possibly aberrant or excessive neuroadaptations to acute substance effects – to biological changes that have some common elements with the abnormalities mediating other mental illnesses, such as depression.
3. Psychoactive substance use may reflect self-medication intended to reverse some of the abnormalities associated with mental illness; these abnormalities may have existed prior to substance use or may have been caused by the substance use. This hypothesis is related closely to, and is not independent of, the second hypothesis.
4. Substance dependence and other mental illnesses have different and independent neurobiological mechanisms, and the observed comorbidity is simply observed by chance. However, this hypothesis is unlikely, considering the extensive epidemiological and neurobiological data indicating the contrary.

There are also other possible non-neurobiological reasons for this comorbidity, such as a common environmental factor; however, a detailed discussion of these factors is beyond the scope of this report, which focuses on neurobiological mechanisms. There is also strong neurobiological and genetic evidence that at least some of the association has a neurobiological basis, as discussed below.

It should be emphasized that the first three hypotheses are not necessarily mutually exclusive: the first hypothesis may be true for one mental disorder and one substance, while the second and third hypotheses may be true for another disorder and another substance. Indeed, current neurobiological and clinical data are consistent with the notion that different hypotheses may be true for different mental disorders, as discussed below. Furthermore, the first three hypotheses may be true in a single patient population. That is, a particular mental illness and substance use disorder originally may be symptomatic expressions of the same underlying neurobiological abnormalities; while at the same time substance use may temporarily relieve some symptoms (i.e. through self-medication), although in the long term the same substance use may worsen the overall severity of the mental disorder. These hypotheses will be explored in the context of schizophrenia and depression.

Schizophrenia

Tobacco smoking and schizophrenia

There is a high degree of comorbidity of schizophrenia with tobacco smoking. Where it has been studied, the prevalence of smoking among individuals with schizophrenia is 2–3 times higher than that in the general population and considerably higher than the prevalence among any other psychiatric population (Masterson & O'Shea, 1984; Goff, Henderson & Amico, 1992; de Leon et al., 1995; Hughes, 1996). Estimates indicate that in some countries, more than 80–90% of patients with schizophrenia smoke, compared to 20–30% in the general population (Masterson & O'Shea, 1984; Goff, Henderson & Amico, 1992; de Leon et al., 1995; Hughes, 1996; Diwan et al., 1998). Furthermore, individuals with schizophrenia are commonly heavy smokers (defined as an individual smoking more than 1.5 packs of cigarettes per day), smoke high-tar cigarettes (which are also high in nicotine content), and extract more nicotine from cigarettes than smokers without schizophrenia (Masterson & O'Shea, 1984; Hughes et al., 1986; Olincy, Young & Freedman, 1997).

Hypotheses to explain the high incidence of cigarette smoking among patients with schizophrenia

The first hypothesis postulates that the high prevalence of cigarette smoking among patients with schizophrenia reflects an attempt to reduce neuroleptic-induced side-effects, such as Parkinsonism (difficulty initiating movements) and tardive dyskinesias (explained below) (Jarvik, 1991). Schizophrenia is associated with excessive activity in mesolimbic and mesocortical dopamine pathways (see Chapter 2). Neuroleptic drugs used to treat schizophrenia block dopamine receptors; however, they block both the affected pathways (mesolimbic, mesocortical) as well as unaffected pathways such as the nigrostriatal pathway which is involved in motor function. Therefore, neuroleptic medications can lead to side-effects such as Parkinsonism. Long-term use of neuroleptics can also lead to side-effects associated with the changes in the brain that occur in response to long-term blockade of dopamine receptors, such as an increase in the number or sensitivity of these receptors. Such changes result in excessive involuntary movements, most often in the mouth and facial area and extremities, called tardive dyskinesias. Anecdotal evidence indicates that a small proportion of patients with schizophrenia report that smoking helps reduce the side-effects of their antipsychotic medication (Glynn & Sussman, 1990). Patients with schizophrenia who are smokers are usually prescribed higher levels of neuroleptic medication compared with nonsmokers (Goff, Henderson & Amico, 1992; Ziedonis et al., 1994) because cigarette smoking increases the metabolism of these medications. This change in metabolism is caused not by nicotine but by the "tar" (polynuclear aromatic hydrocarbons) in cigarettes that induces hepatic microsomal enzymes (Glassman, 1993; Ziedonis et al., 1994). Results from studies on smoking and the side-effects of antipsychotic medications have been mixed, with reports of increased side-effects, decreased side-effects, and no change in side-effects (Binder et al., 1987; Yassa et al., 1987; Decina et al., 1990; Menza et al., 1991; Goff, Henderson & Amico,

1992; Sandyk, 1993; Ziedonis et al., 1994). Nicotine could help to decrease these side-effects through its stimulatory effects on dopamine, and it could also reduce them through its effects on acetylcholine, which acts in the basal ganglia (see Chapter 2) and other brain areas to help coordinate movements. However, the exact mechanism is not currently known. This will be discussed in more detail at the end of this section.

The second hypothesis regarding tobacco dependence and schizophrenia postulates that nicotine administration through tobacco smoking ameliorates the sensory gating deficits and perhaps even more generalized cognitive deficits (Dalack, Healy & Meador-Woodruff, 1998) that are characteristic of patients with schizophrenia. (Freedman et al., 1997). Again, the exact mechanisms responsible for this are not currently known, but the stimulatory effects of nicotine on dopaminergic and cholinergic systems are strong candidates.

The third hypothesis postulates that nicotine administration through tobacco smoking ameliorates the negative symptoms of schizophrenia that are most resistant to the majority of currently available antipsychotic treatments (Marder, Wirshing & Van Putten, 1991; Dalack, Healy & Meador-Woodruff, 1998; Jibson & Tandon, 1998; Moller, 1998). Schizophrenia is characterized by the so-called positive and negative symptoms (American Psychiatric Association, 1994). Positive symptoms reflect an excess or distortion of normal functions, such as hallucinations, delusions and disorganized thought and speech. Negative symptoms reflect a diminution or loss of normal functions, such as loss of pleasure in normally pleasurable activities, loss of motivation, reluctance to speak or impoverished speech, and flattening of emotions. These symptoms appear to result from alterations in reward and motivational processes associated with mesolimbic and mesocortical dopamine. Accruing clinical evidence over the past decade provides some support for the hypothesis that patients with schizophrenia self-medicate negative symptoms with cigarette smoking (Marder, Wirshing & Van Putten, 1991; Dalack, Healy & Meador-Woodruff, 1998; Jibson & Tandon, 1998; Moller, 1998). In a study of 182 patients with schizophrenia, heavy smokers had significantly fewer negative symptoms than non-smokers with schizophrenia (Ziedonis et al., 1994). Further, patients with negative symptoms were less likely to quit smoking than other schizophrenia patients who exhibited few negative symptoms, while no such relationship was shown for positive symptoms and smoking cessation (Hall et al., 1995). Interestingly, patients treated with atypical antipsychotic drugs such as clozapine, risperidone and olanzapine, which are considered to be more effective against the negative symptoms than traditional neuroleptic antipsychotic medications such as haloperidol (Claghorn et al., 1987), reduced their smoking by 25–30% compared with patients who received traditional typical medications (George et al., 1995; McEvoy et al., 1995; McEvoy et al., 1999; George et al., 2000). If indeed atypical antipsychotic drugs are more effective against the negative symptoms than neuroleptic medications (Claghorn et al., 1987), this may reflect diminished need to self-medicate negative symptoms with cigarette smoking after the more efficacious treatment of these symptoms with atypical antipsychotics. This may also be related to the fact that atypical antipsychotics do not stay on the dopamine D2 receptor as long as do the traditional neuroleptics, thereby allowing more physiological dopamine transmission (Kapur & Seeman, 2001). Thus atypical antipsychotics do not have as many side-effects, and the need for nicotine to reduce these side-effects is decreased. Taken together, the above results suggest that nicotine has a beneficial effect on negative symptoms in patients with schizophrenia, and this effect may be one of the reasons why these patients smoke excessively. The most likely neurobiological mechanism for this effect is the increase in dopaminergic and cholinergic function in the brain. Further research on this subject is necessary to determine the exact mechanisms that will provide insight into the etiology and treatment of both schizophrenia and nicotine dependence.

Although the available clinical data do not offer support for one versus the other two interpretations for reduced smoking with atypical antipsychotic medications, such findings have led to promising speculations that these medications "may play a unique role in the treatment of substance-using patients with schizophrenia" for reasons that are poorly understood (Wilkins, 1997; Krystal et al., 1999; McEvoy, Freudenreich & Wilson, 1999). In addition, as indicated above, patients with schizophrenia may smoke for improvement in all three domains, that is negative symptoms, cognitive deficits, and extrapyramidal side-effects induced by neuroleptic medications. Finally, it must be emphasized that the degree of comorbidity between smoking and schizophrenia will also depend on the levels of smoking in the general population of a given country. Comparative international studies are needed to clarify the relative role of neurobiology and environment on comorbidity between smoking and schizophrenia.

Psychostimulant (cocaine and amphetamine) dependence and schizophrenia

There is a high degree of comorbidity between schizophrenia and psychostimulant use in countries with high high rates of cocaine and amphetamine use. Psychostimulant use is 2–5 times higher among patients with schizophrenia compared with the general population, and more prevalent than in other psychiatric populations (LeDuc & Mittleman, 1995). It was estimated that 19–50% of patients with schizophrenia use psychostimulant drugs (Cuffel, 1992; Ziedonis et al., 1992; LeDuc & Mittleman, 1995; Patkar et al., 1999). Interestingly, however, patients with schizophrenia appear to prefer psychostimulants to psychoactive substances with sedative properties, such as opiates, barbiturates and alcohol (Schneier & Siris, 1987; Dixon et al., 1990; Mueser et al., 1990). Certain symptoms of psychostimulant withdrawal also resemble the

negative symptoms of schizophrenia (American Psychiatric Association, 1994; Markou, Kosten & Koob, 1998; Green et al., 1999; Ellenbroek & Cools, 2000). Together, these observations have led to several hypotheses that attempt to explain the high incidence of psychostimulant use among patients with schizophrenia. These hypotheses are not mutually exclusive and parallel those postulated to explain the high incidence of tobacco smoking among patients with schizophrenia. The commonalities in these hypotheses are not surprising considering that cocaine and amphetamine are psychomotor stimulant drugs, and nicotine is considered also to be a relatively mild psychostimulant.

Hypotheses to explain the high rate of psychostimulant use among patients with schizophrenia

The first hypothesis postulates that the high rate of psychostimulant use among patients with schizophrenia reflects an attempt to reduce the unpleasant side-effects of chronic neuroleptic treatment, including the motor side-effects (Schneier & Siris, 1987; Robinson et al., 1991). The reasons for this are likely to be the same as for nicotine. Briefly, since neuroleptic drugs block dopamine, and excessive dopamine blockade results in motor and other side-effects, the use of substances that increase dopamine function may provide relief from such effects.

The second hypothesis postulates that administration of psychostimulants ameliorates the cognitive deficits associated with schizophrenia (Cesarec & Nyman, 1985; Krystal et al., 1999). Again, the mechanism of this effect is likely to be through increasing mesolimbic and mesocortical dopamine transmission; however, there is very little evidence in support of, or against, these two hypotheses.

The third hypothesis postulates that administration of psychostimulants ameliorates the negative symptoms of schizophrenia that are most resistant to the majority of currently available antipsychotic treatments (Khantzian, 1985, 1997; Schneier & Siris, 1987; Dixon et al., 1990; Sevy et al., 1990; Rosenthal, Hellerstein & Miner, 1994; Krystal et al., 1999). Experimental studies over several decades in humans have clearly indicated that although acute amphetamine administration exacerbates the positive symptoms of schizophrenia, chronic administration diminishes the negative symptoms (Angrist, Rotrosen & Gershon, 1980, 1982; Desai et al., 1984; Khantzian, 1985; van Kammen & Boronow, 1988; LeDuc & Mittleman, 1995; Sanfilipo et al., 1996; Krystal et al. 1999). Furthermore, patients with schizophrenia who use psychostimulants exhibit less severe negative symptoms than patients who do not (Dixon et al., 1991; Soni & Brownlee, 1991; Buckley et al., 1994; Lysaker et al., 1994). Interestingly, clozapine, a neuroleptic drug that helps reduce the negative symptoms of schizophrenia, reduced substance use, including psychostimulant use, in more than 85% of the patients, and prevented re-initiation of substance use (Zimmet et al., 2000).

Alcohol use and schizophrenia

Similar links are also observed between schizophrenia and alcohol dependence as those between schizophrenia and nicotine or psychostimulant use. As reported in one large study, an individual with alcohol dependence is 3.3 times more likely to also have schizophrenia, while a patient with schizophrenia is 3.8 times more likely to exhibit alcohol dependence than in the general population (Regier et al., 1990). Nonetheless, it is not clear what the factors leading to this comorbidity are, and few hypotheses have been advanced to explain this association.

Hypotheses to explain the high rate of alcohol use among patients with schizophrenia

As with other psychoactive substances, it has been suggested that alcohol use may be self-medication for symptoms of schizophrenia; however, the available data do not support this self-medication hypothesis. Most clinical studies, patient reports and anecdotal clinical observations indicate that excessive use of alcohol leads to a clear exacerbation of schizophrenia symptomatology (Soyka, 1994; Tsuang & Lohr 1994; Pristach & Smith, 1996; Gerding et al., 1999). Furthermore, it appears that approximately 30% of comorbid patients show harmful use of alcohol before the first signs of schizophrenia emerge (Hambrecht & Hafner, 1996). In terms of schizophrenia and alcohol dependence, the hypothesis that best explains the available data is that alcohol dependence and schizophrenia are different symptomatic expressions of the same underlying neurobiological abnormalities, with alcohol use exacerbating symptoms of schizophrenia. The precise nature of the neurobiological basis of this association is not known, but more research will help to clarify the epidemiology, etiology and treatment of schizophrenia and alcohol dependence. Hypotheses regarding the neurobiological basis of this association are discussed below.

Neurobiological interactions between schizophrenia and the effects of psychoactive substances

There are several brain systems where schizophrenia-related abnormalities and the effects of psychoactive substances may interact to lead to the high degree of comorbidity of schizophrenia with substance dependence. One of these systems is the mesolimbic dopamine system together with its efferent and afferent connections to other brain sites and systems. This system is comprised of dopaminergic projections from an area in the midbrain, called the ventral tegmental area (VTA), to the forebrain region of the nucleus accumbens (also called the ventral striatum) (Mogenson et al., 1980) (see Chapter 2). There is considerable evidence that increased activity of the mesolimbic dopamine system is critically involved in mediating the rewarding effects of most psychoactive substances (Koob, 1992; Koob et al., 1993; Wise, 1998), and possibly drug craving (Markou et al., 1993; Self, 1998; Kilts et al., 2001), although "memory" systems may also be critically involved in craving and dependence (Holden, 2001; Vorel et al., 2001) (see Chapter 3). It has been shown that administration of most psychoactive substances, such as cocaine, amphetamine, nicotine and opioids, increases dopamine levels in the nucleus accumbens (e.g. DiChiara et al., 1999) (see Chapters 3 and 4). Moreover, similar increases in dopamine levels are seen in the amygdala, a limbic brain site believed to be involved in the rewarding effects of psychoactive substances and interconnected with the nucleus accumbens. Increased functioning of the mesolimbic dopamine system has long been implicated in the pathophysiology of schizophrenia (Snyder, 1976; Carlsson, 1977). Neuroleptic antipsychotic medications are dopamine receptor antagonists, and thus, their therapeutic effects are believed to involve dampening of an overactive dopaminergic system (Carlsson, 1978). Consistent with this notion is the finding that administration of high doses of psychostimulant drugs that increase dopamine levels in the nucleus accumbens can induce a transient psychotic state in healthy individuals (Bell, 1965; Angrist & Gershon, 1970; Griffith et al., 1972). Thus it has been argued that the overactive dopamine systems, or hyperdopaminergia, of patients with schizophrenia renders them more likely to seek and use psychoactive substances, and to be more susceptible to their rewarding effects (Chambers, Krystal & Self, 2001).

In addition, developmental abnormalities in the hippocampus and the prefrontal cortex associated with schizophrenia may further contribute to the malfunctioning of the nucleus accumbens system (Chambers, Krystal & Self, 2001). There is accruing evidence that patients with schizophrenia exhibit a disruption in the distribution of cells in the hippocampus (Scheibel & Conrad, 1993; Fatemi, Earle & McMenomy, 2000; Webster et al., 2001), and reductions in hippocampal volume (Bogerts et al., 1993; Razi et al., 1999; Heckers, 2001; Rajarethinam et al., 2001). In the healthy brain, glutamate projections from the hippocampus and the prefrontal cortex have been shown to modulate both the activity of dopamine neurons in the nucleus accumbens (together with inputs from other brain sites such as the amygdala, the thalamus and the entorhinal cortex) and the behavioural output of the nucleus accumbens (Wilkinson et al., 1993; Grace, 1995; Finch, 1996; Blaha et al., 1997; Mittleman, Bratt & Chase, 1998; Legault, Rompre & Wise, 2000). It is hypothesized that in schizophrenia there is malfunction of the normal inhibitory glutamatergic control exerted by projections from the hippocampus and the prefrontal cortex on the nucleus accumbens, resulting in increased drug-seeking and drug-taking behaviour. That is, the neuropathology of schizophrenia may contribute to the vulnerability to substance use, and eventually dependence, by increasing the sensitivity of patients with schizophrenia to the positive rewarding effects of psychoactive substances. In support of this hypothesis preliminary data indicated that patients with schizophrenia exhibited more intense craving for cocaine during the first three days of abstinence compared with cocaine users who do not have schizophrenia (Carol et al., 2001). The above theoretical conceptualization is consistent with the first hypothesis discussed at the beginning of this chapter; that schizophrenia and substance dependence are different symptomatic expressions of the same neuropathology.

In addition to excess dopamine function in mesolimbic and mesocortical brain regions, another neurobiological abnormality that characterizes schizophrenia is decreased functioning of cortical dopaminergic systems. It has been suggested that this hypofrontality contributes to the cognitive deficits associated with schizophrenia (Knable & Weinberger, 1997; Dalack, Healy & Meador-Woodruff, 1998; Hazlett et al., 2000). Atypical antipsychotic medications that are relatively effective in ameliorating the cognitive deficits in patients with schizophrenia also increase dopamine activity in the frontal cortex (Nomikos et al., 1994; Meltzer, Park & Kessler, 1999; Pallanti, Quercioli & Pazzagli, 1999; Rowley et al., 2000; Cuesta, Peralta & Zarzuela, 2001; Harvey & Keefe, 2001). Increases in the functioning of the cortical dopaminergic system can also be induced through administration of a variety of psychoactive substances that are used by patients with schizophrenia. Specifically, psychostimulants such as amphetamine, cocaine and nicotine increase dopamine levels in the frontal cortex (Sorg & Kalivas, 1993; Marshall et al., 1997; Tanda et al., 1997; Beyer & Steketee 2000; Balla et al., 2001). Indeed, it has been shown that nicotine administration through tobacco smoking ameliorated some cognitive deficits of patients with schizophrenia (George et al., 2002), which have been shown to involve activation of the prefrontal cortex (Funahashi & Kubota, 1994; Goldman-Rakic, 1995; Kikuchi-Yorioka & Sawagushi, 2000; Manoach et al., 2000). In conclusion, the above speculation that psychoactive substances increase the functioning of the frontal cortex, and thus lead to improved cognitive function in patients with schizophrenia is consistent with a self-medication hypothesis of comorbidity of schizophrenia with substance dependence.

Another neurotransmitter system that has recently been strongly implicated in both schizophrenia and substance dependence is the glutamatergic system. It has been hypothesized that alterations in glutamatergic neurotransmission are critically involved in the mediation of schizophrenia symptoms, based on the well-established observation that phencyclidine (PCP) administration induces both positive and negative symptoms of schizophrenia in PCP users and human volunteers, and exacerbates both positive and negative symptoms in patients with schizophrenia resembling an acute psychotic episode (Allen & Young, 1978; Snyder, 1980; Javitt & Zukin, 1991; Duncan, Sheitman & Lieberman, 1999; Jentsch & Roth, 1999). PCP is a non-competitive antagonist at the N-methyl-D-aspartate (NMDA) receptor (Lodge & Johnson, 1990) (see Chapter 4). PCP-induced psychosis can last for weeks despite abstinence (Allen & Young, 1978; Luisada 1978). Similarly, ketamine, a PCP analogue that exhibits higher selectivity than PCP for the NMDA receptor (Lodge & Johnson, 1990), also induces psychosis-like effects in healthy volunteers (Newcomer et al., 1999), and exacerbates symptoms in patients with schizophrenia (Lahti et al., 1995; Malhotra et al., 1997). Based on the above, it is speculated that decreased glutamatergic actions at NMDA receptors may mediate symptoms of psychosis. In support of the argument that PCP- and ketamine-induced psychoses are neurobiologically similar to schizophrenia, data exist showing that PCP and ketamine effects are reversed by atypical antipsychotic medications in both humans and in animal subjects (Malhotra et al., 1997), but not by the typical neuroleptic haloperidol (Lahti et al., 1995).

If decreased glutamatergic neurotransmission is involved in schizophrenia, then the administration of psychoactive substances such as cocaine, amphetamine and nicotine would reverse this deficit by acutely enhancing glutamatergic neurotransmission in limbic areas. It has been shown that administration of NMDA receptor antagonists together with psychoactive substances blocks the development of behavioural sensitization (see Chapter 3) to the locomotor-activating effects of psychoactive substances, such as cocaine (Kalivas & Alesdatter, 1993; Wolf & Jeziorski, 1993) and nicotine (Shoaib & Stolerman, 1992); and the development and/or expression of dependence on opioids (Gonzalez et al., 1997), ethanol (Liljequist, 1991) and benzodiazepine (Steppuhn & Turski, 1993). These findings suggest that glutamatergic actions at NMDA receptors are involved in the development of substance dependence. This hypothesis is supported by data demonstrating that acute administration of psychoactive substances, such as cocaine or amphetamine, increases glutamate levels in the VTA and the nucleus accumbens which in turn increases dopaminergic neurotransmission in limbic areas, such as the nucleus accumbens (Smith et al., 1995; Kalivas & Duffy, 1998) that partly mediates the rewarding effects of psychoactive substances (Koob, 1992; Koob et al., 1993; Wise, 1998). In turn, this enhanced glutamatergic neurotransmission would lead to alterations in dopaminergic neurotransmission (increases or decreases depending on the brain site) that would produce rewarding effects, but may potentially worsen some symptoms of schizophrenia if indeed hyperdopaminergia is one of the core abnormalities of schizophrenia.

One brain site where the multiple interactions discussed above may occur is the VTA (Mogenson, Jones & Yim, 1980). Glutamatergic afferents to the VTA, originating in the prefrontal cortex, increase firing of dopamine neurons in the VTA, which results in increased dopamine levels in the nucleus accumbens (Kalivas, Duffy & Barrow, 1989; Suaud-Chagny et al., 1992; Taber & Fibiger, 1995). There are presynaptic $\alpha7$ nicotinic acetylcholine receptors located upon these glutamatergic afferents (Mansvelder & McGehee, 2000), that when stimulated increase glutamate release. This enhanced glutamate release then acts at NMDA and non-NMDA receptor sites on postsynaptic dopamine neurons and increases their firing rate (Fu et al., 2000; Grillner & Svensson, 2000; Mansvelder & McGehee, 2000). These interactions between glutamate and dopamine systems, and nicotinic acetylcholine receptors are particularly relevant because of the extremely high rate of smoking among patients with schizophrenia. In addition to increased glutamate release in the VTA, nicotine also increases glutamate release in other limbic sites, such as the nucleus accumbens (Reid et al., 2000), the prefrontal cortex (Gioanni et al., 1999) and the hippocampus (Gray et al., 1996). Finally, there is preclinical and clinical evidence to suggest that some forms of cognitive deficits that patients with schizophrenia exhibit may depend critically on α7 nicotinic acetylcholine receptors in the hippocampus (Adler et al., 1998). Although nicotine has low affinity for α7 nicotinic acetylcholine receptors (Clarke et al., 1985), it may activate these α7 receptors in the hippocampus, which leads to increased glutamate release to counteract this deficit (Dalack, Healy & Meador-Woodruff, 1998), and thus leads to self-medication through smoking. All of the above data suggest ways by which the use of psychoactive substances would self-medicate symptoms of schizophrenia by enhancing glutamatergic neurotransmission in order to counteract a possible hypoglutamatergia that may characterize this disease.

The above represents a small subset of sites and mechanisms where the effects of psychoactive substances and the neurobiology of schizophrenia may overlap and/or interact to lead to the high degree of comorbidity between the two disorders. Although many of the above neurobiological mechanisms are speculative and most of the studies were conducted in the USA, the recent attention to the issue of comorbidity has led to the initiation of multiple preclinical and clinical studies. These studies will directly investigate the neurobiology of how and why so many patients with schizophrenia use psychoactive substances compared with people without schizophrenia or patients having any other psychiatric disorder, in different countries and settings.

Depression

The comorbidity of depression with substance use is of great importance because of the high overall lifetime prevalence of affective and mood disorders. Approximately 8–13% of the general population experience clinical depression in their lifetime (Regier et al., 1990; Kessler et al., 1994). The comorbidity with substance use is 32% with an odds ratio of 2.6. That is, individuals with an affective disorder are 2.6 times more likely to use psychoactive substances than those without affective disorder (Regier et al., 1990). Considering the various affective disorders separately, bipolar disorder has the highest comorbidity value, with more than 60% of those suffering from this illness using psychoactive substances compared with more than 27% of those suffering from unipolar major depression. The discussion below will focus on unipolar major depression because it is the most common among affective disorders (Regier et al., 1990; Kessler et al., 1994).

Tobacco smoking and depression

There are several close links between major depressive disorder and tobacco smoking. Studies have shown that up to 60% of heavy smokers have a history of mental illness (Hughes et al., 1986; Glassman et al., 1988), and the prevalence of major depressive disorder among smokers is twice that of non-smokers (Glassman et al., 1990). Moreover, smokers who had a history of clinical depression were half as likely to succeed in quitting smoking than smokers without such a history (14% versus 28%) (Glassman et al., 1990).

Cessation of smoking results in an aversive withdrawal syndrome in humans (Shiffman & Jarvik, 1976; Hughes et al., 1991), components of which may be manifest for 1–10 weeks (Hughes, 1992). Depressed mood is one of the core symptoms of the tobacco withdrawal syndrome that is experienced by a large proportion of the people who attempt to quit smoking (Hughes et al., 1984; West et al., 1984; Glassman et al., 1990; Hughes, 1992; Hughes & Hatsukami, 1992; Glassman 1993; Parrott 1993; American Psychiatric Association 1994; Hughes, Higgins & Bickel, 1994). The majority of researchers in the field postulate self-medication of depressive symptoms with tobacco smoking; this depressive symptomatology may have either pre-dated the cigarette smoking or was induced by chronic cigarette smoking (Pomerleau, Adkins & Pertschuk, 1978; Waal-Manning & de Hamel, 1978; Hughes et al., 1986; Glassman, 1993; Markou, Kosten & Koob, 1998; Watkins, Koob & Markou, 2000).

The link between tobacco smoking, the tobacco abstinence syndrome and depression is also supported by the fact that bupropion, an antidepressant compound (Feighner et al., 1984; Caldecott-Hazard & Schneider, 1992) that is a weak norepinephrine and dopamine reuptake inhibitor (Ascher et al., 1995), and a nicotinic acetylcholine receptor antagonist (Fryer & Lukas, 1999; Slemmer, Martin & Damaj, 2000), has been shown to be twice as effective as placebo in clinical smoking cessation trials (Hurt et al., 1997; Jorenby et al., 1999), and has been approved for this indication by the United States Food and Drug Administration (FDA). Bupropion is the only non-nicotine based therapy approved by the FDA as an antismoking agent. Trials have been conducted also using the antidepressants fluoxetine, doxepin, and moclobemide, a monoamine oxidase inhibitor (MAOI) (Robbins, 1993; Ferry & Burchette, 1994; Dalack et al., 1995; Aubin, Tilikete & Barrucand, 1996). These studies demonstrated modest effects of these antidepressants on tobacco withdrawal symptoms. That is, patients treated with antidepressants showed better abstinence rates than those treated with placebo at 4 weeks, although relapse rates at 3 and 6 months remained high. Most interestingly, however, patients with higher baseline depression remained abstinent for longer periods of time than those with no depression when treated with the antidepressant fluoxetine, although their mild depression could not be considered clinically significant (Hitsman et al., 1999).

In conclusion, most antidepressant agents have some usefulness in reducing relapse to smoking after the smoker with depression stops smoking, with bupropion having the highest efficacy overall, and fluoxetine (a selective serotonin reuptake inhibitor) being most effective in people with depression. The efficacy of antidepressant drugs, particularly bupropion and fluoxetine, as anti-smoking agents supports the hypothesis that pre-existing depressive symptomatology or depression associated with protracted nicotine abstinence contributes to the perpetuation of substance dependence (West et al., 1984; Glassman et al., 1990; Hughes et al., 1991; Hughes & Hatsukami, 1992; Parrott, 1993; West & Gossop, 1994; Markou, Kosten & Koob, 1998).

From most of the studies reviewed above, it is unclear whether individuals who suffer from depressive symptomatology are more likely to initiate smoking or whether depressive symptoms are induced or exacerbated by long-term smoking and withdrawal from smoking (Markou, Kosten & Koob, 1998). Epidemiological data support both processes (Breslau, Kilbey & Andreski, 1993, 1998), suggesting that smoking and depression share the same neurobiological substrates (Breslau et al., 1998). Although the mechanisms are not currently known, candidate neurotransmitter systems are serotonin and dopamine, both of which may be dysregulated in depression, and are increased by nicotine. The mesolimbic dopamine pathway is strongly associated with reward and dependence (see Chapter 3), but is also a candidate pathway that is dysregulated in depression (Nestler et al., 2002).

Other clinical evidence that supports a linkage between smoking and depression comes from a potential familial aggregation. It was shown that dizygotic twin pairs, who share only about half of their genes, had an intermediate level of association of smoking and depression, which fell between that of the monozygotic twin pairs (which had a higher level) and that of the general population (which had a lower level) (Kendler et al., 1993b). These data are consistent with the hypothesis that common or shared genes are a source of the association between depression and smoking.

Psychostimulant dependence and depression

Epidemiological data from the USA indicate that the lifetime rates of major depression were 32% in cocaine users, and only 8–13% among non-cocaine users (Robins et al., 1984; Regier et al., 1990; Robins & Reiger, 1991; Rounsaville et al., 1991; Kessler et al., 1994). Similar to tobacco smoking, antidepressant treatment of people with substance dependence results in greater improvement in both mood and reduction in the use of psychostimulants in those who also suffer from depression, than among those who do not.

Treatment with antidepressants appears to decrease cocaine use, as well as depression. Treatment with the tricyclic antidepressant desmethyli-mipramine resulted in a 90% reduction in cocaine use in users with depression, while users who were not depressed showed a 50% reduction in their use of cocaine (Ziedonis & Kosten, 1991). Similarly, 26% of cocaine users with depression who were treated with imipramine (another tricyclic antidepressant) had at least three consecutive cocaine-free weeks compared with only 5% of those treated with placebo (Nunes et al., 1995). These results suggest that psychostimulant users may consume psychostimulants in an attempt to self-medicate an underlying negative affective state (Khantzian, 1997; Markou, Kosten & Koob, 1998).

In humans psychostimulant withdrawal is characterized by severe mood disturbances including depressive symptoms combined with irritability and anxiety (Gawin & Kleber, 1986; Weddington et al., 1990; Satel et al., 1991; American Psychiatric Association, 1994). These symptoms last from several hours to days, one of the most salient being anhedonia (i.e. diminished interest or pleasure), which is also a core symptom of depression.This anhedonia may be one of the motivating factors in the etiology and maintenance of the cycle of psychostimulant dependence. Thus, the similarity between a major depressive episode and psychostimulant withdrawal further supports the hypothesis that there are overlapping neurobiological substrates that mediate these depressive symptoms that are common to the two disorders. Again, the mesolimbic dopamine system seems to be a likely candidate that mediates both the reward of substance use, and the lack of pleasure associated with substance withdrawal and depression. In the case of psychostimulant dependence, it is clear that, at least in some cases, the depressive symptoms are drug-induced. Substance use may also reflect an attempt to self-medicate a pre-existing depression.

Alcohol use and depression

Studies in the United States over the past 20 years indicated that lifetime rates of major depressive disorder were 38–44% in people with alcohol dependence compared with only 7% in non-dependent individuals (Rounsaville et al., 1982; Myers et al., 1984; Robins et al., 1984; Rounsaville, 1987; Robins & Reiger, 1991; Rounsaville et al., 1991; Kessler et al., 1994; Miller et al., 1996b; Schuckit et al., 1997a, 1997b). Furthermore, approximately 80% of people with alcohol dependence had symptoms of depression (Schuckit, 1985; Regier et al., 1990; Roy et al., 1991; Kessler et al., 1996). Thus, there is substantial data indicating that the rates of depression among people with alcohol dependence and the rates of alcohol use among people with depression are substantially higher than expected from the individual rates of these disorders.

Although not consistent, other evidence supporting the hypothesis that depression and alcohol dependence are linked disorders comes from clinical studies indicating that in some cases antidepressant treatment resulted in both improvement in mood and reduction in alcohol use. People with depression who are dependent on alcohol show lower rates of relapse to alcohol use when treated with antidepressants (e.g. imipramine or fluoxetine), compared with subjects who were given a placebo, either with or without depression (Nunes et al., 1993; Cornelius et al., 1995; McGrath et al., 1996; Mason et al., 1996). These observations in people with depression and alcohol dependence are significant considering that 80% of people with alcohol dependence have symptoms of depression, one-third of whom meet the criteria for a major depressive episode (Schuckit, 1985; Regier et al., 1990; Roy et al., 1991; Kessler et al., 1996).

In summary, epidemiological and clinical evidence suggests that depression and alcohol dependence are associated. Nevertheless, the majority of these clinical and epidemiological studies were unable to determine whether the depression was primary (i.e. appearing before the onset of alcohol dependence) or secondary (i.e. appearing after the initiation of alcohol use) and thus potentially alcohol-induced. Such a distinction is critical in establishing whether alcohol dependence and depression are different symptomatic expressions of the same neurobiological abnormalities, or whether the depression is alcohol-induced, and how self-medication may lead to the observed comorbidity. A recent study designed to examine this issue suggested that alcohol dependence and depression were divided nearly evenly between primary and secondary disorders (Compton et al., 2000a). Other data suggest that alcohol dependence leads to depression (i.e. that depression is secondary) and that once the alcohol use ceases then the symptoms of depression remit (Schuckit, 1994).

Considering the above summarized data and the various hypotheses put forward that attempt to explain the comorbidity of psychiatric disorders with substance use, in the case of alcohol and depression it appears that there is some familiar aggregation that would support the first hypothesis of common neurobiological substrates with different symptomatic expressions, although there is much data that are not supportive of this genetic linkage. A self-medication hypothesis is not supported because alcohol does not improve symptoms of depression (Hendrie, Sairally & Starkey, 1998). In fact, there are ample data to suggest that excessive alcohol use leads to depression (Schuckit, 1994), supporting the hypothesis of drug-induced depression that explains the high degree of comorbidity observed between alcohol dependence and depression.

Neurobiological interactions between depression and the effects of psychoactive substances

Substance withdrawal, one of the syndromes that may be associated with substance dependence (Himmelsbach, 1943; Wikler, 1973; Koob & LeMoal, 2001) (see Chapter 1), exhibits similarities with depression. Cessation of chronic drug use induces the behavioural and physical expression of the neuroadaptations that develop as a response to drug exposure. These are expressed as withdrawal syndromes that are distinct for each class of psychoactive substances (Koob et al., 1993; Markou, Kosten & Koob, 1998) (see Chapter 4). Interestingly, however, depression is a common symptom of withdrawal from substances from a variety of pharmacological classes including psychostimulants (Gawin & Kleber, 1986; Weddington et al., 1990;

Satel et al., 1991), opioids (Haertzen & Hooks, 1969; Henningfield, Johnson & Jasinski, 1987; Jaffe, 1990), ethanol (Jaffee, 1990; Edwards, 1990; Bokstrom & Balldin, 1992; Goodwin, 1992; West & Gossop, 1994; Schuckit et al., 1997) and nicotine (West et al., 1984; West & Gossop, 1994). This depressive symptomatology is conceptualized to reflect alterations in reward and motivational processes (Markou, Kosten & Koob, 1998). This similarity and neurobiological evidence (reviewed below) suggest several commonalities in the neurobiology of the symptomatology of depression and substance dependence that support either of the first two hypotheses described at the beginning of this chapter.

Alterations in the neurotransmission of serotonin, norepinephrine, acetylcholine, dopamine, GABA, corticotropin-releasing factor (CRF), neuropeptide Y(NPY) and somatostatin have been observed in individuals with depression (Caldecott-Hazard et al., 1991; Markou, Kosten & Koob, 1998). In animals most of these neurotransmitter systems are also modulated by antidepressant treatment, suggesting their involvement in the mode of action of antidepressant drugs. Many of these same systems have also been implicated in withdrawal from psychoactive substances, though not all systems have been implicated in withdrawal from every psychoactive substance. Furthermore, some of these systems are implicated directly in the affective/depressive aspects of substance withdrawal that constitute the common symptomatology of substance dependence and depression (Markou, Kosten & Koob, 1998).

Serotonin

Decreased serotonergic neurotransmission is one of the most consistent changes occurring during withdrawal from a variety of substances, such as stimulants (Parsons, Smith & Justice, 1991; Imperato et al., 1992; Rossetti, Hmaidan & Gessa, 1992; Weiss et al., 1992; Parsons, Koob & Weiss, 1995), ethanol (Rossetti, Hmaidan & Gessa, 1992; Weiss et al., 1996) and benzodiazepines (Lima, Salazar & Trejo, 1993). Interestingly, in the case of stimulant withdrawal, the decreases in serotonin levels in the nucleus accumbens were larger and appeared earlier than the decreases in dopamine (Parsons, Smith & Justice, 1995); and during ethanol withdrawal, the decreases in serotonin levels were more resistant to reversal by further ethanol self-administration than the decreases in dopamine (Weiss et al., 1996).

Serotonin appears to be critically involved in depression and it is hypothesized that reduced serotonegic neurotransmission mediates depression (Schildkraut, 1965; Coppen, 1967). Cerebrospinal fluid measures reflecting central serotonin activity in humans with depression provided evidence of reduced serotonergic activity (Caldecott-Hazard et al., 1991). Accordingly, some of the most effective antidepressants are serotonin selective reuptake inhibitors (SSRIs), with almost all SSRIs thus far tested being effective in treating depression (Caldecott-Hazard & Schneider, 1992).

Altering levels of serotonin produces dysphoric mood in both healthy individuals (Young et al., 1985; Benkelfat et al., 1994; Ellenbogen et al., 1996) and those with depression (Shopsin et al., 1975; Shopsin, Friedman & Gershon, 1976; Delgado et al., 1990, 1991, 1993; Lam et al., 1996; Miller et al., 1996a), suggesting a role of serotonin in depression (however, not all studies have reported such effects (Delgado et al., 1994; Heninger et al., 1996). Finally, chronic treatment with a variety of antidepressant treatments, such as tricyclics, MAOIs, electroconvulsive therapy, atypical antidepressants and SSRIs, produce robust changes in serotonin function through both presynaptic and postsynaptic mechanisms (Willner, 1985; Green, 1987; Blier, de Montigny & Chaput, 1990; Caldecott-Hazard et al., 1991; Blier & de Montigny, 1994). The neurochemical changes observed in the serotonin system consist primarily of changes at the serotonin$_{1A}$ and serotonin$_{2A}$ receptors (Blier & de Montigny, 1994; Stahl, 1994).

Recent experiments with rats provided strong evidence for a link between psychostimulant and nicotine withdrawal, and depression. The reward deficits observed during either amphetamine or nicotine withdrawal were reversed by a drug treatment that increased serotonin function (Allen et al., 1997), with no effect on the somatic aspects of withdrawal (Harrison, Liem & Markou, 2001). The reversal of the depression-like aspects of withdrawal from two different substances (i.e. amphetamine and nicotine) with different primary mechanisms of action, by a clinically-proven antidepressant serotonergic drug treatment supports the hypothesis of overlapping neurobiological abnormalities mediating depressive symptomatology as observed across psychiatric diagnostic categories (Geyer & Markou, 1995; Markou, Kosten & Koob, 1998; Geyer & Markou, 2002).

In the case of substance dependence, most available evidence emphasizes the critical role of dopamine neurotransmission, rather than serotonin, in the mediation of the acute rewarding effects of several psychoactive substances, such as stimulants, opioids, nicotine and ethanol (Koob & Le Moal, 2001). By contrast, a critical role for dopamine in depression has not been persuasively shown (Markou, Kosten & Koob, 1998), because direct and indirect dopaminergic agonists do not appear to be effective antidepressant treatments (Caldecott-Hazard et al., 1991; Caldecott-Hazard & Schneider, 1992; Kapur & Mann, 1992). It may be hypothesized that decreased dopaminergic neurotransmission may lead to some symptoms of depression, but that most of the symptoms may be mediated by other neurotransmitter systems.

Peptide systems

Another intriguing commonality between the neurobiology of depression and substance dependence is the consistent observation of increased CRF neurotransmission in both depression (Post et al., 1982; Nemeroff et al., 1984) and withdrawal from all psychoactive substances investigated thus far

(Richter & Weiss, 1999; Koob & Le Moal, 2001). Further, there is evidence indicating blunted neurotransmission of neuropeptide Y (NPY) and somatostatin in depression (Heilig & Widerlov, 1990; Rubinow, 1986), and blunted neurotransmission of NPY in psychostimulant withdrawal (Wahlestedt et al., 1991). Based on the hypothesis that NPY and somatostatin systems act in opposition to the CRF system (Heilig et al., 1994), there is heuristic value in further investigating the role of NPY and somatostatin in substance dependence. One hypothesis is that NPY and somatostatin may be endogenous "buffers" against the stressor-induced release of CRF. Given the role of CRF and NPY in behavioural responses to stress (Heilig et al., 1994), it is conceivable that neurotransmission of CRF, NPY and somatostatin is mostly related to the anxiety or stress-like symptomatology seen in both a subgroup of people with depression and in those in substance withdrawal. The same argument can also be made about the GABA system that has also been implicated in depression (Lloyd et al., 1989; Petty, 1995), and alcohol and benzodiazepine dependence (Andrews & File, 1993; Roberts, Cole & Koob, 1996), considering that benzodiazepines that enhance GABAergic neurotransmission are anxiolytics. Administration of psychoactive substances, such as cocaine and alcohol, modulate neurotransmission of CRF (Goeders, Bienvenu & de Souza, 1990; Merlo Pich et al., 1995; Richter et al., 1995; Richter & Weiss, 1999) and NPY (Wahlestedt et al., 1991), and thus could potentially restore temporarily the hypothesized imbalance between the two systems.

Role of limbic structures in depression and substance dependence

Another common element between depression and substance dependence is that most changes observed following antidepressant treatment or administration of psychoactive substances are seen in limbic-related structures, such as the frontal cortex, nucleus accumbens, olfactory tubercle, hippocampus, amygdala, and the hypothalamus. For instance, in the frontal cortex antidepressants alter the numbers of serotonin$_{1A}$ receptors (Peroutka & Snyder, 1980), and increase serotonin levels (Bel & Artigas, 1993). Antidepressants also produce supersensitive serotonin$_{1A}$ receptors in the amygdala (Wang & Aghajanian, 1980) and the hippocampus (de Montigny & Aghajanian, 1978; Chaput, de Montigny & Blier, 1991). Chronic antidepressant treatments also enhance dopaminergic activity in the nucleus accumbens (Nomikos et al., 1991) and upregulate GABA$_A$ receptors in the frontal cortex (Lloyd, Thuret & Pilc, 1985). In addition, CRF receptors are decreased in the frontal cortex of individuals with depression (Nemeroff et al., 1988); electroconvulsive shock increases NPY brain levels in the frontal cortex, the hypothalamus and the hippocampus (Wahlestedt et al., 1990); and desmethylimipramine increases the numbers of somatostatin receptors in the nucleus accumbens (Gheorvassaki et al., 1992).

Similarly, considerable evidence suggests an important role for limbic-related structures in substance dependence and withdrawal. For example, during withdrawal from psychostimulants (Parsons, Smith & Justice, 1995; Richter & Weiss, 1999) or ethanol (Rossetti, Hmaidan & Gessa, 1992; Merlo Pich et al., 1995; Weiss et al., 1996) dopamine and serotonin levels are decreased in the nucleus accumbens, while CRF levels are elevated in the amygdala. Furthermore, blockade of opioid receptors in the nucleus accumbens or the amygdala readily induces some affective signs of opioid withdrawal (Koob, Wall & Bloom, 1989; Stinus, Le Moal & Koob, 1990), while blockade of dopamine receptors in the nucleus accumbens produces at least the somatic signs of opioid withdrawal (Harris & Aston-Jones, 1994). Limbic structures, such as the VTA, nucleus accumbens, hippocampus and the frontal cortex are also critically involved in nicotine dependence (Dani & Heinemann, 1996; Kenny & Markou, 2001). Taken together, these data suggest that alterations in several neurotransmitter systems implicated in depression may also mediate dependence on psychoactive substances, and these commonalities may underlie the comorbidity between these psychiatric disorders.

Discussion and conclusions

In summary, clinical, epidemiological and neurobiological evidence, together with theoretical considerations, suggest several commonalities in the neurobiology of substance dependence, and of schizophrenia and depression that support the first three hypotheses discussed at the beginning of this chapter. The most likely neurobiological substrate underlying mental illnesses and substance dependence in general is dysfunction in the mesolimbic dopamine system. However, the many neurochemical effects of psychoactive substances, and the many behavioural expressions of mental illnesses suggest that there may be a number of causative factors. Research into the comorbidity of substance dependence and mental illness will illuminate common causative, preventative, and treatment factors. Few epidemiological studies directly address this issue and international research is lacking. Breslau and colleagues determined that in terms of depression and tobacco smoking, it appears that both processes are operating, i.e. depression predisposes to tobacco smoking and tobacco smoking predisposes to depression (Breslau, Kilbey & Andreski, 1993; Breslau, 1995; Breslau et al., 1998). In terms of other psychiatric disorders and substance dependence in general, a retrospective study concluded that antisocial personality disorder (see Box 6.1) and phobias generally appeared before the onset of substance dependence, while for all other psychiatric disorders, the disorder appeared before the onset of substance dependence for almost half of the cases, and for the remaining half the reverse was true. Finally, a study on schizophrenia and substance dependence concluded that a unidirectional causality for the two disorders was not supported by the data (Hambrecht & Hafner, 1996). These investigators found that 30% of patients with both schizophrenia and substance dependence use alcohol or illicit drugs before the first signs of

BOX 6.1

Substance use and the development of antisocial personality disorder (ASPD)

Adolescents with depression often develop substance use disorders (SUD), probably through efforts at self-medication. Substance use effects such as impulsivity and aggressive or irresponsible behaviours, and substance use consequences such as failure at school, and impairment of social functioning, and the subsequent exposure to antisocial models of social cognition and behaviour, may contribute to the development of antisocial personality disorder (ASPD). Substance use may be the major mediator between depression and ASPD during adolescence and young adulthood.

Recent research showed some evidence that SUD is a correlate of major depressive disorders in adolescents and ASPD in young adults. Other correlates may include poor social functioning or failure at school. Comparable correlates support causal relationships between heterotypic disorders and, in the case of ASPD, may provide useful leads for understanding the mechanisms involved in the development of personality disorders.

Source: Chabrol & Armitage, 2002.

schizophrenia, while the rest start substance use around or after the first signs of schizophrenia. In conclusion, although a clear association is indicated between schizophrenia and depression, and substance dependence, there are insufficient data to favour any specific hypothesis of shared neurobiology; it is also possible that all three hypotheses are true. Future longitudinal epidemiological studies are needed to directly address these questions.

An extension of the three hypotheses of shared neurobiology is that substance dependence may involve, at least in some cases, self-medication to reverse some of the neurotransmitter abnormalities associated with depression or schizophrenia that either existed before or were induced by substance use. None of the psychoactive substances are considered as clinically effective antidepressant or antipsychotic medications by practising clinicians. Nevertheless, the possibility remains that simultaneous or sequential use of various substances – as "self-prescribed" by the emotional or cognitive needs of the individual – leads to an adequate therapeutic effect for specific symptoms, while the substance use may simultaneously worsen other symptoms or the self-medicated symptoms in the long term. There are indeed reports that substance dependence is associated with poorer outcome and worse prognosis for patients with schizophrenia compared with patients who are not users (Khantzian, 1985; Dixon, 1999). Thus, it may be possible that psychoactive substances may provide short-term relief from some symptoms but that the long-term outcome is worse than if the patient did not use any drugs (Kosten & Ziedonis, 1997).

The best clinical support for the self-medication hypothesis is provided by evidence that:

— antidepressant treatment is more effective in reducing substance use in users suffering from depression than in users who are not, suggesting that antidepressant medication may replace the need for consumption of psychoactive substances;

— atypical antipsychotic medications that are most effective against the negative symptoms and cognitive deficits associated with schizophrenia reduce substance use as though the need for self-medication has been reduced;

— these studies emphasize the importance of treating comorbid psychiatric illness, and show that this treatment can be efficacious in managing substance dependence.

The preclinical and clinical investigations of the factors that may lead to the high degree of comorbidity are likely to provide valuable information about the neurobiology of schizophrenia and depression which in turn would lead to the development of better treatments for these debilitating disorders. If indeed patients with schizophrenia and depression self-medicate various symptoms with psychoactive substances, then insights could be gained from the patients' patterns of substance use in terms of novel medications that can be developed that may have beneficial effects for these disorders. Accordingly, owing to the recent awareness of the comorbidity of substance dependence with psychiatric disorders, preclinical animal studies have been initiated to investigate the neurobiological substrates that may explain this comorbidity.

Future studies should continue to directly address the hypotheses of shared neurobiological substrates using animal models of depression, schizophrenia and substance dependence, based on the current understanding of the neurobiology of these three psychiatric disorders. Generally, it would be fruitful to design research programmes that would explicitly test, with similar experimental approaches, hypotheses generated in the field of depression and schizophrenia in animal models of substance dependence and vice versa. Considering that all psychiatric disorders, including depression, schizophrenia and substance dependence, involve primarily behavioural symptoms that reflect underlying neurobiological abnormalities, progress in understanding these diseases at any level of analysis will certainly involve a multidisciplinary approach to research. Emphasis should be placed on both clinical and preclinical studies in the study of specific behavioural dimensions or psychological processes (e.g. specific symptoms) that are thought to be affected by the disorder of interest (Geyer & Markou, 1995, 2002). Long-term prospective studies that follow individuals from an early age would also be very informative, though difficult in practice.

Another area that requires greater research attention is the role of gender in the presence of comorbidity among people with substance use disorders.

Though this is an area with practical implications for treatment, few sytematic studies of gender specific prevalence of substance dependence and psychiatric disorders have been conducted. Findings from available studies show that gender differences in the prevalence of psychiatric disorders among people with substance dependence tend be consistent with findings from general population surveys (Compton et al., 2000b; Frye et al., 2003). In one of these studies (Frye et al., 2003), the risk of alcohol dependence in patients with bipolar disorder was shown to be higher among women than among men, when compared to risk in the general population. Escamilla et al. (2002) also showed that among patients with bipolar disorder in Costa Rica, gender was strongly associated with substance use disorders, primarily alcohol dependence. Among adolescents with substance use problems, there were no gender differences in the rate of bipolar disorder, but female users exhibited a higher rate of major depression than male users (Latimer et al., 2002).

Crosscultural studies are urgently needed to better assess and understand the association between the use of psychoactive substances and the various other mental disorders. The availability and increasing use of different substances in various cultures, and specific policies related to these substances are likely to influence the rates of comorbidity. Understanding cultural differences that might be present will help to clarify the role of neurobiology in the etiology of concurrent disorders.

Finally, the comorbidity of psychiatric disorders with substance dependence, and the apparent neurobiological link between these disorders has important implications for both the treatment of these diseases and for public health policy. It is important for the community, health care practitioners and policy-makers to recognize that this neurobiological link clearly indicates that psychiatric disorders and substance dependence are diseases stemming from underlying neuropathologies. Furthermore, comorbidity indicates that many heavy users of psychoactive substances have active mental disorders that would greatly benefit from psychiatric or psychological services and treatments. There are several effective treatments for depression and schizophrenia. Providing pharmacological and behavioural therapies to patients with mental disorders would facilitate abstinence or reduction of substance use, which would eventually improve the patients' prognosis. It should also be recognized that many of the patients with substance dependence who are refractory to current interventions may be so because abstinence worsens their psychiatric symptoms. Thus, more intensive interventions may be required for people with comorbidity to facilitate abstinence, including pharmacological treatment to help with withdrawal symptoms. In conclusion, understanding that there is a high degree of comorbidity of substance dependence with psychiatric disorders will greatly facilitate the implementation of medical treatments and public health policies that would directly address this social and medical issue.

References

Adler LE et al. (1998) Schizophrenia, sensory gating and nicotinic receptors. *Schizophrenia Bulletin*, **24**:189–202.

Allen AR et al. (1997) The 5-HT1ᵃ receptor antagonist p-MPPI blocks responses mediated by postsynaptic and presynaptic 5-HT1ᵃ receptors. *Pharmacology, Biochemistry and Behavior*, **57**:301–307.

Allen RM, Young SJ (1978) Phencyclidine-induced psychosis. *American Journal of Psychiatry*, **135**:1081–1084.

American Psychiatric Association (1994) *Diagnostic and statistical manual of mental disorders- Fourth Editon*Washington, DC, American Psychiatric Press.

Andrews N, File SE (1993) Increased 5-HT release mediates the anxiogenic response during benzodiazepine withdrawal: a review of supporting neurochemical and behavioural evidence. *Psychopharmacology*, **112**:21–25.

Angrist B, Gershon S (1970) The phenomenology of experimentally-induced amphetamine psychosis: preliminary observations. *Biological Psychiatry*, **2**:95–107.

Angrist B, Rotrosen J, Gershon S (1980) Differential effects of amphetamine and neuroleptics on negative and positive symptoms in schizophrenia. *Psychopharmacology*, **72**:17–19.

Angrist B et al. (1982) Partial improvement in negative schizophrenic symptoms after amphetamine. *Psychopharmacology*, **78**:128–130.

Ascher JA et al. (1995) Bupropion: a review of its mechanisms of antidepressant activity. *Journal of Clinical Psychiatry*, **56**:395–401.

Aubin HJ, Tilikete S, Barrucand D (1996) Depression and smoking. *Encephale*, **22**:17–22.

Balla A et al. (2001) Phencyclidine-induced dysregulation of dopamine response to amphetamine in prefrontal cortex and striatum. *Neurochemistry Research*, **26**:1001–1006.

Bel N, Artigas F (1993) Chronic treatment with fluvoxamine increases extracellular serotonin in the frontal cortex but not in raphe nuclei. *Synapse*, **15**:243–245.

Bell DS (1965) Comparison of amphetamine psychosis and schizophrenia. *British Journal of Psychiatry*, **111**:701–707.

Benkelfat C et al. (1994) Mood-lowering effect of tryptophan depletion: enhanced susceptibility in young men at genetic risk for major affective disorders. *Archives of General Psychiatry*, **51**:687–697.

Beyer CE, Steketee JD (2000) Intra-medial prefrontal cortex injection of quinpirole, but not SKF 38393, blocks the acute motor-stimulant response to cocaine in the rat. *Psychopharmacology*, **151**:211–218.

Binder RL et al. (1987) Smoking and tardive dyskinesia. *Biological Psychiatry*, **22**:1280–1282.

Blaha CD et al. (1997) Stimulation of the ventral subiculum of the hippocampus evokes glutamate receptor-mediated changes in dopamine efflux in the rat nucleus accumbens. *European Journal of Neuroscience*, **9**:902–911.

Blier P, de Montigny C (1994) Current advances and trends in the treatment of depression. *Trends in Pharmacological Sciences*, **15**:220–226.

Blier P, de Montigny C, Chaput Y (1990) A role for the serotonin system in the mechanism of action of antidepressant treatments: preclinical evidence. *Journal of Clinical Psychiatry*, **51** Suppl: S14–S20.

Bogerts B (1993) Hippocampus-amygdala volumes and psychopathology in chronic schizophrenia. *Biological Psychiatry*, **33**:236–246.

Bokstrom K, Balldin J (1992) A rating scale for assessment of alcohol withdrawal psychopathology (AWIP). *Alcoholism: Clinical and Experimental Research*, **16**:241–249.

Breslau N (1995) Psychiatric comorbidity of smoking and nicotine dependence. *Behavior Genetics*, **25**:95–101.

Breslau N, Kilbey MM, Andreski P (1993) Nicotine dependence and major depression: new evidence from a prospective investigation. *Archives of General Psychiatry*, **50**:31–35.

Breslau N et al. (1998) Major depression and stages of smoking: a longitudinal investigation. *Archives of General Psychiatry*, **55**:161–166.

Buckley P et al. (1994) Substance abuse among patients with treatment-resistant schizophrenia: characteristics and implications for clozapine therapy. *American Journal of Psychiatry*, **151**:385–389.

Caldecott-Hazard S, Schneider LS (1992) Clinical and biochemical aspects of depressive disorders. III. Treatment and controversies. *Synapse*, **10**:141–168.

Caldecott-Hazard S et al. (1991) Clinical and biochemical aspects of depressive disorders. II. Transmitter/receptor theories. *Synapse*, **9**:251–301.

Carlsson A (1977) Does dopamine play a role in schizophrenia? *Psychological Medicine*, **7**:583–597.

Carlsson A (1978) Mechanism of action of neuroleptic drugs. In: Lipton MA, Di Mascio A, Killian KF, eds. *Psychopharmacology: a generation in progress*. New York, NY, Raven Press:1057–1070.

Carol G et al. (2001) A preliminary investigation of cocaine craving among persons with and without schizophrenia. *Psychiatry Services*, **52**:1029–1031.

Cesarec Z, Nyman AK (1985) Differential response to amphetamine in schizophrenia. *Acta Psychiatrica Scandinavica*, **71**:523–538.

Chabrol H, Armitage J (2002) Substance use and the development of antisocial personality in depressed adolescents. *Archives of General Psychiatry*, **59**:665.

Chambers RA, Krystal JH, Self DW (2001) A neurobiological basis for substance abuse comorbidity in schizophrenia. *Biological Psychiatry*, **50**:71–83.

Chaput Y, de Montigny C, Blier P (1991) Presynaptic and postsynaptic modifications of the serotonin system by long-term administration of antidepressant treatments: an in vivo electrophysiologic study in the rat. *Neuropsychopharmacology*, **5**:219–229.

Claghorn J et al. (1987) The risks and benefits of clozapine versus chloromazine. *Journal of Clinical Psychopharmacology*, **7**:377–384.

Clarke PB et al. (1985) Nicotine binding in rat brain: autoradiographic comparison of [3H]acetylcholine, [3H]nicotine, and [125I]-alpha-bungarotoxin. *Journal of Neuroscience*, **5**:1307–1315.

Compton III WM et al. (2000a) Psychiatric disorders among drug dependent subjects: are they primary or secondary? *American Journal on Addictions*, **9**:126–134.

Compton III WM et al. (2000b) Substance dependence and other psychiatric disorders among drug dependent subjects: race and gender correlates. *American Journal on Addictions*, **9**:113-125.

Coppen A (1967) The biochemistry of affective disorders. *British Journal of Psychiatry*, **113**:1237–1264.

Cornelius JR et al. (1995) Preliminary report: double-blind, placebo-controlled study of fluoxetine in depressed alcoholics. *Psychopharmacology Bulletin*, **31**:297–303.

Cuesta MJ, Peralta V, Zarzuela A (2001) Effects of olanzapine and other antipsychotics on cognitive function in chronic schizophrenia: a longitudinal study. *Schizophrenia Research*, **48**:17–28.

Cuffel BJ (1992) Prevalence estimates of substance abuse in schizophrenia and their correlates. *Journal of Nervous and Mental Disorders*, **180**:589–592.

Dalack GW, Healy DJ, Meador-Woodruff JH (1998) Nicotine dependence in schizophrenia: clinical phenomena and laboratory findings. *American Journal of Psychiatry*, **155**:1490–1501.

Dalack GW et al. (1995) Mood, major depression, and fluoxentine response in cigarette smokers. *American Journal of Psychiatry*, **152**:398–403.

Dani JA, Heinemann S (1996) Molecular and cellular aspects of nicotine abuse. *Neuron*, **16**:905–908.

Decina P et al. (1990) Cigarette smoking and neuroleptic-induced parkinsonism. *Biological Psychiatry*, **28**:502–508.

de Leon J et al. (1995) Schizophrenia and smoking: an epidemiological survey in a state hospital. *American Journal of Psychiatry*, **152**:453–455.

Delgado PL et al. (1990) Serotonin function and the mechanism of antidepressant action: reversal of antidepressant-induced remission by rapid depletion of plasma tryptophan. *Archives of General Psychiatry*, **47**:411–418.

Delgado PL et al. (1991) Rapid serotonin depletion as a provocative challenge test for patients with major depression: relevance to antidepressant action and the neurobiology of depression. *Psychopharmacology Bulletin*, **27**:321–330.

Delgado PL et al. (1993) Monoamines and the mechanism of antidepressant action: effects of catecholamine depletion on mood of patients treated with antidepressants. *Psychopharmacology Bulletin*, **29**:389–396.

Delgado PL et al. (1994) Serotonin and the neurobiology of depression: effects of tryptophan depletion in drug-free depressed patients. *Archives of General Psychiatry*, **51**:865–874.

de Montigny C, Aghajanian GK (1978) Tricyclic antidepressants: long-term treatment increases responsivity of rat forebrain neurons to serotonin. *Science*, **202**:1303–1306.

Desai NG et al. (1984) Treatment of negative schizophrenia with d-amphetamine. *American Journal of Psychiatry*, **141**:723–724.

Di Chiara G et al. (1999) Drug addiction as a disorder of associative learning: role of nucleus accumbens shell/extended amygdala dopamine. *Annals of the New York Acadamy of Sciences*, **877**:461–485.

Diwan A et al. (1998) Differential prevalence of cigarette smoking in patients with schizophrenic vs mood disorders. *Schizophrenia Research*, 33:113–118.

Dixon L (1999) Dual diagnosis of substance abuse in schizophrenia: prevalence and impact outcomes. *Schizophrenia Research*, **35** Suppl: S93–S100.

Dixon L et al. (1990) Acute effects of drug abuse in schizophrenic patients: clinical observations and patients' self-reports. *Schizophrenia Bulletin*, 16:69–79.

Dixon L et al. (1991) Drug abuse in schizophrenic patients: clinical correlates and reasons for use. *American Journal of Psychiatry*, **148**:224–230.

Duncan GE, Sheitman BB, Lieberman JA (1999) An integrated view of pathophysiological models of schizophrenia. *Brain Research Reviews*, **29**:250–264.

Edwards G (1990) Withdrawal symptoms and alcohol dependence: fruitful mysteries. *British Journal of Addiction*, **85**:447–461.

Ellenbogen MA et al. (1996) Mood response to acute tryptophan depletion in healthy volunteers: sex differences and temporal stability. *Neuropsychopharmacology*, **15**:465–474.

Ellenbroek BA, Cools AR (2000) Animal models for the negative symptoms of schizophrenia. *Behavioural Pharmacology*, **11**:223–233.

Escamilla MA et al. (2002) Comorbidity of bipolar disorder and substance abuse in Costa Rica: pedigree- and population-based studies. *Journal of Affective Disorders*, **71**:71-83.

Fatemi SH, Earle JA, McMenomy T (2000) Reduction in Reelin immunoreactivity in hippocampus of subjects with schizophrenia, bipolar disorder and major depression. *Molecular Psychiatry*, **5**:654–663.

Feighner JP et al. (1984) A double-blind study of bupropion and placebo in depression. *American Journal of Psychiatry*, **141**:525–529.

Ferry LH, Burchette RJ (1994) Evaluation of buproprion versus placebo for treatment of nicotine dependence. In: *American Psychiatric Association New Research*, Washington, DC, American Psychiatric Press:199–200.

Finch DM (1996) Neurophysiology of converging synaptic inputs from the rat prefrontal cortex, amygdala, midline thalamus, and hippocampal formation onto single neurons of the caudate/putamen and nucleus accumbens. *Hippocampus*, **6**:495–512.

Freedman R et al. (1997) Linkage of a neurophysiological deficit in schizophrenia to a chromosome 15 locus. *Proceedings of the National Academy of Sciences of the United States of America*, **94**:587–592.

Frye MA et al. (2003) Gender differences in prevalence, risk, and clinical correlates of alcoholism comorbidity in bipolar disorder. *American Journal of Psychiatry*, **160**:883-889.

Fryer JD, Lukas RJ (1999) Noncompetitive functional inhibition at diverse, human nicotinic acetylcholine receptor subtypes by bupropion, phencyclidine, and ibogaine. *Journal of Pharmacology and Experimental Therapeutics*, **288**:88–92.

Fu Y et al. (2000) Systemic nicotine stimulates dopamine release in nucleus accumbens: re-evaluation of the role of *N*-methyl-D-aspartate receptors in the ventral tegmental area. *Journal of Pharmacology and Experimental Therapeutics*, **294**:458–465.

Funahashi S, Kubota K (1994) Working memory and prefrontal cortex. *Neuroscience Research*, **21**:1–11.

Gawin FH, Kleber HD (1986) Abstinence symptomatology and psychiatric diagnosis in cocaine abusers: clinical observations. *Archives of General Psychiatry*, 43**:107–113.**

George TP et al. (1995) Effects of clozapine on smoking in chronic schizophrenic outpatients. *Journal of Clinical Psychiatry*, **56**:344–346.

George TP et al. (2000) Nicotine transdermal patch and atypical antipsychotic medications for smoking cessation in schizophrenia. *American Journal of Psychiatry*, **157**:1835–1842.

George TP et al. (2002) Effects of smoking abstinence on visuospatial working memory function in schizophrenia. *Neuropsychopharmacology*, **26**:75–85.

Gerding LB et al. (1999) Alcohol dependence and hospitalization in schizophrenia. *Schizophrenia Research*, **38**:71–75.

Geyer MA, Markou A (1995) Animal models of psychiatric disorders. In: Bloom FE, Kupfer DJ, eds. *Psychopharmacology: the fourth generation of progress*. New York, NY, Raven Press:787–798.

Geyer MA, Markou A (2002) The role of preclinical models in the development of psychotropic drugs. In: Charney D et al., eds. *Psychopharmacology: the fifth generation of progress*. Hagerstown, MD: Lippincott, Williams & Wilkins:445–455.

Gheorvassaki EG et al. (1992) Effects of acute and chronic desipramine treatment on somatostatin receptors in brain. *Psychopharmacology*, **108**:363–366.

Gioanni Y et al. (1999) Nicotinic receptors in the rat prefrontal cortex: increase in glutamate release and facilitation of mediodorsal thalamo-cortical transmission. *European Journal of Neuroscience*, **11**:18–30.

Glassman AH (1993) Cigarette smoking: implications for psychiatric illness. *American Journal of Psychiatry*, **150**:546–553.

Glassman AH et al. (1988) Heavy smokers, smoking cessation, and clonidine: results of a double-blind, randomized trial. *Journal of the American Medical Association*, **259**:2863–2866.

Glassman AH et al. (1990) Smoking, smoking cessation, and major depression. *Journal of the American Medical Association*, **264**:1546–1549.

Glynn SM, Sussman S (1990) Why patients smoke. *Hospital and Community Psychiatry*, **41**:1027–1028.

Goeders NE, Bienvenu OJ, de Souza EB (1990) Chronic cocaine administration alters corticotropin-releasing factor receptors in the rat brain. *Brain Research*, **531**:322–328.

Goff DC, Henderson DC, Amico E (1992) Cigarette smoking in schizophrenia: relationship to psychopathology and medication side effects. *American Journal of Psychiatry*, **149**:1189–1194.

Goldman-Rakic PS (1995) Cellular basis of working memory. *Neuron*, **14**:477–485.

Gonzalez P et al. (1997) Decrease of tolerance to, and physical dependence on, morphine by glutamate receptor antagonists. *European Journal of Pharmacology*, **332**:257–262.

Goodwin DW (1992) Alcohol: clinical aspects. In: Lowinson JH et al., eds. *Substance abuse: a comprehensive textbook*, 2nd ed. Baltimore, MD, Williams & Wilkins:144–151.

Grace AA (1995) The tonic/phasic model of dopamine system regulation: its relevance for understanding how stimulant abuse can alter basal ganglia function. *Drug and Alcohol Dependence*, **37**:111–129.

Gray R et al. (1996) Hippocampal synaptic transmission enhanced by low concentrations of nicotine. *Nature*, **383**:713–716.

Green AI et al. (1999) Clozapine for comorbid substance use disorder and schizophrenia: do patients with schizophrenia have a reward-deficiency syndrome that can be ameliorated by clozapine? *Harvard Review of Psychiatry*, **6**:287–296.

Green AR (1987) Evolving concepts on the interactions between antidepressant treatments and monoamine neurotransmitters. *Neuropharmacology*, **26**:815–822.

Griffith JD et al. (1972) Dextroamphetamine: evaluation of psychotomimetic properties in man. *Archives of General Psychiatry*, **26**:97–100.

Grillner P, Svensson TH (2000) Nicotine-induced excitation of mid-brain dopamine neurons in vitro involves ionotropic glutamate receptor activation. *Synapse*, **38**:1–9.

Haertzen CA, Hooks NT Jr (1969) Changes in personality and subjective experience associated with the chronic administration and withdrawal of opiates. *Journal of Nervous and Mental Disorders*, **148**:606–614.

Hall RG et al. (1995) Level of functioning, severity of illness, and smoking status among chronic psychiatric patients. *Journal of Nervous and Mental Disorders*, **183**:468–471.

Hambrecht M, Hafner H (1996) Substance abuse and the onset of schizophrenia. *Biological Psychiatry*, **40**:1155–1163.

Harris GC, Aston-Jones G (1994) Involvement of D2 dopamine receptors in the nucleus accumbens in the opiate withdrawal syndrome. *Nature*, **371**:155–157.

Harrison AA, Liem YT, Markou A (2001) Fluoxetine combined with a serotonin-1A receptor antagonist reversed reward deficits observed during nicotine and amphetamine withdrawal in rats. *Neuropsychopharmacology*, **25**:55–71.

Harvey PD, Keefe RS (2001) Studies of cognitive change in patients with schizophrenia following novel antipsychotic treatment. *American Journal of Psychiatry*, **158**:176–184.

Hazlett EA et al. (2000) Hypofrontality in unmedicated schizophrenia patients studied with PET during performance of a serial verbal learning task. *Schizophrenia Research*, **43**:33–46.

Heckers S (2001) Neuroimaging studies of the hippocampus in schizophrenia. *Hippocampus*, **11**:520–528.

Heilig M, Widerlov E (1990) Neuropeptide Y: an overview of central distribution, functional aspects, and possible involvement in neuropsychiatric illnesses. *Acta Psychiatrica Scandinavica*, **82**:95–114.

Heilig M et al. (1994) Corticotropin-releasing factor and neuropeptide Y: role in emotional integration. *Trends in Neuroscience*, **17**:80–85.

Hendrie CA, Sairally J, Starkey N (1998) Self-medication with alcohol appears not to be an effective treatment for the control of depression. *Journal of Psychopharmacology*, **12**:108.

Heninger GR, Delgado PL, Charney DS (1996) The revised monoamine theory of depression: a modulatory role for monoamines, based on new findings from monoamine depletion experiments in humans. *Pharmacopsychiatry*, **29**:2–11.

Henningfield JE, Johnson RE, Jasinski DR (1987) Clinical procedures for the assessment of abuse potential. In: Bozarth MA, ed. *Methods of assessing the reinforcing properties of abused drugs.* New York, NY, Springer-Verlag:573–590.

Himmelsbach CK (1943) Can the euphoric, analgetic, and physical dependence effects of drugs be separated? IV. With reference to physical dependence. *Federation Proceedings*, **2**:201–203.

Hitsman B et al. (1999) Antidepressant pharmacotherapy helps some cigarette smokers more than others. *Journal of Consulting and Clinical Psychology*, **67**:547–554.

Holden C (2001) Drug addiction: zapping memory center triggers drug craving. *Science*, **292**:1039.

Hughes JR (1992) Tobacco withdrawal in self-quitters. *Journal of Consulting and Clinical Psychology*, **60**:689–697.

Hughes JR (1996) The future of smoking cessation therapy in the United States. *Addiction*, **91**:1797–1802.

Hughes JR, Hatsukami D (1992) The nicotine withdrawal syndrome: a brief review and update. *International Journal on Smoking Cessation*, **1**:21–26.

Hughes JR, Higgins ST, Bickel WK (1994) Nicotine withdrawal versus other drug withdrawal syndromes: similarities and dissimilarities. *Addiction*, **89**:1461–1470.

Hughes JR et al. (1984) Effect of nicotine on the tobacco withdrawal syndrome. *Psychopharmacology*, **83**:82–87.

Hughes JR et al. (1986) Prevalence of smoking among psychiatric outpatients. *American Journal of Psychiatry*, **143**:993–997.

Hughes JR et al. (1991) Symptoms of tobacco withdrawal: a replication and extension. Archives of General Psychiatry, **48**:52–59.

Hurt RD et al. (1997) A comparison of sustained-release buproprion and placebo for smoking cessation. *New England Journal of Medicine*, **337**:1195–1202.

Imperato A et al. (1992) Chronic cocaine alters extracellular dopamine: neurochemical basis for addiction. *European Journal of Pharmacology*, **212**:299–300.

Jaffe JH (1990) Drug addiction and drug abuse. In: Goodman AG et al., eds. *Goodman and Gilman's pharmacological basis of therapeutics*, 8th ed. New York, NY, Pergamon Press:522–573.

Jarvik ME (1991) Beneficial effects of nicotine. *British Journal of Addiction*, **86**:571–575.

Javitt DC, Zukin SR (1991) Recent advances in the phencyclidine model of schizophrenia. *American Journal of Psychiatry*, **148**:1301–1308.

Jentsch JD, Roth RH (1999) The neuropsychopharmacology of phencyclidine: from NMDA receptor hypofunction to the dopamine hypothesis of schizophrenia. *Neuropsychopharmacology*, **20**:201–225.

Jibson MD, Tandon R (1998) New atypical antipsychotic medications. *Journal of Psychiatric Research*, **32**:215–228.

Jorenby DE et al. (1999) A controlled trial of sustained-release buproprion, a nicotine patch, or both for smoking cessation. *New England Journal of Medicine*, 340:685–691.

Kalivas PW, Alesdatter JE (1993) Involvement of *N*-methyl-D-aspartate receptor stimulation in the ventral tegmental area and amygdala in behavioral sensitization to cocaine. *Journal of Pharmacology and Experimental Therapeutics*, **267**:486–495.

Kalivas PW, Duffy P (1998) Repeated cocaine administration alters extracellular glutamate in the ventral tegmental area. *Journal of Neurochemistry*, **70**:1497–1502.

Kalivas PW, Duffy P, Barrow J (1989) Regulation of the mesocorticolimbic dopamine system by glutamic acid receptor subtypes. *Journal of Pharmacology and Experimental Therapeutics*, **251**:378–387.

Kapur S, Mann JJ (1992) Role of the dopaminergic system in depression. *Biological Psychiatry*, **32**:1–17.

Kapur S, Seeman P (2001) Does fast dissociation from the dopamine d(2) receptor explain the action of atypical antipsychotics: a new hypothesis. *American Journal of Psychiatry*, **158**:360–369.

Kendler KS et al. (1993) Smoking and major depression: a causal analysis. *Archives of General Psychiatry*, **50**:36–43.

Kenny PJ, Markou A (2001) Neurobiology of the nicotine withdrawal syndrome. *Pharmacology, Biochemistry and Behavior*, **70**:531–549.

Kessler RC et al. (1994) Lifetime and 12-month prevalence of DSM-III-R psychiatric disorders in the United States: results from the National Comorbidity Survey. *Archives of General Psychiatry*, **51**:8–19.

Kessler RC et al. (1996) The epidemiology of co-occurring addictive and mental disorders: implications for prevention and service utilization. *American Journal of Orthopsychiatry*, **66**:17–31.

Khantzian EJ (1985) The self-medication hypothesis of addictive disorders: focus on heroin and cocaine dependence. *American Journal of Psychiatry*, **142**:1259–1264.

Khantzian EJ (1997) The self-medication hypothesis of substance use disorders: a reconsideration and recent applications. *Harvard Review of Psychiatry*, **4**:231–244.

Kikuchi-Yorioka Y, Sawaguchi T (2000) Parallel visuospatial and audiospatial working memory processes in the monkey dorsolateral prefrontal cortex. *Nature Reviews in Neuroscience*, 3:1075–1076.

Kilts CD et al. (2001) Neural activity related to drug craving in cocaine addiction. *Archives of General Psychiatry*, **58**:334–341.

Knable MB, Weinberger DR (1997) Dopamine, the prefrontal cortex and schizophrenia. *Journal of Psychopharmacology*, 11:123–131.

Koob GF (1992) Drugs of abuse: anatomy, pharmacology and function of reward pathways. *Trends in Pharmacological Sciences*, **13**:177–184.

Koob GF, Le Moal M (2001) Drug addiction, dysregulation of reward, and allostasis. *Neuropsychopharmacology*, 24:97–129.

Koob GF, Wall TL, Bloom FE (1989) Nucleus accumbens as a substrate for the aversive stimulus effects of opiate withdrawal. *Psychopharmacology*, **98**:530–534.

Koob GF et al. (1993) Opponent process and drug dependence: neurobiological mechanisms. *Seminars in Neuroscience*, 5:351–358.

Kosten TR, Ziedonis DM (1997) Substance abuse and schizophrenia: editors' introduction. *Schizophrenia Bulletin*, 23:181–186.

Kosten TR, Markou A, Koob GF (1998) Depression and stimulant dependence: neurobiology and pharmacotherapy. *Journal of Nervous and Mental Disorders*, **186**:737–745.

Krystal JH et al. (1999) Toward a rational pharmacotherapy of comorbid substance abuse in schizophrenic patients. *Schizophrenia Research*, **35**(Suppl.):S35–S49.

Lahti AC et al. (1995) Subanesthetic doses of ketamine stimulate psychosis in schizophrenia. *Neuropsychopharmacology*, **13**:9–19.

Lam RW et al. (1996) Effects of rapid tryptophan depletion in patients with seasonal affective disorder in remission after light therapy. *Archives of General Psychiatry*, **53**:41–44.

Latimer WW et al. (2002) Gender differences in psychiatric comorbidity among adolescents with substance use disorders. *Experimental & Clinical Psychopharmacology*, **10**:310-315.

Le Duc PA, Mittleman G (1995) Schizophrenia and psychostimulant abuse: a review and re-analysis of clinical evidence. *Psychopharmacology*, **121**:407–427.

Legault M, Rompre PP, Wise RA (2000) Chemical stimulation of the ventral hippocampus elevates nucleus accumbens dopamine by activating dopaminergic neurons of the ventral tegmental area. *Journal of Neuroscience*, **20**:1635–1642.

Liljequist S (1991) NMDA receptor antagonists inhibit ethanol-produced locomotor stimulation in NMRI mice. *Alcohol*, **8**:309–312.

Lima L, Salazar M, Trejo E (1993) Modulation of 5-HTIA receptors in the hippocampus and the raphe area of rats treated with clonazepam. *Progress in Neuropsychopharmacology and Biological Psychiatry*, 17:663–677.

Lloyd KG, Thuret F, Pilc A (1985) Upregulation of gamma-aminobutyric acid (GABA) B binding sites in rat frontal cortex: a common action of repeated administration of different classes of antidepressants and electroshock. *Journal of Pharmacology and Experimental Therapeutics*, **235**:191–199.

Lloyd KG et al. (1989) The GABAergic hypothesis of depression. *Progress in Neuropsychopharmacology and Biological Psychiatry*, **13**:341–351.

Lodge D, Johnson KM (1990) Noncompetitive excitatory amino acid receptor antagonists. *Trends in Pharmacological Sciences*, **11**:81–86.

Luisada PV (1978) The phencyclidine psychosis: phenomenology and treatment. *NIDA Research Monograph*, **21**:241–253.

Lysaker P et al. (1994) Relationship of positive and negative symptoms to cocaine abuse in schizophrenia. *Journal of Nervous and Mental Disorders*, **182**:109–112.

McEvoy JP, Freudenreich O, Wilson WH (1999) Smoking and therapeutic response to clozapine in patients with schizophrenia. *Biological Psychiatry*, **46**:125–129.

McEvoy J et al. (1995) Clozapine decreases smoking in patients with chronic schizophrenia. *Biological Psychiatry*, **37**:550–552.

McGrath PJ et al. (1996) Imipramine treatment of alcoholics with primary depression: a placebo-controlled clinical trial. *Archives of General Psychiatry*, **53**:232–240.

Malhotra AK et al. (1997) Ketamine-induced exacerbation of psychotic symptoms and cognitive impairment in neuroleptic-free schizophrenics. *Neuropsychopharmacology*, **17**:141–150.

Manoach DS et al. (2000) Schizophrenic subjects show aberrant fMRI activation of dorsolateral prefrontal cortex and basal ganglia during working memory performance. *Biological Psychiatry*, **48**:99–109.

Mansvelder HD, McGehee DS (2000) Long-term potentiation of excitatory inputs to brain reward areas by nicotine. *Neuron*, **27**:349–357.

Marder SR, Wirshing WC, Van Putten T (1991) Drug treatment of schizophrenia: overview of recent research. *Schizophrenia Research*, **4**:81–90.

Markou A, Kosten TR, Koob GF (1998) Neurobiological similarities in depression and drug dependence: a self-medication hypothesis. *Neuropsychopharmacology*, **18**:135–174.

Markou A et al. (1993) Animal models of drug craving. *Psychopharmacology*, **112**:163–182.

Marshall DL, Redfern PH, Wonnacott S (1997) Presynaptic nicotinic modulation of dopamine release in the three ascending pathways studied by in vivo microdialysis: comparison of naïve and chronic nicotine-treated rats. *Journal of Neurochemistry*, **68**:1511–1519.

Mason BJ et al. (1996) A double-blind, placebo-controlled trial of desipramine for primary alcohol dependence stratified on the presence or absence of major depression. *Journal of the American Medical Association*, **275**:761–767.

Masterson E, O'Shea B (1984) Smoking and malignancy in schizophrenia. *British Journal of Psychiatry*, **145**:429–432.

Mauskopf JA et al. (1999) Annual health outcomes and treatment costs for schizophrenia populations. *Journal of Clinical Psychiatry*, **60** Suppl: S14–S19.

Meltzer HY (1999) Outcome in schizophrenia: beyond symptom reduction. *Journal of Clinical Psychiatry*, **60** Suppl: S3–S7.

Meltzer HY, Park S, Kessler R (1999) Cognition, schizophrenia, and the atypical antipsychotic drugs. *Proceedings of the National Academy of Sciences of the United States of America*, **96**:13 591–13 593.

Menza MA et al. (1991) Smoking and movement disorders in psychiatric patients. *Biological Psychiatry*, **30**:109–115.

Merlo Pich E et al. (1995) Increase of extracellular corticotropin-releasing factor-like immunoreactivity levels in the amygdala of awake rats during restraint stress and ethanol withdrawal as measured by microdialysis. *Journal of Neuroscience*, **15**:5439–5447.

Miller HL et al. (1996a) Clinical and biochemical effects of catecholamine depletion on antidepressant-induced remission of depression. *Archives of General Psychiatry*, **53**:117–128.

Miller NS et al. (1996b) Prevalence of depression and alcohol and other drug dependence in addictions treatment populations. *Journal of Psychoactive Drugs*, **28**:111–124.

Mittleman G, Bratt AM, Chase R (1998) Heterogeneity of the hippocampus: effects of subfield lesions on locomotion elicited by dopaminergic agonists. *Behavioural Brain Research*, **92**:31–45.

Mogenson GJ, Jones DL, Yim CY (1980) From motivation to action: functional interface between the limbic system and the motor system. *Progress in Neurobiology*, **14**:69–97.

Moller HJ (1998) Novel antipsychotics and negative symptoms. *International Clinical Psychopharmacology*, **13** Suppl: S43–S47.

Mueser KT et al. (1990) Prevalence of substance abuse in schizophrenia: demographic and clinical correlates. *Schizophrenia Bulletin*, **16**:31–56.

Myers JK et al. (1984) Six-month prevalence of psychiatric disorders in three communities, 1980 to 1982. *Archives of General Psychiatry*, **41**:959–967.

Nemeroff CB et al. (1984) Elevated concentrations of CSF corticotropin-releasing factor-like immunoreactivity in depressed patients. *Science*, **226**:1342–1344.

Nemeroff CB et al. (1988) Reduced corticotropin-releasing factor binding sites in the frontal cortex of suicide victims. *Archives of General Psychiatry*, **45**:577–579.

Nestler EJ et al. (2002) Neurobiology of depression. *Neuron*, **34**:13–25.

Newcomer JW et al. (1999) Ketamine-induced NMDA receptor hypofunction as a model of memory impairment and psychosis. *Neuropsychopharmacology*, **20**:106–118.

Nomikos GG et al. (1991) Electroconvulsive shock produces large increases in the interstitial concentrations of dopamine in the rat striatum: an in vivo microdialysis study. *Neuropsychopharmacology*, **4**:65–69.

Nomikos GG et al. (1994) Systemic administration of amperozide, a new atypical antipsychotic drug, preferentially increases dopamine release in the rat medial prefrontal cortex. *Psychopharmacology*, **115**:147–156.

Nunes EV et al. (1993) Imipramine treatment of alcoholism with comorbid depression. *American Journal of Psychiatry*, **150**:963–965.

Nunes EV et al. (1995) Imipramine treatment of cocaine abuse: possible boundaries of efficacy. *Drug and Alcohol Dependence*, **39**:185–195.

Olincy A, Young DA, Freedman R (1997) Increased levels of the nicotine metabolite cotinine in schizophrenic smokers compared to other smokers. *Biological Psychiatry*, **42**:1–5.

Pallanti S, Quercioli L, Pazzagli A (1999) Effects of clozapine on awareness of illness and cognition in schizophrenia. *Psychiatry Research*, **86**:239–249.

Parrott AC (1993) Cigarette smoking: effects upon self-rated stress and arousal over the day. *Addictive Behaviors*, **18**:389–395.

Parsons LH, Smith AD, Justice JB Jr (1991) Basal extracellular dopamine is decreased in the rat nucleus accumbens during abstinence from chronic cocaine. *Synapse*, **9**:60–65.

Parsons LH, Koob GF, Weiss F (1995) Serotonin dysfunction in the nucleus accumbens of rats during withdrawal after unlimited access to intravenous cocaine. *Journal of Pharmacology and Experimental Therapeutics*, **274**:1182–1191.

Patkar AA et al. (1999) Changing patterns of illicit substance use among schizophrenic patients: 1984–1996. *American Journal on Addictions*, **8**:65–71.

Peroutka SJ, Snyder SH (1980) Long-term antidepressant treatment decreases spiroperidol-labelled serotonin receptor binding. *Science*, **210**:88–90.

Petty F (1995) GABA and mood disorders: a brief review and hypothesis. *Journal of Affective Disorders*, **34**:275–281.

Pomerleau O, Adkins D, Pertschuk M (1978) Predictors of outcome and recidivism in smoking cessation treatment. *Addictive Behaviors*, **3**:65–70.

Post RM et al. (1982) Peptides in the cerebrospinal fluid of neuropsychiatric patients: an approach to central nervous system peptide function. *Life Sciences*, **31**:1–15.

Pristach CA, Smith CM (1996) Self-reported effects of alcohol use on symptoms of schizophrenia. *Psychiatric Services*, **47**:421–423.

Rajarethinam R et al. (2001) Hippocampus and amygdala in schizophrenia: assessment of the relationship of neuroanatomy to psychopathology. *Psychiatry Research*, **108**:79–87.

Razi K et al. (1999) Reduction of the parahippocampal gyrus and the hippocampus in patients with chronic schizophrenia. *British Journal of Psychiatry*, **174**:512–519.

Regier DA et al. (1990) Comorbidity of mental disorders with alcohol and other drug abuse: results from the Epidemiological Catchment Area (ECA) Study. *Journal of the American Medical Association*, **264**:2511–2518.

Reid MS et al. (2000) Nicotine stimulation of extracellular glutamate levels in the nucleus accumbens: neuropharmacological characterization. *Synapse*, **35**:129–136.

Richter RM, Weiss F (1999) In vivo CRF release in rat amygdala is increased during withdrawal after cocaine withdrawal in self-administering rats. *Synapse*, **32**:254–261.

Richter RM et al. (1995) Sensitization of cocaine-stimulated increase in extracellular levels of corticotropin-releasing factor from the rat amygdala after repeated administration as determined by intracranial microdialysis. *Neuroscience Letters*, **187**:169–172.

Robbins AS (1993) Pharmacological approaches to smoking cessation. *American Journal of Preventive Medicine*, **9**:31–33.

Roberts AJ, Cole M, Koob GF (1996) Intra-amygdala muscimol decreases operant ethanol self-administration in dependent rats. *Alcoholism: Clinical and Experimental Research*, **20**:1289–1298.

Robins LN et al. (1984) Lifetime prevalence of specific psychiatric disorders in three sites. *Archives of General Psychiatry*, **41**:949–958.

Robins LN, Regier DA, eds (1991) *Psychiatric disorders in America: the Epidemiologic Catchment Area Study*. New York, NY, The Free Press.

Robinson D et al. (1991) Mood responses of remitted schizophrenics to methylphenidate infusion. *Psychopharmacology*, **105**:247–252.

Rosenthal RN, Hellerstein DJ, Miner CR (1994) Positive and negative syndrome typology in schizophrenic patients with psychoactive substance use disorders. *Comprehensive Psychiatry*, **35**:91–98.

Rossetti ZL, Hmaidan Y, Gessa GL (1992) Marked inhibition of mesolimbic dopamine release: a common feature of ethanol, morphine, cocaine and amphetamine abstinence in rats. *European Journal of Pharmacology*, **221**:227–234.

Rounsaville BJ et al. (1982) Heterogeneity of psychiatric disorders in treated opiate addicts. *Archives of General Psychiatry*, **39**:161–168.

Rounsaville BJ et al. (1987) Psychopathology as a predictor of treatment outcome in alcoholics. *Archives of General Psychiatry*, **44**:505–513.

Rounsaville BJ et al. (1991) Psychiatric diagnoses of treatment-seeking cocaine abusers. *Archives of General Psychiatry*, **48**:43–51.

Rowley HL et al. (2000) A comparison of the acute effects of zotepine and other antipsychotics on rat cortical dopamine release, in vivo. *Naunyn-Schmiedebergs Archives of Pharmacology*, **361**:187–192.

Roy A et al. (1991) Depression among alcoholics: relationship to clinical and cerebrospinal fluid variables. *Archives of General Psychiatry*, **48**:428–432.

Rubinow DR (1986) Cerebrospinal fluid somatostatin and psychiatric illness. *Biological Psychiatry*, **21**:341–365.

Rupp A, Keith S (1993) The costs of schizophrenia. *Psychiatric Clinics of North Am*, **16**:413–423.

Sandyk R (1993) Cigarette smoking: effects on cognitive functions and drug-induced parkinsonism in chronic schizophrenia. *International Journal of Neuroscience*, **70**:193–197.

Sanfilipo M et al. (1996) Amphetamine and negative symptoms of schizophrenia. *Psychopharmacology*, **123**:211–214.

Satel SL et al. (1991) Clinical phenomenology and neurobiology of cocaine abstinence: a prospective inpatient study. *American Journal of Psychiatry*, **148**:1712–1716.

Scheibel AB, Conrad AS (1993) Hippocampal dysgenesis in mutant mouse and schizophrenic man: is there a relationship? *Schizophrenia Bulletin*, **19**:21–33.

Schildkraut JJ (1965) The catecholamine hypothesis of affective disorders: a review of supporting evidence. *American Journal of Psychiatry*, **122**:509–522.

Schneier FR, Siris SG (1987) A review of psychoactive substance use and abuse in schizophrenia: patterns of drug choice. *Journal of Nervous and Mental Disorders*, **175**:641–652.

Schuckit MA (1985) The clinical implications of primary diagnostic groups among alcoholics. *Archives of General Psychiatry*, **42**:1043–1049.

Schuckit MA (1994) Alcohol and depression: a clinical perspective. *Acta Psychiatrica Scandinavica*, **377**:28–32.

Schuckit MA et al. (1997a) Comparison of induced and independent major depressive disorders in 2,945 alcoholics. *American Journal of Psychiatry*, **154**:948–957.

Schuckit MA et al. (1997b) The life-time rates of three major mood disorders and four major anxiety disorders in alcoholics and controls. *Addiction*, **92**:1289–1304.

Self DW (1998) Neural substrates of drug craving and relapse in drug addiction. *Annals of Medicine*, **30**:379–389.

Sevy S et al. (1990) Significance of cocaine history in schizophrenia. *Journal of Nervous and Mental Disorders*, **178**:642–648.

Shiffman SM, Jarvik ME (1976) Smoking withdrawal symptoms in two weeks of abstinence. *Psychopharmacology*, **50**:35–39.

Shoaib M, Stolerman IP (1992) MK801 attenuates behavioural adaptation to chronic nicotine administration in rats. *British Journal of Pharmacology*, **105**:514–515.

Shopsin B, Friedman E, Gershon S (1976) Parachlorophenylalanine reversal of tranylcypromine effects in depressed patients. *Archives of General Psychiatry*, **33**:811–819.

Shopsin B et al. (1975) Use of synthesis inhibitors in defining a role for biogenic amines during imipramine treatment in depressed patients. *Psychopharmacology Communications*, **1**:239–249.

Slemmer JE, Martin BR, Damaj MI (2000) Bupropion is a nicotinic antagonist. *Journal of Pharmacology and Experimental Therapeutics*, **295**:321–327.

Smith JA et al. (1995) Cocaine increases extraneuronal levels of aspartate and glutamate in the nucleus accumbens. *Brain Research*, **683**:264–269.

Snyder SH (1976) Dopamine and schizophrenia. *Psychiatric Annals*, **6**:53–64.

Snyder SH (1980) Phencyclidine. *Nature*, **285**:355–356.

Soni SD, Brownlee M (1991) Alcohol abuse in chronic schizophrenics: implications for management in the community. *Acta Psychiatrica Scandinavica*, **84**:272–276.

Sorg BA, Kalivas PW (1993) Effects of cocaine and footshock stress on extracellular dopamine levels in the medial prefrontal cortex. *Neuroscience*, **53**:695–703.

Soyka M (1994) Alcohol dependence and schizophrenia: what are the interrelationships? *Alcohol and Alcoholism*, Suppl 2: S473–S478.

Stahl S (1994) 5-HT receptors and pharmacotherapy: is serotonin receptor down-regulation linked to the mechanism of action of antidepressant drugs? *Psychopharmacology Bulletin*, **30**:39–43.

Steppuhn KG, Turski L (1993) Diazepam dependence prevented by glutamate antagonists. *Proceedings of the National Academy of Sciences of the United States of America*, **90**:6889–6893.

Stinus L, Le Moal M, Koob GF (1990) The nucleus accumbens and amygdala are possible substrates for the aversive stimulus effects of opiate withdrawal. *Neuroscience*, **37**:767–773.

Suaud-Chagny MF et al. (1992) Relationship between dopamine release in the rat nucleus accumbens and the discharge activity of dopaminergic neurons during local *in vivo* application of amino acids in the ventral tegmental area. *Neuroscience*, **49**:63–72.

Taber MT, Fibiger HC (1995) Electrical stimulation of the prefrontal cortex increases dopamine release in the nucleus accumbens of the rat: modulation by metabotropic glutamate receptors. *Journal of Neuroscience*, **15**:3896–3904.

Tanda G et al. (1997) Contribution of blockade of the noradrenaline carrier to the increase of extracellular dopamine in the rat prefrontal cortex by amphetamine and cocaine. *European Journal of Neuroscience*, **9**:2077–2085.

Tsuang JW, Lohr JB (1994) Effects of alcohol on symptoms in alcoholic and nonalcoholic patients with schizophrenia. *Hospital and Community Psychiatry*, **45**:1229–1230.

Van Kammen DP, Boronow JJ (1988) Dextro-amphetamine diminishes negative symptoms in schizophrenia. *International Clinical Psychopharmacology*, **3**:111–121.

Vorel SR et al. (2001) Relapse to cocaine-seeking after hippocampal theta burst stimulation. *Science*, **292**:1175–1178.

Waal-Manning HJ, de Hamel FA (1978) Smoking habit and psychometric scores: a community study. *New Zealand Medical Journal*, **88**:188–191.

Wahlestedt C et al. (1990) Electroconvulsive shocks increase the concentration of neocortical and hippocampal neuropeptide Y (NPY)-like immunoreactivity in the rat. *Brain Research*, **507**:65–68.

Wahlestedt C et al. (1991) Cocaine-induced reduction of brain neuropeptide Y synthesis dependent on medial prefrontal cortex. *Proceedings of the National Academy of Sciences of the United States of America*, **88**:2078–2082.

Wang RY, Aghajanian GK (1980) Enhanced sensitivity of amygdaloid neurons to serotonin and norepinephrine after chronic antidepressant treatment. *Communications in Psychopharmacology*, **4**:83–90.

Watkins SS, Koob GF, Markou A (2000) Neural mechanisms underlying nicotine addiction: acute positive reinforcement and withdrawal. *Nicotine and Tobacco Research*, **2**:19–37.

Webster MJ et al. (2001) Immunohistochemical localization of phosphorylated glial fibrillary acidic protein in the prefrontal cortex and hippocampus from patients with schizophrenia, bipolar disorder, and depression. *Brain Behavior and Immunology*, **15**:388–400.

Weddington WW et al. (1990) Changes in mood, craving, and sleep during short-term abstinence reported by male cocaine addicts: a controlled, residential study. *Archives of General Psychiatry*, **47**:861–868.

Weiss F et al. (1992) Basal dopamine levels in the nucleus accumbens are decreased during cocaine withdrawal after unlimited-access self-administration. *Brain Research*, **593**:314–318.

Weiss F et al. (1996) Ethanol self-administration restores withdrawal-associated deficiencies in accumbal dopamine and 5-hydroxytryptamine release in dependent rats. *Journal of Neuroscience*, **16**:3474–3485.

West RJ, Gossop M (1994) Overview: a comparison of withdrawal symptoms from different drug classes. *Addiction*, **89**:1483–1489.

West RJ et al. (1984) Effect of nicotine replacement on the cigarette withdrawal syndrome. *British Journal of Addiction*, **79**:215–219.

Wikler A (1973) Dynamics of drug dependence: implications of a conditioning theory for research and treatment. *Archives of General Psychiatry*, **28**:611–616.

Wilkins JN (1997) Pharmacotherapy of schizophrenia patients with comorbid substance abuse. *Schizophrenia Bulletin*, **23**:215–228.

Wilkinson LS et al. (1993) Enhancement of amphetamine-induced locomotor activity and dopamine release in nucleus accumbens following excitotoxic lesions of the hippocampus. *Behavioural Brain Research*, **55**:143–150.

Willner P (1985) Antidepressants and serotonergic neurotransmission: an integrative review. *Psychopharmacology*, **85**:387–404.

Wise RA (1998) Drug-activation of brain reward pathways. *Drug and Alcohol Dependence*, **51**:13–22.

Wolf ME, Jeziorski M (1993) Co-administration of MK-801 with amphetamine, cocaine or morphine prevents rather than transiently masks the development of behavioral sensitization. *Brain Research*, **613**:291–294.

Wong ML, Licinio J (2001) Research and treatment approaches to depression. *Nature Reviews in Neuroscience*, **2**:343–351.

Yassa R et al. (1987) Nicotine exposure and tardive dyskinesia. *Biological Psychiatry*, **22**:67–72.

Young SN et al. (1985) Tryptophan depletion causes a rapid lowering of mood in normal males. *Psychopharmacology*, **87**:173–177.

Ziedonis DM, Kosten TR (1991) Depression as a prognostic factor for pharmacological treatment of cocaine dependence. *Psychopharmacology Bulletin*, **27**:337–343.

Ziedonis DM et al. (1992) Adjunctive desipramine in the treatment of cocaine abusing schizophrenics. *Psychopharmacology Bulletin*, **28**:309–314.

Ziedonis DM et al. (1994) Nicotine dependence and schizophrenia. *Hospital and Community Psychiatry*, **45**:204–206.

Zimmet SV et al. (2000) Effects of clozapine on substance use in patients with schizophrenia and schizoaffective disorder: a retrospective survey. *Journal of Clinical Pharmacology*, **20**:94–98.

CHAPTER 7

Ethical Issues in Neuroscience Research on Substance Dependence Treatment and Prevention

Introduction

Previous chapters have presented the latest findings in neuroscience research, and have pointed to potential treatment and prevention strategies. However, there are many ethical implications of the research itself, as well as the treatment and prevention strategies, that must be considered. The rapid pace of change in the field of neuroscience brings with it a host of new ethical issues, which need to be addressed. This chapter considers the important ethical and human rights issues that are raised by neuroscience research on psychoactive substance dependence.

Types of research on the neuroscience of substance dependence

Neuroscience research on substance dependence is classified here into five broad categories: animal experiments; epidemiological research on substance dependence; human experiments; clinical trials of pharmacological treatments for substance dependence; and trials of preventive pharmacological interventions.

Animal experiments

Animal experiments investigate the biological processes underlying substance dependence using animal models of human substance dependence. The major reasons for carrying out these studies are that much greater experimental control is possible with animals, and more invasive experiments can be done on animals than would be permitted in humans.

Epidemiological research on substance dependence

Although not strictly neuroscience research per se, epidemiological research informs and complements neuroscience research. Epidemiological research on patterns of substance use and dependence includes: surveys in the general population and within the special population of drug users and dependent persons (Anthony & Helzer, 1991; Kessler et al., 1994; Andrews, Henderson & Hall, 2001), family studies (Swendsen et al., 2002), adoption studies (Hjern,

Lindblad & Vinnerljung, 2002), twin studies of the genetics of substance dependence (Heath, 1995) and longitudinal studies of substance use and its consequences (Fergusson & Horwood, 2000; Kandel & Chen, 2000) and among persons who have been treated for substance dependence (Hser et al., 2001). The findings of such studies inform neuroscience research by describing substance dependence phenomena that need to be explained by neuroscience theories, for example, the individual characteristics that predict substance use and the development of substance dependence and other drug-related problems, and the genetic epidemiology of substance dependence found in twin and adoption studies. The distinction between epidemiological and neuroscience research on substance dependence is also likely to become blurred when epidemiological studies include biological measures, such as DNA, from which specific susceptibility genes can be tested, as well as other biological markers of risk.

Experimental studies in humans

Human neuroscience experiments typically involve laboratory studies under controlled conditions of the effects of chronic drug exposure on current brain function or the acute effects of exposure to drugs, drug analogues, or drug-related cues (e.g. the presence of injecting equipment) on behaviour and brain function (Adler, 1995). An increasingly common type of study involves the use of brain imaging technologies, such as PET, SPECT and fMRI (Gilman, 1998; Fu & McGuire, 1999) to study the acute effects of drugs and the neurobiological consequences of chronic substance use and dependence (Sell et al., 1999; Kling et al., 2000; Martin-Soelch et al., 2001) (see Chapters 2 and 4).

Clinical trials of pharmacotherapy for substance dependence

Clinical trials of pharmacotherapies for substance dependence compare the effects of different drug treatments, and sometimes placebos, on the patterns of drug use, on health, social adjustment and well-being of persons who are dependent on drugs (Brody, 1998). The drugs that are trialed are increasingly identified as potential treatments for substance dependence as a result of neuroscience research on the biological mechanisms underlying substance dependence. These may include trials of drugs that assist in completing the withdrawal from a psychoactive substance; drugs that are intended to reduce relapse to substance dependence after withdrawal; and drugs that are intended to provide long-term maintenance of abstinence or psychosocial stability.

Clinical trials have some chance of benefiting participants in the study (Brody, 1998). This may be by obtaining access to good-quality treatment for substance dependence (in the event of their receiving standard treatment or a placebo) or access to a promising experimental treatment for substance dependence (if they are assigned to the new treatment). As with participants in experimental studies, they may also be exposed to risks of the drug treatment, such as side-effects and toxicity (Brody, 1998; Gorelick et al., 1999).

Trials of pharmacotherapies to prevent substance dependence

Preventive trials involve controlled evaluations of pharmacological treatments that aim to prevent the development of substance dependence. This might be achieved by using a drug to treat a condition that increases a person's risks of developing substance dependence (e.g. attention deficit hyperactivity disorder (ADHD), see Chapter 4). It could conceivably involve the administration of a drug immunotherapy (e.g. against nicotine or cocaine) to young people who are at risk of substance dependence in order to reduce their chances of developing substance dependence.

Trials of preventive pharmacotherapies are more a prospect on the horizon than a major undertaking at present; however, two research developments suggest that such trials may soon be advocated. One is the development of immunotherapies against cocaine and nicotine (see Chapter 4). The initial motive for developing these immunotherapies has been to reduce relapse to substance use in persons who have been treated for substance dependence (Fox, 1997). However, these immunotherapies could be administered to children and adolescents with the intention of reducing their likelihood of becoming dependent. The second development is that of "early interventions", which so far have involved persons at high risk of developing schizophrenia, but it is likely that the same could be proposed for substance dependence. These involve a combination of psychosocial and pharmacological interventions. Because this work has been controversial in the field of psychiatry, neuroscience researchers on substance dependence would benefit from discussions of issues that may arise in trials of preventive pharmacological treatments for substance dependence.

Approach to ethical analysis

Over the past 30 years or so, an influential set of moral principles has emerged in Anglo-American analyses of the ethics of biomedical research (Brody, 1998; Jonsen, 1998). These are the principles of autonomy, non-maleficence, beneficence, and justice (Beauchamp & Childress, 2001). They have also been included in influential international statements of ethical principles for medical research, such as the Helsinki Declaration (see Box 7.1) and the declarations of United Nations organizations (Brody, 1998). These principles can be regarded as a moral baseline for the ethical analysis of neuroscience research on substance dependence; with the proviso that they may need to be supplemented to deal with newly-emerging issues.

BOX 7.1

Declaration of Helsinki[1]

Ethical principles for medical research involving human subjects

A. Introduction

1. The World Medical Association has developed the Declaration of Helsinki as a statement of ethical principles to provide guidance to physicians and other participants in medical research involving human subjects. Medical research involving human subjects includes research on identifiable human material or identifiable data.

2. It is the duty of the physician to promote and safeguard the health of the people. The physician's knowledge and conscience are dedicated to the fulfillment of this duty.

3. The Declaration of Geneva of the World Medical Association binds the physician with the words, "The health of my patient will be my first consideration", and the International Code of Medical Ethics declares that, "A physician shall act only in the patient's interest when providing medical care which might have the effect of weakening the physical and mental condition of the patient".

4. Medical progress is based on research which ultimately must rest in part on experimentation involving human subjects.

5. In medical research on human subjects, considerations related to the well-being of the human subject should take precedence over the interests of science and society.

6. The primary purpose of medical research involving human subjects is to improve prophylactic, diagnostic and therapeutic procedures and the understanding of the aetiology and pathogenesis of disease. Even the best proven prophylactic, diagnostic, and therapeutic methods must continuously be challenged through research for their effectiveness, efficiency, accessibility and quality.

7. In current medical practice and in medical research, most prophylactic, diagnostic and therapeutic procedures involve risks and burdens.

8. Medical research is subject to ethical standards that promote respect for all human beings and protect their health and rights. Some research populations are vulnerable and need special protection. The particular needs of the economically and medically disadvantaged must be recognized. Special attention is also required for those who cannot give or refuse consent for themselves, for those who may be subject to giving consent under duress, for those who will not benefit personally from the research and for those for whom the research is combined with care.

9. Research Investigators should be aware of the ethical, legal and regulatory requirements for research on human subjects in their own countries as well as applicable international requirements. No national ethical, legal or regulatory requirement should be allowed to reduce or eliminate any of the protections for human subjects set forth in this Declaration.

B. Basic principles for all medical research

10. It is the duty of the physician in medical research to protect the life, health, privacy, and dignity of the human subject.

11. Medical research involving human subjects must conform to generally accepted scientific principles, be based on a thorough knowledge of the scientific literature, other relevant sources of information, and on adequate laboratory and, where appropriate, animal experimentation.

12. Appropriate caution must be exercised in the conduct of research which may affect the environment, and the welfare of animals used for research must be respected.

13. The design and performance of each experimental procedure involving human subjects should be clearly formulated in an experimental protocol. This protocol should be submitted for consideration, comment, guidance, and where appropriate, approval to a specially appointed ethical review committee, which must be independent of the investigator, the sponsor or any other kind of undue influence. This independent committee should be in conformity with the laws and regulations of the country in which the research experiment is performed. The committee has the right to monitor ongoing trials. The researcher has the obligation to provide monitoring information to the committee, especially any serious adverse events. The researcher should also submit to the committee, for review, information regarding funding, sponsors, institutional affiliations, other potential conflicts of interest and incentives for subjects.

14. The research protocol should always contain a statement of the ethical considerations involved and should indicate that there is compliance with the principles enunciated in this Declaration.

15. Medical research involving human subjects should be conducted only by scientifically qualified persons and under the supervision of a clinically competent medical person. The responsibility for the human subject must always rest with a medically qualified person and never rest on the subject of the research, even though the subject has given consent.

16. Every medical research project involving human subjects should be preceded by careful assessment of predictable risks and burdens in comparison with foreseeable benefits to the subject or to others. This does not preclude the participation of healthy volunteers in medical research. The design of all studies should be publicly available.

17. Physicians should abstain from engaging in research projects involving human subjects unless they are confident that the risks involved have been adequately assessed and can be satisfactorily managed. Physicians should cease any investigation if the risks are found to outweigh the potential benefits or if there is conclusive proof of positive and beneficial results.

18. Medical research involving human subjects should only be conducted if the importance of the objective outweighs the inherent risks and burdens to the subject. This is especially important when the human subjects are healthy volunteers.

19. Medical research is only justified if there is a reasonable likelihood that the populations in which the research is carried out stand to benefit from the results of the research.

20. The subjects must be volunteers and informed participants in the research project.

21. The right of research subjects to safeguard their integrity must always be respected. Every precaution should be taken to respect the privacy of the subject, the confidentiality of the patient's information and to minimize the impact of the study on the subject's physical and mental integrity and on the personality of the subject.

22. In any research on human beings, each potential subject must be adequately informed of the aims, methods, sources of funding, any possible conflicts of interest, institutional affiliations of the researcher, the anticipated benefits and potential risks of the study and the discomfort it may entail. The subject should be informed of the right to abstain from participation in the study or to withdraw consent to participate at any time without reprisal. After ensuring that the subject has understood the information, the physician should then obtain the subject's freely-given informed consent, preferably in writing. If the consent cannot be obtained in writing, the non-written consent must be formally documented and witnessed.

23. When obtaining informed consent for the research project the physician should be particularly cautious if the subject is in a dependent relationship with the physician or may consent under duress. In that case the informed consent should be obtained by a well-informed physician who is not engaged in the investigation and who is completely independent of this relationship.

24. For a research subject who is legally incompetent, physically or mentally incapable of giving consent or is a legally incompetent minor, the investigator must obtain informed consent from the legally authorized representative in accordance with applicable law. These groups should not be included in research unless the research is necessary to promote the health of the population represented and this research cannot instead be performed on legally competent persons.

25. When a subject deemed legally incompetent, such as a minor child, is able to give assent to decisions about participation in research, the investigator must obtain that assent in addition to the consent of the legally authorized representative.

26. Research on individuals from whom it is not possible to obtain consent, including proxy or advance consent, should be done only if the physical/

mental condition that prevents obtaining informed consent is a necessary characteristic of the research population. The specific reasons for involving research subjects with a condition that renders them unable to give informed consent should be stated in the experimental protocol for consideration and approval of the review committee. The protocol should state that consent to remain in the research should be obtained as soon as possible from the individual or a legally authorized surrogate.

27. Both authors and publishers have ethical obligations. In publication of the results of research, the investigators are obliged to preserve the accuracy of the results. Negative as well as positive results should be published or otherwise publicly available. Sources of funding, institutional affiliations and any possible conflicts of interest should be declared in the publication. Reports of experimentation not in accordance with the principles laid down in this Declaration should not be accepted for publication.

C. Additional principles for medical research combined with medical care

28. The physician may combine medical research with medical care, only to the extent that the research is justified by its potential prophylactic, diagnostic or therapeutic value. When medical research is combined with medical care, additional standards apply to protect the patients who are research subjects.

29. The benefits, risks, burdens and effectiveness of a new method should be tested against those of the best current prophylactic, diagnostic, and therapeutic methods. This does not exclude the use of placebo, or no treatment, in studies where no proven prophylactic, diagnostic or therapeutic method exists.

30. At the conclusion of the study, every patient entered into the study should be assured of access to the best proven prophylactic, diagnostic and therapeutic methods identified by the study.

31. The physician should fully inform the patient which aspects of the care are related to the research. The refusal of a patient to participate in a study must never interfere with the patient-physician relationship.

32. In the treatment of a patient, where proven prophylactic, diagnostic and therapeutic methods do not exist or have been ineffective, the physician, with informed consent from the patient, must be free to use unproven or new prophylactic, diagnostic and therapeutic measures, if in the physician's judgement it offers hope of saving life, re-establishing health or alleviating suffering. Where possible, these measures should be made the object of research, designed to evaluate their safety and efficacy. In all cases, new information should be recorded, and, where appropriate, published. The other relevant guidelines of this Declaration should be followed.

Note of clarification on Paragraph 29

The WMA hereby reaffirms its position that extreme care must be taken in making use of a placebo-controlled trial and that in general this methodology should only be used in the absence of existing proven therapy. However, a placebo-controlled trial may be ethically acceptable, even if proven therapy is available, under the following circumstances:

— Where for compelling and scientifically sound methodological reasons its use is necessary to determine the efficacy or safety of a prophylactic, diagnostic or therapeutic method; or

— Where a prophylactic, diagnostic or therapeutic method is being investigated for a minor condition and the patients who receive placebo will not be subject to any additional risk of serious or irreversible harm.

All other provisions of the Declaration of Helsinki must be adhered to, especially the need for appropriate ethical and scientific review.

---

[1] The Declaration of Helsinki is an official policy document of the World Medical Association, the global representative body for physicians. It was first adopted in 1964 (Helsinki, Finland) and revised in 1975 (Tokyo, Japan), 1983 (Venice, Italy), 1989 (Hong Kong), 1996 (Sommerset-West, South Africa) and 2000 (Edinburgh, Scotland). Note of clarification on Paragraph 29 added by the WMA General Assembly, Washington, 2002.

Source: World Medical Association, 2002 (available on web site http://www.wma.net/e/policy17-e_e.html).

Principles of biomedical ethics

i. Respect for autonomy

Respecting autonomy means that people respect and do not interfere with the actions of rational persons that have a capacity for autonomous action, that is, adults who are able to freely decide upon a course of action without influence, coercion or force (Beauchamp & Childress, 2001). In the context of biomedical research, the principle of respect for autonomy is usually taken to require the following: informed consent to treatment or research participation, voluntariness in research participation, and maintenance of confidentiality and privacy of information provided to a researcher (Beauchamp & Childress, 2001).

ii. Non-maleficence

The principle of non-maleficence simply means, *do no harm* (Beauchamp & Childress, 2001). Following the principle of non-maleficence requires people to refrain from causing harm or injury, or from placing others at risk of harm or injury. In the context of biomedical research, the principle of non-maleficence requires researchers to minimize the risks associated with participation in research (Brody, 1998; Beauchamp & Childress, 2001).

iii. Beneficence

Beauchamp and Childress have identified "positive beneficence" and "utility" as two elements of the principle of beneficence (Beauchamp & Childress, 2001). Positive beneficence requires people to perform actions that result in benefit. Utility requires that the benefits of peoples' actions outweigh the burdens they impose upon others. The principle of beneficence therefore requires that an action produces benefits and that its benefits outweigh its burdens. In the context of biomedical research, this means that the benefits of the research to society should outweigh its risks to participants.

iv. Distributive justice

Justice is probably the most controversial of the four moral principles. For the purpose of this discussion, "justice" refers to "distributive justice" rather than retributive (criminal) or rectificatory (compensatory) justice (Beauchamp & Childress, 2001). In bioethics, the principle of distributive justice has been central to debates about how to ensure equitable access to health care and to reduce unequal health outcomes. In the case of research, the principle of distributive justice refers to the equitable distribution of the risks, as well as the benefits of research participation (Brody, 1998). A fair and just research policy would aim to achieve a distribution of the benefits and burdens of research participation that is as fair and equitable as possible.

Human rights

In 1948 the Universal Declaration of Human Rights (UDHR) set out an international set of human rights that would be honoured by all nations which signed the declaration (United Nations General Assembly, 10 December, 1948). The UDHR recognised that all people have rights by virtue of being human and that these were universal in the sense of applying equally to all people around the world, regardless of who they are or where they live (International Federation of Red Cross and Red Crescent Societies and François-Xavier Bagnoud Center for Health and Human Rights, 1999; Mann et al., 1999). The UDHR enjoined nations to treat all people as equal and to promote and protect the right to life, liberty and security of person. It included "negative rights" such as the rights not to be enslaved or in servitude, not be to be tortured or subject to cruel, inhuman and degrading treatment or punishment. It also obliged signatory states to afford people equal treatment before the law and the equal protection of the law, without discrimination, by requiring that everyone charged with a penal offence should be presumed innocent until proved guilty (UDHR, 1948, article 11).

Ethical principles in medicine and human rights both embody injunctions to behave in specific ways but they differ in to whom they apply (Mann, 1999). Ethical principles typically apply to individuals, usually health care workers and researchers, whereas human rights impose obligations on states and governments to promote and protect the rights of their citizens from infringements by the state or by others (Mann, 1999). Human rights are most relevant to the way in which treatments and interventions derived from neuroscience research are used to treat and prevent substance dependence. This is because treatment and prevention may involve the use of the coercive powers of the state to threaten the human rights of persons who are dependent on psychoactive substances (Gostin & Mann, 1999).

Ethics of animal experimentation in neuroscience research

The use of animals in biomedical research has traditionally been justified by the argument that the harm inflicted upon animals in the course of research is outweighed by the gains in scientific knowledge to humans (and animals) (Resnik, 1998). The scientific community has generally accepted this defence, but it has not received similar support from the public as a result of media reporting of controversial examples of animal experimentation (Brody, 1998).

Animal research has provided some significant benefits to humans, for example, the identification of mechanisms that cause disease and the improvement of treatments (Naquet, 1993).

Although there are alternatives to animal models in some situations, such as tissue cultures and computer simulation (Resnik, 1998), these models cannot replace the use of animals in research because they cannot model the rich behavioural and physiological environment of live animals (American Psychological Association Science Directorate, 2001).

A criticism of animal experimentation is that the animals used do not provide good models of human biology, physiology and psychology (Resnik, 1998). For example, research has shown that cortical organization in the brain varies between species and that some primates lack characteristics found in humans (Preuss, 2000). It has also been argued that the psychology and neurobiology of substance dependence are not well-modelled in commonly used animals such as mice and rats (Resnik, 1998), and that non-human primate models are more desirable because the cortical anatomy and behavioural repertoire of primates more closely resembles those of humans (National Academy of Science, 1996). However, much of the current knowledge regarding the neuroscience of substance dependence has come from animal experimentation using a number of different species. Genetically engineered mice, for example, have been used to identify initial targets for drugs, such as the CB1 cannabinoid receptor, and biochemical pathways involved in cocaine metabolism have been investigated (Nestler, 2000). Rats and other non-primate species have provided good models for certain aspects of the psychology and neurobiology of substance dependence, thus reducing the number of primates needed in research.

It seems that a societal compromise exists between those who oppose animal experimentation and those who deem it necessary (Varner, 1994). The moral objections to animal experimentation have increased the burden of proof that defenders of research must meet (Varner, 1994). This is a reasonable outcome as long as the burden of proof is not insurmountable.

In most countries, legislation adopts one of two perspectives which acknowledge the need for animal experimentation while placing restrictions on the practice (Brody, 1998). Legislation in Europe and America takes a "human priority" position in which animal suffering and loss are minimized but the interests of humans take precedence over those of animals when they conflict (Brody, 1998). In contrast, legislation in Australia and the United Kingdom is based on a "balancing" position in which the interests of humans are generally regarded as more important than those of animals but they can sometimes be overridden in order to protect animals (Brody, 1998). Unlike legislation in America and Europe, legislation in Australia and the United Kingdom requires that during the ethical review process, the benefits of the proposed experiments be weighed against the harm that will be inflicted on the animals (Brody, 1998).

Ethical principles in human biomedical research

Since the Nuremberg trials of German medical researchers after World War II, a consensus has been developed about the basic ethical requirements for biomedical research on humans (Brody, 1998; Jonsen, 1998). In most developed countries, national ethical codes set out obligations that investigators must adhere to if their research is to be ethically and scientifically legitimate. Although specific conditions for ethical approval may differ from country to country the same basic set of ethical principles is found in most national guidelines (Brody, 1998). These include independent ethical review of research proposals, respect for patient privacy, informed consent to participate in research, and protection of privacy and confidentiality of information (Brody, 1998).

Independent ethical review of risks and benefits

In order for any human research to gain approval, investigators must obtain ethical approval from an independent ethical review committee, usually an institutional ethical review committee. An external review of a study protocol provides an independent assessment of whether the benefits of the proposed trial outweigh any risks that it poses to participants (Brody, 1998).

Informed consent

Informed consent to participate in a research study is usually a matter of asking the research participant to consent to their participation after a detailed discussion of what it will entail and a description of any adverse events that may occur (Brody, 1998). The participation of persons under the age of 18 years would normally require the consent of a parent or guardian, along with the assent of the participant. Any uncertainty about the risks of participation must be accurately communicated and there must be close monitoring of any adverse events, with medical care promptly provided for any adverse outcomes. The inclusion of persons with cognitive impairments in a study may require special consideration (see below). Consent may need to be obtained from a surrogate who makes a decision on behalf of the impaired research participant (Brody, 1998). This has implications for research involving persons with substance dependence if the person has long-term cognitive, psychiatric, or neurological dysfunction as a result of substance use (see Chapter 4), or if the person has a concurrent psychiatric illness (see Chapter 6).

All forms of consent must be given after the participants are informed of what their involvement in the research will require of them. Research participants should have time to reflect on and consider their obligations at each stage of the consent procedure. Ideally, the consent process should include a third party, usually a clinician not involved in the study, to ensure the integrity of the process. Participants must be allowed to withdraw from the study at any time. If they decide to withdraw, their decision must be respected and they must be informed that they will not suffer any consequences, such as refusal of routine counselling or medical care (Brody, 1998). If any participant withdraws from the study, the data collected from them must be omitted from the final results.

Recruitment of subjects

The conditions under which persons are recruited into a study must not involve any form of coercion or the use of excessive inducements to participate (Brody, 1998). In recent years, it has become common to reimburse participants for their involvement in some research studies. The most common justification is that reimbursements maximize initial recruitment and retention of participants in a study. Small reimbursements are offered to compensate participants for the time spent participating in a trial or for their travel expenses. Reimbursements may be interpreted by some potential subjects as rewards for participation, and by researchers as a way of increasing the number of trial participants. Ashcroft argues that inducements are ethically acceptable if the inducement serves to recompense a participant for the inconvenience, as long as it is not seen as a payment for any harm caused (Ashcroft, 2001). In Australia, for example, it has been common practice since the early 1980s for drug researchers to pay drug users A$20 if they participate in research interviews. The money is intended to compensate participants for their time, travel expenses and inconvenience. Payment of research participants is also standard practice in drug research in Canada and the USA.

In Australia this strategy has proved to be a successful way of recruiting illicit drug users for research studies of risk factors for the transmission of HIV, hepatitis C and other infectious blood-borne diseases; patterns of illicit amphetamine use (including injecting use, the reasons for making the transition to injecting, and the prevalence of psychological and health problems caused by injecting use); the prevalence and correlates of drug overdoses among heroin users; and national monitoring of trends in illicit drug use since 1996. The information collected in these studies could not be easily obtained in any other way. Interviewing drug users in treatment, for example, would be of limited use because many drug users do not seek treatment, and those who do usually do so after several years of problem drug use. Obtaining information in this way provides advance warning of emerging trends in illicit drug use. It also creates an opportunity to provide drug users with information about the risks of their drug use, and such information may also help in the design of educational campaigns aimed at illicit drug users. The findings of these studies are also regularly presented to staff at treatment centres to alert them to problems emerging among persons seeking their help.

A concern expressed by critics of this practice of paying participants is that the money will serve as an inducement because of its potential for buying drugs. The first question is whether drug users have the same rights as anyone else to be compensated for the time and inconvenience of being interviewed. The money may well be used to pay for tobacco, alcohol or illicit drugs, but so may any income that drug users obtain by employment, social welfare, or crime. In terms of the daily pattern of drug use of most injecting drug users, $20 buys only a very small amount of the street drugs normally used per day. This issue is controversial and remains unresolved.

Privacy and confidentiality

Researchers are obligated to protect the privacy of study participants. Participants' personal information must not be divulged to any individual or group of individuals without their direct consent, and they should not be identifiable from the published results of the study (Brody, 1998). These rules are especially important when study participants have a stigmatized condition such as mental illness or substance dependence.

Protecting the privacy of participants and the confidentiality of the information that they provide is critical in research where data are collected on substance use. The use of some psychoactive substances (e.g. cannabis, cocaine and heroin) is illegal, as is the use of alcohol by persons who are under the minimum legal drinking age. Surveys of drug use may also ask about illicit drug use and the commission of other illegal acts, such as driving while intoxicated, selling illicit drugs or engaging in theft, fraud or violence to finance drug use. If such data were linked to an identified individual and given to the police then the participant could face criminal charges. In the USA researchers can obtain certificates of confidentiality that provide subjects with an assurance that this will not happen. However, the legal status of these certificates is unclear, given that the certificate is issued federally; it is unclear if it would have legal status in state courts. Furthermore, the threat of access to these documents from civil law suits is also unclear. The legal situation in most other countries is similarly unclear.

Confidentiality is much less of a problem when data are collected in a single cross-sectional interview. The information provided usually does not contain participants name or other identifiers because this information need not be collected. Confidentiality becomes more of an issue if interviews are recorded (e.g. on tape) because this could be used in a court of law. Confidentiality becomes a potentially serious issue in longitudinal studies in which data that permit identification of subjects (e.g. the participant's name and address, and the names and addresses of their family and friends) are collected so that individuals may be recontacted for further interviews at a later date. A standard precaution is to store names and identifiers so that they are secure, and to keep them separate from the survey data. Confidentiality will become an even more important issue when DNA samples (or biological tissues from which DNA can be obtained) are collected because DNA provides a unique way of identifying all individuals (except identical twins). When linked with questionnaire or interview data, DNA permits information on self-reported illegal acts to be reliably linked to an individual. Special precautions will therefore be necessary to protect privacy in epidemiological studies of illicit drug use that also collect biological samples. This may require legislation similar to that which applies in the USA.

Emerging ethical issues in neuroscience research

Research on vulnerable persons

Research involving persons who have cognitive or physical impairments requires special ethical consideration (Brody, 1998). A major ethical issue is whether vulnerable persons are capable of providing informed consent, specifically whether they are able understand the rationale behind a clinical trial (Mora, 2000), understand exactly what is required of them and why (Stahl, 1996), and give their free and informed consent to participate in the study (Anthony & Helzer, 1991).

A person may be vulnerable for one or more of the following three reasons: personal limitations to their freedom (intrinsic), environmental factors that limit their freedom (extrinsic), and limitations on their freedom by virtue of a relationship with another person or group (relational) (Roberts & Roberts, 1999).

Are substance dependent people vulnerable persons?

Few studies have been conducted on whether persons who are substance dependent have an impaired capacity to consent to participation in research (Adler, 1995; Gorelick et al., 1999). Most of the recent controversy about neuroscience research on vulnerable populations has been about research on persons with schizophrenia (Shamoo, 1998) and stroke (Alves & Macciocchi, 1996). In these cases, there are serious doubts about the capacity of some patients to give free and informed consent because they are cognitively impaired, either intermittently or chronically. There are some analogies between these cases and issues concerning experimental research on persons who are substance dependent. There are long-term neurological, cognitive and psychiatric consequences of some types of substance use (see Chapter 4), which may affect the ability of some individuals to give informed consent.

Drug dependent persons may be vulnerable to coercion and inducement to participate in research when they are intoxicated or when they are experiencing acute withdrawal symptoms (Adler, 1995; Gorelick et al., 1999). Persons who are severely intoxicated by alcohol and cocaine, for example, suffer similar impairments to a person who is acutely psychotic. Similarly, a person who is experiencing acute withdrawal symptoms could be induced to consent to participate in research studies by offering them the substance on which they are dependent, or medication to relieve their withdrawal symptoms (Adler, 1995; Gorelick et al., 1999). Intoxicated persons should normally be excluded from experimental studies on the grounds of good research design, apart from the ethical problems associated with their inclusion. Issues of informed consent arise in conducting controlled trials of drugs that are used to treat symptoms of drug toxicity or overdose. In such cases where a person is unable to give consent, proxy consent may be required.

Provocation studies

Provocation studies in neuroscience research on dependence often use neuroimaging to study the effects of a psychoactive substance on brain function in substance users and substance dependent persons. For example, persons dependent on heroin may be injected with a radioactively-labelled substance, placed in a PET or SPECT scan (Fu & McGuire, 1999), and then given an opioid drug or exposed to drug-related stimuli, with the aim of identifying sites in the brain at which the drug acts (Sell et al., 1999; Kling et al., 2000; Martin-Soelch et al., 2001). These provocation studies involve little or no immediate prospect of therapeutic gain to participants. Their most likely benefits are an improved understanding of substance dependence that may benefit future patients by improving treatment outcome.

Informed-consent procedures for provocation studies on substance dependence need to make clear to potential participants the absence of any therapeutic gain, and the risks of participation. Participants who were seeking treatment should be actively referred to a treatment service (Gorelick et al., 1999). Steps also need to be taken to ensure that the capacity to give voluntary consent is not impaired because participants are intoxicated or experiencing withdrawal symptoms. This may require screening for symptoms of intoxication and withdrawal at the time of recruitment (Adler, 1995).

Drug administration in these studies is considerably less risky than drug use that occurs outside the laboratory setting. Significantly lower doses of pharmaceutically pure drugs are used in laboratory studies, in the absence of concurrent drug use which occurs in the community. In addition, the drug is administered under medical supervision with protocols in place to deal with any adverse events (Adler, 1995). The risks of drug administration can be further reduced by screening out persons who have experienced adverse effects from drugs such as the psychostimulants. The use of stimuli associated with substance use is much less invasive and poses fewer risks than exposure to drugs. The radioactively-labelled substances used in some forms of neuroimaging pose very little risk to participants, and the newer imaging methods, such as fMRI, do not involve exposure to radiation or radioactive substances (Gilman, 1998).

Ethical issues in epidemiological research on substance dependence

The major ethical issues in epidemiological research are: ensuring that participants give free and informed consent, and protecting their privacy and the confidentiality of any information that is collected. There are also considerations unique to epidemiological studies. Since no experimental procedures are involved, the major risks that research participants face arise from the possible mis-use of any information that they provide. These risks may potentially include social ostracism and stigmatization, if their drug use becomes known to family, friends or neighbours; and criminal prosecution, if any information that they provide about illegal drug use or other criminal behaviour becomes known to the police in a way that can be linked to the individual.

Justice and the criteria for good epidemiological research both require that a representative sample of the population at risk is recruited into studies of patterns of substance use and dependence in the population. There may be issues raised by poorer retention in longitudinal studies of the indigent and homeless, who may be at higher risk of developing substance dependence. Justice may also be an issue if there is a preponderance of studies of persons entering publicly-funded treatment for substance dependence, and a lack of representation of those who are treated by private health services or private specialist physicians and psychiatrists. It is also possible that the results of a study may potentially lead to stigmatization of a group, if for example, a study identifies a high rate of substance dependence in a particular social, cultural or ethnic group.

Ethical issues in clinical trials of pharmacological treatments for substance dependence

Clinical trials of new therapeutic drugs are required for drug registration in most developed countries and are a now widely accepted part of medical practice. There is international agreement on the criteria for the ethical conduct of such studies. In addition to the previously discussed issues of independent ethical review – i.e. free and informed consent by study participants; an acceptable risk–benefit ratio for participants; and protection of patient privacy and confidentiality (Brody, 1998) – there are also issues of trial design, conflict of interest and distributive justice.

Trial design

A randomized controlled trial is widely accepted as the "gold standard" for treatment evaluation in medicine because it minimizes bias in determining which patients receive which treatments (Cochrane, 1972). Random assignment to treatment is ethically acceptable if there is genuine uncertainty about the comparative worth of the two treatments; if trial participants are aware that they will be randomized; and if they are informed about the type of treatment to which they may be assigned (e.g. active or placebo), and the risks of these treatments in the course of obtaining their informed consent to participate in the trial.

The choice of a comparison condition for a randomized controlled trial raises the issue of when is it ethically acceptable to compare the effectiveness of a new drug treatment for substance dependence with a placebo. Some authors have argued that it is unethical to provide only a placebo treatment, if there is an existing treatment that is effective for the condition (Brody, 1998). This argument is relevant in the case of substance dependence, some forms of which can be life-threatening in the absence of treatment. It would be ethically acceptable, however, to use a placebo comparison condition if there was no effective pharmacotherapy for the condition, and if both treatment groups received the best available psychosocial treatment (Gorelick et al., 1999). In this case, the clinical trial would answer the question: does adding pharmacotherapy to good quality psychosocial care improve outcome by comparison with adding a placebo? Since it is likely that any pharmacotherapy will ultimately be used in combination with good quality psychosocial treatment (Fox, 1997), this is usually the most relevant question to ask in a randomized controlled trial of a new pharmacotherapy for drug dependence.

Distributive justice

Justice and the criteria for sound clinical trials both require that a representative sample of the population at risk is recruited into such studies (Brody, 1998). Special efforts may need to be made to ensure that women, children and minority groups are included in clinical trials to ensure that they have access to the benefits of research participation and that the results of research studies can be applied to these groups if drugs that are trialed are eventually approved and registered for clinical use (Brody, 1998).

Conflicts of interest

An ethical issue of increasing significance, given the extent of funding of clinical trials by pharmaceutical companies, is ensuring public confidence in the results (Davidoff et al., 2001; DeAngelis, Fontanarosa & Flanagin, 2001). Public trust has been undermined in recent years because investigators have failed to disclose their personal financial interests in the outcomes of clinical trials (e.g. as a result of being paid large consultancy fees for promoting pharmaceuticals or shares in a pharmaceutical company). This has become an increasingly larger problem as public funding for medical research and universities has declined and pharmaceutical companies have become a major source of research funds. Moreover, research funded by these companies has been conducted by contract research organizations, with the conditions in which data can be published being controlled by pharmaceutical sponsors (DeAngelis, Fontanarosa & Flanagin, 2001; Anon, 2001).

No matter how scientifically rigorous and ethically conducted a study may be, its findings are of limited use if the public does not have confidence in their validity (Davidoff et al., 2001; DeAngelis, Fontanarosa & Flanagin, 2001). A number of policies have been implemented by editors of leading medical journals in an effort to restore trust in clinical research. One is the decision by these editors to require that authors disclose funding sources and potential conflicts of interest, and assert that they have had complete control over the study data and their analysis (Davidoff et al., 2001; DeAngelis, Fontanarosa & Flanagin, 2001). Another policy has been the creation of a register of clinical trial protocols before the start of the study to minimize the suppression of unfavourable results or ex post facto selection of results and methods of analysis in order to make a drug look its best (Horton, 1997).

Additional policy recommendations have been made that have not so far been implemented. These include: independent monitoring of compliance with the study protocol, especially with reporting of any adverse events experienced by participants; and a requirement that investigators and the sponsors of a trial commit to publishing its results within two years of completing data collection, as a condition of the study protocol being approved by an ethics committee (Reidenberg, 2001). The latter seems well based given that the major ethical justification for undertaking research studies is to contribute to scientific knowledge (Brody, 1998), and this cannot happen if trial results are not published (Reidenberg, 2001).

Trials of preventive pharmacological interventions for substance dependence

Psychosocial and educational interventions have been widely used with the aim of preventing young people from using drugs (Spooner & Hall, 2002). Universal interventions are aimed at all young people, while indicated, targeted or selective interventions are aimed at those young people who are identified as being at higher risk of initiating drug use. The impact of both universal and selective educational interventions on rates of drug use has often been modest (National Research Council, 2001).

Psychosocial preventive interventions raise ethical issues. Universal interventions (those directed at all young people) raise concerns about unintended adverse consequences, such as encouraging drug experimentation in young people. Targeted or indicated interventions raise additional ethical issues because they require the identification of young people who are at increased risk of using drugs. Their consent and that of their parents is required for them to participate in preventive interventions. In the process of obtaining such consent, the parents and their children may become acquainted with their risk status. Participation in trials of preventive interventions may also expose the children to social stigmatization and discrimination, if it becomes known to their teachers, peers and their peers' parents. For example, parents whose children are judged to be at "low risk" may actively discourage their children from associating with "high-risk" children, or they may insist that high-risk children be excluded or removed from schools.

The same ethical issues of stigmatization and discrimination are also raised by pharmacological or immunological interventions that aim to prevent substance dependence. Two such interventions are discussed below: early pharmacological interventions in persons at risk of substance dependence that may be inspired by similar efforts to prevent psychoses (McGorry, Yung & Phillips, 2001); and the preventive use of immunotherapies against drug effects to reduce risk of substance dependence (Cohen, 1997).

Early intervention studies

Early interventions for substance dependence have been discussed which would be analogous to studies of schizophrenia that identify persons who are at increased risk of developing the disorder because they have a family history of schizophrenia or they have psychological symptoms that may be early or "prodromal" symptoms of the disorder. The aim of this approach is to prevent the development of schizophrenia by a combination of good quality psychosocial care and low doses of the neuroleptic drugs that are used to treat schizophrenia (McGorry, Yung & Phillips, 2001). Studies in Australia and the USA have shown that it is possible, using standardized criteria, to identify a group of young people who have a high risk (30–40%) of developing schizophrenia in the ensuing 6 to 12 months (McGlashan, 2001; McGorry, Yung & Phillips, 2001). A number of quasi-experiments and randomized controlled trials suggest that the combined intervention reduces the rate at which schizophrenia occurs and reduces its severity (McGorry, Yung & Phillips, 2001). Similar trials can be foreseen for substance dependence, once research clarifies the risk and protective factors, genetic predisposition, and treatment options.

Critics of these studies have raised a number of ethical issues (Cornblatt, Lencz & Kane, 2001; DeGrazia, 2001). These include the fact that there is a high false positive rate: 60% of those who are identified as being at risk of developing schizophrenia do not develop the disorder. This can also be seen to apply to the development of substance dependence. There is also the potential for stigmatization and discrimination against those who are identified as being at risk. Even if there is no discrimination, there is the possibility that there will be adverse effects on individuals of being labelled as at risk. There is also concern about the capacity of children and adolescents to consent to participate in such studies, and doubts about the acceptability of using proxy parental consent. Long-term preventive treatment with drugs may have health consequences. McGorry, Yung & Phillips (2001) have countered, with respect to schizophrenia, that the potential benefits (the prevention of schizophrenia and early treatment of cases that do occur) outweigh the potential risks of neuroleptic medication and stigmatization, both of which they suggest (on the basis of controlled studies) have been exaggerated.

Analogous approaches to early interventions could be taken for substance dependence, although to date no trials have been explicitly undertaken with the aim of using pharmacotherapies as preventive interventions for substance dependence. It is likely that many of the same ethical issues would arise. Psychostimulant drugs, such as methylphenidate and dexamphetamine, have been used to treat children and adolescents with attention deficit hyperactivity disorder (ADHD), an intervention that is controversial (Levy, 1997). Since ADHD in combination with conduct disorders increases the risks of developing substance use disorders (Lynskey & Hall, 2001), and psychostimulant drugs reduce symptoms of ADHD (Swanson et al., 1998), an unintended by-product of psychostimulant medication may be the prevention of substance use disorders. However, no one has so far argued for the use of psychostimulant medication to prevent substance dependence, and it is unlikely that anyone would do so. Public concern about the long-term use of stimulant drugs to treat ADHD suggests that any such proposal will be opposed and support for the chronic use of drugs in late childhood or adolescence to prevent the development of substance dependence would seem to be even less likely.

Preventive use of drug immunotherapies

Animal studies have shown that it is possible to induce the formation of antibodies to substances such as cocaine (Fox et al., 1996; Carrera et al., 2000). These antibodies in the blood combine with the substance to prevent it reaching the brain to exert its effects (Fox et al., 1996) (see Chapter 4). Animal studies show that antibodies against cocaine markedly attenuate its stimulant effects and block self-administration in rats (Carrera et al., 1995; Johnson & Ettinger, 2000). If cocaine immunotherapies prove safe and effective in treating persons with cocaine dependence, they could be used to prevent cocaine dependence in adolescents and young adults, as well as in adults and in legally coerced treatment. Such possibilities have been raised and briefly discussed (Cohen, 1997, 2000). Similar arguments will no doubt arise with the proposed preventive use of nicotine immunotherapies.

If a controlled clinical trial demonstrates that nicotine and cocaine immunotherapies are safe and effective treatments of these types of substance dependence, then a number of ethical issues concerning their use in voluntary treatment of substance dependent adults need to be addressed (Cohen, 1997; Hall & Carter, 2002). The preventive use of cocaine and nicotine immunotherapies would be ethical in the case of adults who voluntarily decided to use them after being informed of any risks. The immunotherapies would need to be shown to be safe and effective for this purpose, with higher standards of proof generally required for the safety and efficacy of preventive measures (Hall & Carter, 2002). The foreseeable risks of using the immunotherapy would have to be communicated to the person, who would have given informed consent to its use, and steps would need to be taken to protect the person's privacy. Under these conditions, the voluntary administration of a cocaine immunotherapy to consenting adults who considered themselves to be susceptible to cocaine dependence would be ethically acceptable (Hall & Carter, 2002). However, such use is likely to be unusual.

A potentially unique feature of active immunization against cocaine is that it may, in principle, have long-lasting consequences, namely, creating antibodies that can be detected in the blood of treated patients for some months or years. These antibody levels may not be sufficiently high to be therapeutic but the fact that they could be detected raises the ethical issues of privacy and discrimination (Cohen, 1997).

Of special concern is the possible loss of privacy by recovering cocaine-dependent individuals if employers and insurance companies had access to this information. Employers and insurance companies often obtain detailed personal medical information and, on occasion, blood samples from potential employees or clients. Because the community often strongly disapproves of cocaine dependence, the loss of privacy by a recovering cocaine-dependent individual may lead to embarrassment, at best, and to social stigmatization and ostracism by people in their social environment and in the wider community. In the future, increasing social stigmatization of smokers, and the possibility of discrimination by employers and the health insurance industry, may raise similar issues for smokers who use nicotine immunization to stop smoking.

Discrimination may arise if workplace-based drug testing were to screen for cocaine antibodies before and during employment. A recovering cocaine-dependent person would be at risk of losing an employment opportunity or his or her job if cocaine antibodies were detected in a blood sample. If this information were more widely disseminated to other workers it could have a devastating effect on the employment prospects and recovery of the individual (Cohen, 1997).

One way of avoiding these outcomes may be to accept Cohen's proposal that a society that wishes to have the benefits of a cocaine immunotherapy "must institute legal and behavioural changes that preserve privacy and confidentiality" (Cohen, 1997). This requires a culture that encourages and supports the recovery of persons with substance dependence. Legislation that punishes discriminatory behaviour towards recovering persons has been adopted in the case of HIV-infected persons. The adoption of a similar approach to people who have been treated for cocaine dependence would be an important step towards reducing discrimination and protecting privacy.

The risks of loss of privacy and discrimination could also be minimized by using "passive" rather than "active" immunization to prevent relapse (e.g. by administering antibodies to cocaine rather than an immunization). This approach would not produce an enduring change in the person's immune system and the antibodies would disappear over a period of weeks. These advantages would be gained at the expense of a shorter period of protection (without a booster injection) that may reduce treatment effectiveness. This may be a trade-off that a patient concerned about privacy would be prepared to make, but it is a choice that they should be offered (Hall & Carter, 2002).

The preventive "immunization" of children and adolescents against cocaine dependence is a much more ethically complex issue. Children would presumably be immunized against cocaine dependence at the request of their parents. Their parents would consent on behalf of their children who, as minors, would not be legally able to give informed consent. Parents already make choices on behalf of their children that will affect their future (e.g. regarding diet and education). Some have argued, therefore, that immunization against cocaine dependence would simply be another decision that some parents would make for their children (Cohen, 1997). On the basis of this argument, a parent would have the right to immunize their children against cocaine dependence in much the same way as they have the right to immunize them against measles or other infectious diseases (Kaebnick, 2000).

Cocaine use may begin in adolescence. Adolescents under the age of majority have sufficient capacity to be involved in decisions about their future, such as whether they want to be immunized against cocaine dependence. Even if it is ethically acceptable for parents to consent on behalf of their children, the assent of an adolescent or an older child should be sought, and if they fail to give it, their decision should rarely be overridden and only if there is a strong reason for doing so (Brody, 1998). It must be remembered that not everyone who uses cocaine for the first time goes on to become dependent.

Implications of neuroscience research for models of substance dependence

There has been a long-standing conflict between moral and medical models of substance dependence (Gerstein & Harwood, 1990; Leshner, 1997). A moral model of substance dependence sees it as largely a voluntary behaviour in which people freely engage. Drug users who offend against the criminal code are therefore to be prosecuted and imprisoned if found guilty (Szasz, 1985). A medical model of substance dependence, by contrast, recognizes that, while many people use certain psychoactive drugs without developing substance dependence, a small proportion of users develop substance dependence that requires specific treatment (Leshner, 1997).

Medical models of substance dependence may not be a wholly positive development if they lead to over-simplified social policies. For example, the idea that substance dependence is a categorical disease entity lends itself to a simplification in the case of alcohol, namely, that if people who are genetically vulnerable to alcohol dependence are identified, then there may be an assumption that the rest of the population can use alcohol without developing dependence (Hall & Sannibale, 1996). This view does not take into account the adverse public health effects of alcohol intoxication. It is also at odds with the multi-dimensional nature of alcohol and illicit drug use and symptoms of substance dependence, and with the genetic evidence that multiple genes are involved in vulnerability to substance dependence (see Chapter 5). It can also lead users to abdicate responsibility for their behaviour (Nelkin & Lindee, 1996), and to a preoccupation with individual explanation of behaviour with a corresponding lack of attention towards remediable social causes and social policy options for reducing the prevalence of substance dependence, including drug control policies.

The implications of a neuroscience view of substance dependence for drug control policy (discussed below) are also not as simple as they may seem. Exposure to drug use remains a necessary condition for the development of substance dependence. Thus societal efforts still need to be made (whether by criminal law or public health measures) to limit access to drugs by young people (Leshner, 1997). Social disapproval remains a potent means of discouraging drug use. It is hoped that neuroscience explanations of substance dependence may temper social stigmatization and ostracism of people with substance dependence. Demonstrations of the greater cost-effectiveness of treatment compared with imprisonment may also provide an economic justification for a more humane, as well as a more effective and efficient, societal response to substance dependence.

The challenge for the neuroscience community in the field of substance dependence is to explain substance dependence in biological terms without depicting people with substance dependence as automatons under the control of receptors in their brains (Valenstein, 1998). This means viewing substance dependence as the result, in part, of choices that are made by individuals, not always independently. In the case of young people, many of them operate with a short-term view, a sense of personal invulnerability, and with scepticism towards their elders' warnings about the risks of substance use. Adolescents are particularly vulnerable to marketing pressures, especially with regard to tobacco and alcohol use. It will also mean viewing substance dependence as a matter of degree, with dependent drug users retaining the capacity to choose to become abstinent and to seek help to do so. It will also mean acknowledging that pharmacological treatment is only the beginning of the process of recovery and reintegration of the drug dependent person into the community. Moreover it will require attention to a broader range of social policies in seeking to prevent drug use by young people (Spooner & Hall, 2002).

Implications of neuroscience research for the treatment of substance dependence

Access to treatment

If pharmacological treatments derived from neuroscience research prove to be effective, the issue of ensuring equal access to treatment for all those who may need it is an ethical issue that needs to be addressed. If a substantial proportion of substance-dependent persons are unable to access treatment because they cannot afford it, public funding may be needed (Gerstein & Harwood, 1990). Public provision of such treatment will require economic justification, especially in the case of persons who are dependent on illicit drugs, many of whom will be indigent and unable to pay for their treatment. Advocates for publicly subsidized drug treatment will need to make clear the comparative economic and social costs of treating drug dependent people, as against the current policy in many countries of dealing with substance dependence solely through the criminal justice system (Gerstein & Harwood, 1990; National Research Council, 2001).

Legally coerced treatment

The potential use of a pharmacological treatment for substance dependence or a drug immunotherapy under legal coercion needs to be considered (Cohen, 1997). It is often the first possible use raised when the concept of a drug immunotherapy is mentioned; community concern about this way of using drug immunotherapies may also adversely affect attitudes towards other therapeutic uses. The issue accordingly needs to be discussed, even if it is a long way from being realized. There are good reasons for caution about any coerced use of a pharmacological treatment or a drug immunotherapy. The community has little sympathy for drug dependent offenders who engage in property-related and other crimes, so particular attention must be paid to protecting the legal and human rights of drug offenders.

The rationale for treatment under legal coercion

Legally coerced drug treatment is entered into by persons charged with or convicted of an offence to which their substance dependence has contributed. It is most often provided as an alternative to imprisonment, and usually under the threat of imprisonment if the person fails to comply with treatment (Hall, 1997; Spooner et al., 2001).

One of the major justifications for treatment under coercion is that it is an effective way of treating offenders' substance dependence that will reduce the likelihood of their re-offending (Gerstein & Harwood, 1990; Inciardi & McBride, 1991). This approach has historically been most often used in the treatment of offenders who are dependent on heroin (Leukefeld & Tims, 1988) although it has most recently been used with cocaine-dependent offenders in "drug courts" in the USA (National Research Council, 2001). One issue is whether there should be a higher standard of proven effectiveness for coerced rather than for voluntary treatment. Another issue is that if the treatment is court-mandated, there may be a tendency for the treatment period to last at least as long as would the jail term. Thus, the form and duration of the treatment are being set by criteria which relate to the judicial system, and not necessarily to therapeutic best practice.

The advent of HIV/AIDS has provided an additional argument for treating rather than imprisoning drug-dependent offenders. Prisoners who inject drugs are at higher risk of having contracted HIV and hepatitis C virus by needle-sharing prior to imprisonment (Dolan, 1996). They are at risk of transmitting these infectious diseases to other inmates by needle-sharing and penetrative sexual acts while they are in prison (Vlahov & Polk, 1988) and also to their sexual partners before or after imprisonment. Providing drug treatment under coercion in the community is one way of reducing HIV transmission. The correctional and public health arguments for drug treatment under coercion are reinforced by the economic argument that it is less costly to treat offenders who are drug dependent in the community than it is to imprison them (Gerstein & Harwood, 1990).

Forms of legal coercion

Offenders may be coerced into drug treatment in a variety of ways (Gostin, 1991; Spooner et al., 2001). After an offence has been detected the police may decide not to charge the offender if he or she agrees to enter drug treatment. This form of coercion is not generally favoured because it is not under judicial oversight and thus is open to abuse. Coercion into treatment may also occur after an offender has been charged and before being processed by the court. This is the case in USA drug courts, where adjudication may be postponed until treatment has been completed (General Accounting Office, 1995).

An offender may be coerced into treatment after conviction. If this is done before sentencing, the court may make completion of treatment a condition of a suspended sentence. Alternatively, an offender may be encouraged to enter drug treatment to help him or her to remain abstinent while a sentence is suspended. Drug treatment may also be required after part of a sentence has been served: enrolment in drug treatment may be made a condition of release on parole. Alternatively, enrolment in drug treatment may be encouraged as a way of remaining free of illicit drugs while on parole.

Ethical issues in coerced treatment

Coerced treatment involves the use of state power to force people to receive treatment and so unavoidably raises ethical and human rights issues (Mann, 1999). Evidence from the USA suggests that treatment for heroin dependence, such as methadone maintenance, therapeutic communities and drug free counselling, is of benefit to those who receive it (Gerstein & Harwood, 1990). However, the benefits for any individual are still uncertain since treatment assists only about 50% of those who receive it (Gerstein & Harwood, 1990), and relapse to heroin use after treatment is high. The treatment of cocaine dependence is much less effective than treatment for opioid dependence (Platt, 1997). This weakens the ethical justification for "civil commitment" for cocaine dependence but it may not rule out less coercive forms of treatment.

A consensus view on drug treatment under coercion prepared for WHO (Porter, Arif & Curran, 1986) concluded that such treatment was legally and ethically justified only if the rights of the individuals were protected by "due process" (in accordance with human rights principles) (Mora, 2000), and if effective and humane treatment was provided (Stahl, 1996).

The uncertain benefits of coerced treatment have led some proponents to argue that offenders should be allowed two "constrained choices" (Fox, 1992). The first constrained choice would be whether they participate in drug treatment or not. If they declined to be treated, they would be dealt with by the criminal justice system in the same way as anyone charged with the same offence. The second constrained choice would be given to those who agreed to participate in drug treatment: they would be given the choice of the type of treatment that they received. There is some empirical support for these recommendations in that there is better evidence for the effectiveness of coerced treatment that requires some "voluntary interest" by the offender (Gerstein & Harwood, 1990).

The most ethically defensible form of legally coerced treatment for drug dependent offenders is the use of imprisonment as an incentive for treatment entry, and fear of return to prison as a reason for complying with drug treatment. Offenders should have a constrained choice as to whether they take up treatment or not, and, if they choose to do so, they should be able to choose from a range of treatment options. Moreover, the process should be subject to judicial oversight and review.

If drug immunotherapies and pharmacological treatments are used under legal coercion, their safety, effectiveness and cost-effectiveness should be rigorously evaluated (National Research Council, 2001). Any such use should be cautiously trialed and evaluated, and only after considerable experience has been acquired in their therapeutic use with voluntary patients.

Summary and conclusions

Substance dependence is a serious personal and public health issue throughout the world. Many forms of substance dependence are difficult to treat because of a lack of effective psychosocial or pharmacological treatments.

Experimental studies on humans of the neurobiological basis of substance dependence raise a number of ethical issues, one of which is the capacity of dependent persons to give their consent to participate in such studies. As long as participants are not intoxicated or suffering acute withdrawal symptoms at the time they give consent, there is no compelling reason for believing that persons who are substance dependent cannot give free and informed consent. The risks of administration of drugs, and the use of neuroimaging methods in these experiments, generally do not pose a serious risk to participants.

The ethical issues raised by clinical trials of new pharmacotherapies have been extensively debated and a consensus has evolved on the conditions that must be met. These include free and informed consent, an acceptable risk–benefit ratio, and protection of participant privacy and confidentiality. Trials with substance dependent persons require special attention to informed consent in order to ensure that persons are not intoxicated or experiencing withdrawal symptoms when deciding to participate in trials. Placebo comparisons may be ethically acceptable in such trials if there is no effective pharmacotherapy and if participants are also offered good quality psychosocial care.

Preventive pharmacological interventions for substance dependence do not yet exist and are likely to be highly controversial if they are developed. It is a possibility that may loom larger in the future with the development of interventions that have a potential preventive use, foremost among which are drug immunotherapies. The ethical issues raised by these approaches need to be debated now. The risks of stigmatization and discrimination that are raised by any preventive intervention that identifies high-risk subjects will need to be dealt with. So too will issues of consent in minors, and the potential risks to participants of immunological interventions.

The use of pharmacotherapies and drug immunotherapies under legal coercion is likely to be contentious. It is an arguably ethical policy if the process is under judicial oversight and if offenders are offered constrained choices of whether or not to accept treatment, and of the type of treatment that they accept. Any coerced use of a cocaine immunotherapy should be done cautiously and only after considerable clinical experience of its use with voluntary patients. It should be trialed, and its safety, effectiveness and cost-effectiveness should be rigorously evaluated. Such an evaluation also needs to examine any adverse social or ethical consequences.

References

Adler MW (1995) Human subject issues in drug abuse research: college on problems of drug dependence. *Drug and Alcohol Dependence*, **37**:167–175.

Alves WA, Macciocchi SN (1996) Ethical considerations in clinical neuroscience: current concepts in neuroclinical trials. *Stroke*, **27**:1903–1909.

American Psychological Association Science Directorate (2001) *Research with animals in psychology*. Washington, DC, American Psychological Association.

Andrews G, Henderson S, Hall W (2001) Prevalence, comorbidity, disability and service utilisation: overview of the Australian national mental health survey. *British Journal of Psychiatry*, **178**:145–153.

Anon (2001) The tightening grip of big pharma. *Lancet*, **357**:1141.

Anthony JC, Helzer J (1991) Syndromes of drug abuse and dependence. In: Robins LN, Regier DA, eds. *Psychiatric disorders in America*. New York, NY, Academic Press:116–154.

Ashcroft R (2001) Selection of human research subjects. In: Chadwick R, Ed. *The concise encyclopedia of the ethics of new technologies*. New York, NY, Academic Press:255–266.

Beauchamp TL, Childress JF (2001) *Principles of biomedical ethics*. Oxford, Oxford University Press.

Brody BA (1998) *The ethics of biomedical research: an international perspective*. Oxford, Oxford University Press.

Carrera MR et al. (1995) Suppression of psychoactive effects of cocaine by active immunization. *Nature*, **378**:727–730.

Carrera MR et al. (2000) Cocaine vaccines: antibody protection against relapse in a rat model. *Proceedings of the National Academy of Sciences of the United States of America*, **97**:6202–6206.

Cochrane AL (1972) *Effectiveness and efficiency: random reflections on health services*. Abingdon, Berkshire, Nuffield Provincial Hospitals Trust.

Cohen PJ (1997) Immunization for prevention and treatment of cocaine abuse: legal and ethical implications. *Drug and Alcohol Dependence*, **48**:167–174.

Cohen PJ (2000) No more kicks. *New Scientist*, **166**:23–36.

Cornblatt BA, Lencz T, Kane JM (2001) Treatment of the schizophrenia prodrome: is it presently ethical? *Schizophrenia Research*, **51**:31–38.

Davidoff F et al. (2001) Sponsorship, authorship, and accountability. *New England Journal of Medicine*, **345**:825–827.

de Angelis CD, Fontanarosa PB, Flanagin A (2001) Reporting financial conflicts of interest and relationships between investigators and research sponsors. *Journal of the American Medical Association*, **286**:89–91.

de Grazia D (2001) Ethical issues in early-intervention clinical trials involving minors at risk for schizophrenia. *Schizophrenia Research*, **51**:77–86.

Dolan K (1996) HIV risk behaviour of IDUs before, during and after imprisonment in New South Wales. *Addiction Research*, **4**:151–160.

Fergusson DM, Horwood LJ (2000) Cannabis use and dependence in a New Zealand birth cohort. *New Zealand Medical Journal*, **113**:156–158.

Fox BS (1997) Development of a therapeutic vaccine for the treatment of cocaine addiction. *Drug and Alcohol Dependence*, **48**:153–158.

Fox BS et al. (1996) Efficacy of a therapeutic cocaine vaccine in rodent models. *Nature Medicine*, **2**:1129–1132.

Fox RG (1992) The compulsion of voluntary treatment in sentencing. *Criminal Law Journal*, **16**:37–54.

Fu CH, McGuire PK (1999) Functional neuroimaging in psychiatry. *Philosophical Transactions of the Royal Society of London* (Series B: Biological Sciences), **354**:1359–1370.

General Accounting Office (1995) *Drug courts: information on a new approach to address drug-related crime*. Washington, DC, United States General Accounting Office.

Gerstein DR, Harwood HJ (1990) *Treating drug problems. Vol. 1. A study of effectiveness and financing of public and private drug treatment systems*. Washington, DC, National Academy Press.

Gilman S (1998) Imaging the brain: first of two parts. *New England Journal of Medicine*, **338**:812–820.

Gorelick D et al. (1999) Clinical research in substance abuse: human subjects issues. In: Pincus HA et al., eds. *Ethics in psychiatric research: a resource manual for human subjects protection*. Washington, DC, American Psychiatric Association:177–218.

Gostin LO (1991) Compulsory treatment for drug-dependent persons: justifications for a public health approach to drug dependency. *Milbank Quarterly*, **69**:561–593.

Gostin LO, Mann JM (1999) Toward the development of a human rights impact assessment for the formulation and evaluation of public health policies. In: Mann JM et al., eds. *Health and human rights: a reader*. London, Routledge:54–71.

Hall W (1997) The role of legal coercion in the treatment of offenders with alcohol and heroin problems. *Australian and New Zealand Journal of Criminology*, **30**:103–120.

Hall W, Sannibale C (1996) Are there two types of alcoholism? *Lancet*, **348**:1258.

Hall W, Carter L (2002) Ethical and policy issues in trialing and using a cocaine vaccine to treat and prevent cocaine dependence. *Bulletin of the World Health Organization*, (in press).

Heath AC (1995) Genetic influences on alcoholism risk: a review of adoption and twin studies. *Alcohol Health and Research World*, **19**:166–171.

Hjern A, Lindblad F, Vinnerljung B (2002) Suicide, psychiatric illness, and social maladjustment in intercountry adoptees in Sweden: a cohort study. *Lancet*, **360**:443–448.

Horton R (1997) Medical editors trial amnesty. *Lancet*, **350**:756.

Hser YI et al. (2001) A 33-year follow up of narcotic addicts. *Archives of General Psychiatry*, **58**:503–508.

Inciardi JA, McBride DC (1991) *Treatment alternatives to street crime: history, experiences and issues*. Rockville, MD, National Institute of Drug Abuse.

International Federation of Red Cross and Red Crescent Societies and Francois-Xavier Bagnoud Center for Health and Human Rights (1999) Human rights: an introduction. In: Mann JM et al., eds. *Health and human rights: a reader*. London, Routledge:21–28.

Johnson MW, Ettinger RH (2000) Active cocaine immunization attenuates the discriminative properties of cocaine. *Experimental and Clinical Psychopharmacology*, **8**:163–167.

Jonsen AR (1998) *The birth of bioethics*. Oxford, Oxford University Press.

Kaebnick GE (2000) Vaccinations against bad habits. *Hastings Center Report*, **30**:48.

Kandel DB, Chen K (2000) Types of marijuana users by longitudinal course. *Journal of Studies on Alcohol*, **61**:367–378.

Kessler RC et al. (1994) Lifetime and 12-month prevalence of DSM-III-R psychiatric disorders in the United States: results from the National Comorbidity Survey. *Archives of General Psychiatry*, **51**:8–19.

Kling MA et al. (2000) Opioid receptor imaging with positron emission tomography and [(18)F]cyclofoxy in long-term, methadone-treated former heroin addicts. *Journal of Pharmacology and Experimental Therapeutics*, **295**:1070–1076.

Leshner AI (1997) Addiction is a brain disease, and it matters. *Science*, **278**:45–47.

Leukefeld CG, Tims FM (1988) Compulsory treatment: a review of the findings. In: Leukefeld CG, Tims FM, eds. *Compulsory treatment of drug abuse*. Rockville, MD, National Institute of Drug Abuse:236–251.

Levy F (1997) Attention deficit hyperactivity disorder. *British Medical Journal*, **315**:894–895.

Lynskey MT, Hall W (2001) Attention deficit hyperactivity disorder and substance use disorders: is there a causal link? *Addiction*, **96**:815–822.

McGlashan TH (2001) Psychosis treatment prior to psychosis onset: ethical issues. *Schizophrenia Research*, **51**:47–54.

McGorry PD, Yung A, Phillips L (2001) Ethics and early intervention in psychosis: keeping up the pace and staying in step. *Schizophrenia Research*, **51**:17–29.

Mann JM (1999) Medicine and public health, ethics and human rights. In: Mann JM et al., eds. *Health and human rights: a reader*. London, Routledge:439–452.

Mann JM et al. (1999) Health and human rights. In: Mann JM et al., eds. *Health and human rights: a reader*. London, Routledge:7–20.

Martin-Soelch C et al. (2001) Reward mechanisms in the brain and their role in dependence: evidence from neurophysiological and neuroimaging studies. *Brain Research Reviews*, **36**:139–149.

Mora F (2000) The brain and the mind. In: Gelder MG, Lopez-Ibor JJ, eds. *The new Oxford textbook of psychiatry*. Oxford, Oxford University Press:153–157.

Naquet R (1993) Ethical and moral considerations in the design of experiments. *Neuroscience*, **57**:183–189.

National Academy of Science (1996) *Pathways of addiction: opportunities in drug abuse research*. Washington, DC, National Academy Press.

National Bioethics Advisory Commission (1999) *Research involving persons with mental disorders that may affect decision-making capacity*. Rockville, MD, National Bioethics Advisory Commission.

National Research Council (2001) *Informing America's policy on illegal drugs: what we don't know keeps hurting us*. Washington, DC, National Academy Press.

Nelkin D, Lindee MS (1996) "Genes made me do it": the appeal of biological explanations. *Politics and Life Sciences*, **15**:95–97.

Nestler EJ (2000) Genes and addiction. *Nature Genetics*, **26**:277–281.

Platt JJ (1997) *Cocaine addiction: theory, research, and treatment*. Cambridge, MA, Harvard University Press.

Porter L, Arif AE, Curran WJ (1986) *The law and the treatment of drug- and alcohol-dependent persons: a comparative study of existing legislation*. Geneva, World Health Organization.

Preuss TM (2000) Taking the measure of diversity: comparative alternatives to the model-animal paradigm in cortical neuroscience. *Brain Behavior and Evolution*, **55**:287–299.

Reidenberg MM (2001) Releasing the grip of big pharma. *Lancet*, **358**:664.

Resnik DB (1998) *The ethics of science: an introduction*. London, Routledge.

Roberts LW, Roberts B (1999) Psychiatric research ethics: an overview of evolving guidelines and current ethical dilemmas in the study of mental illness. *Biological Psychiatry*, **46**:1025–1038.

Sell LA et al. (1999) Activation of reward circuitry in human opiate addicts. *European Journal of Neuroscience*, **11**:1042–1048.

Shamoo AE (1998) *Ethics in neurobiological research with human subjects: the Baltimore Conference on Ethics*. Amsterdam, Gordon & Breach.

Spooner C, Hall W (2002) Preventing substance misuse among young people: we need to do more than "just say no". *Addiction,* **97**:478-481.

Spooner C et al. (2001) An overview of diversion strategies for drug-related offenders. *Drug and Alcohol Review*, **20**:281–294.

Stahl SM (1996) *Essential psychopharmacology: neuroscientific basis and practical applications*. Cambridge, Cambridge University Press.

Swanson JM et al. (1998) Attention-deficit hyperactivity disorder and hyperkinetic disorder. *Lancet*, **351**:429–433.

Swendsen JD et al. (2002) Are personality traits familial risk factors for substance use disorders: results of a controlled family study. *American Journal of Psychiatry*, **159**:1760–1766.

Szasz TS (1985) *Ceremonial chemistry*. Holmes Beach, FL, Holmes Learning Publications.

Valenstein ES (1998) *Blaming the brain: the truth about drugs and mental health*. New York, NY, The Free Press.

Varner GE (1994) The prospects for consensus and convergence in the animal rights debate. *Hastings Center Report*, **24**:24–28.

Vlahov D, Polk BF (1988) Intravenous drug use and human immunodeficiency virus (HIV) infection in prison. *AIDS Public Policy Journal*, **3**:42–46.

World Medical Organization (1996) Declaration of Helsinki. *British Medical Journal*, **313**:1448–1449.

CHAPTER 8

Conclusion and Implications for Public Health Policy

Introduction

There is now a much better understanding of the mechanisms of action of different psychoactive substances in the brain, and of why people experience pleasure or the relief of pain from using the substances. Substances differ with respect to the particular class of receptors they affect in the brain, but there are also considerable commonalities between them. The neural pathways that psychoactive substances affect are also those which are affected by many other human behaviours, including eating a meal, having sex, and gambling for money. In this sense, the use of psychoactive substances, at least initially, is one part of the spectrum of human behaviours which potentially bring pleasure or avoid pain. Depending on the route of administration, the substances may have an especially intense effect and high concentrations of some of them are lethal.

Advances in the neuroscience of psychoactive substance use and dependence and their implications

Psychoactive substances also differ in their non-neural biological effects. The form and means of administration of the substance are important in this dimension. Thus the potential for adverse health effects from nicotine taken in as cigarette smoke is high compared with that from nicotine in chewing gum. There is thus a strong public health interest in differentiating the availability of different forms of the substance according to their adverse health effects.

Apart from their toxic biological effects, there are two other mechanisms by which psychoactive substances may have adverse health and social effects, as outlined in Chapter 1 (Fig. 1.2). One is through their psychoactive effects, and particularly through intoxication. Different psychoactive substances differ in the nature and severity of their intoxicating effects. Those of alcohol, for instance, are great, and the potential for adverse casualty consequences accordingly large, while the effects of nicotine as usually consumed are small. Limiting the harm from intoxication, not only to the substance user but also to others, is an important objective for public health-oriented controls of the use of psychoactive substances.

The third major mechanism by which psychoactive substances may have adverse effects is through dependence. As technically defined, the concept of dependence includes elements which are directly biologically measurable, such as tolerance and withdrawal and those which are cognitive and experiential, such as craving and impairment or loss of control. These latter elements can be modelled in or inferred from biological measurements, but cannot yet be directly measured. Thus, while neuroscience research can directly measure states and effects which are relevant to concepts of dependence it cannot measure dependence itself. Dependence is seen as a major contributor to the health and social harm from psychoactive substance use according to its definition as the motor of continuing use. In fact, one element of the definition of dependence is by imputation back from the occurrence of harm: that use has continued despite knowledge of the harm (Chapter 1, Box 1.2, Criterion 3). The strength of effect on the various components of dependence differs between different psychoactive substances, and according to the dosage and dosage schedule. The potential of a given substance to produce various aspects of dependence is also affected by the sociocultural circumstances in which it is used and by individual genetic inheritance.

Dependence is a complex disorder; how an individual becomes dependent on drugs is probably as complex as the brain itself. Some aspects of the syndrome are clear, but much remains to be learned, for instance in the areas of craving and loss of control. There is no linear relationship between the amount of a substance used and the severity of dependence, no single relationship between pattern of use and onset of dependence, and no fixed relationship between experimentation and dependence. Thus, despite our knowledge about such matters as vulnerability, mechanisms of tolerance, withdrawal and craving, we presently cannot predict who will lose control over use and become dependent. A lot thus remains to be learned about these processes when studying the neuroscience and social science of dependence-related behaviours.

Thus far, one side of the findings from neuroscience has been emphasized: how psychoactive substances act in terms of the common biological inheritance shared by all humans. The other side of the neuroscience research, reflected in Chapter 5 and partly in Chapter 6, is to some extent a counterpoint to this. The genetic research focuses on the differences in action of the substances between one human and another which are attributable to different genetic inheritances. The findings from this literature suggest that genetics modulates many aspects of the actions of psychoactive substances in humans. Thus genetic differences can make the use of the substance more or less pleasurable or aversive to a particular individual and can affect the toxicity of the substance, both in terms of overdose and of chronic health effects. Genetics can also affect the intensity of psychoactive effects of a given formulation and dose of a substance, as well as the likelihood of the occurrence of different aspects of dependence, i.e. tolerance and withdrawal, and those aspects which are not directly biologically measurable.

As with our knowledge of mechanisms of dependence, much remains to be learned about the genetics of dependence. We are far from genetically identifying which individuals will become dependent or will experiment with drugs. Genetic vulnerability tells little about the individual probability of psychoactive substance use and its related problems.

There is a need for governments to support, to whatever extent possible, neuroscience research, to develop a cadre of expertise, and to facilitate linking neuroscience with social science. Governments in developed countries should provide support for international collaborations and aid to developing countries to build local capacity.

Potential advances in policy, prevention and treatment from the neuroscience findings

Neuroscience findings in recent years have transformed our understanding of the actions of psychoactive substances. This knowledge should be used not only for the prevention and treatment of disorders and problems arising from acute and long-term use of these substances, but also for updating how they are controlled both under international drug conventions and in national and local laws and policies.

In the light of the neuroscience findings, there is increasing understanding that substance use disorders are like many other disorders in having biological, psychological and social determinants. However, a major difference in the case of substance dependence is the extreme stigma with which the disorder is regarded in many societies. A WHO study of attitudes to 18 disabilities in 14 countries found that "drug addiction" ranked at or near the top in terms of social disapproval or stigma, and that "alcoholism" ranked closely behind in most of the societies (Room et al., 2001). Reintegrating back into society persons treated for problems with psychoactive substance use will require developing and disseminating effective approaches to reducing this stigma.

With respect to prevention strategies, the main potential application of neuroscience findings so far would be from the genetic studies. Genetic screening, based on the research findings, can potentially identify subgroups of the population with a greater susceptibility to dependence or harm from a particular psychoactive substance. At present, such identification is in terms of probabilities rather than certainties. Actions which could be taken on the basis of a positive screen might include notification of the affected person (or of the person's parents or guardian, in the case of a child), and preventive interventions such as therapeutic education, or those targeted at reducing vulnerability to substance use and dependence. Possible preventive measures resulting from other neuroscientific research include preventive immunotherapies, e.g. against cocaine or nicotine, performed either on the general population or on those identified genetically or otherwise as being at high risk. As discussed in

Chapter 7 and below, there are important ethical considerations in any such genetic screening or preventive immunotherapy.

With respect to treatment strategies deriving from neuroscience research, immunotherapies could also presumably be applied to cases coming to treatment. Future developments in neuroscience may produce genetic modifications which would alter susceptibility to use of or dependence on particular classes of substances, though such developments presently seem quite far in the future.

Apart from the above, there seem to be two main choices in terms of biological interventions. Both of these are already on the scene, and the main pay-off from the neuroscience research is likely to be in improvements in the particular medication or formulation used. The first choice is the use of medications or procedures which interfere in one way or another with the action of the substance in the body, taking away the positive rewards from using the substance or making its use aversive. Such medications have been in use for more than half a century. Extensive experience suggests that the main problem with these interventions is lack of patient compliance, where those with a history of extensive use of a substance often prove unable to keep to any commitment they have made to continual use of the antagonist or aversive substance.

The other choice is the use of substances which are wholly or partially agonists, replacing the problematic substance or mode of administration with another which produces at least some of the same biological and experiential effects. This choice has been most widely explored and used for opioids, with codeine, methadone, buprenorphine and other substances substituting for heroin or other opiates. Nicotine replacement therapy, which substitutes for cigarettes, is now widely used thereby eliminating most of the public health harm.

Ethical issues in the application of the neuroscience findings

In the broadest sense, ethical issues have always been important in the use of psychoactive substances, and in societal responses to their use. Whether they should be used at all continues to be a contentious issue. Thus, for instance, Islam and some branches of other major world religions forbid the use of alcohol to faithful adherents. Ethical judgements are written into the major international drug control conventions (see Box 1.1). On the other hand, arguments against the criminalization of substance use are also frequently couched in ethical terms (e.g. Husak, 2002).

Within the somewhat narrower frame of ethics in health and human services, research and interventions, Chapter 7 has considered in some detail many of the ethical issues which are relevant to neuroscience research and the application of its findings. Only a few of these are emphasized here, with particular reference to their potential applications mentioned above.

Perhaps the most urgent ethical considerations arise around the issue of genetic screening, which is already on the horizon. A person identified by a genetic screen as being vulnerable or at risk is potentially disadvantaged by that identification in a number of ways. In the first place, the person's self-esteem may be reduced; as a minimum requirement, a substantial tangible benefit from the identification would be needed to balance this risk. The person's financial and status interests may be adversely affected if the identification is available to anyone else; for example, an insurance company may refuse insurance, an employer may choose not to employ, a person may refuse to marry. At present, in many countries, these adverse effects of such identification are not at all theoretical: for instance, insurance companies may have routine access to health records, or may require such access as a condition for issuing an insurance (thereby coercing consent).

There is an urgent need to consider the ethical issues raised by such genetic identifications in the course of providing health services in an international context, as well as at national and local levels. The issue is not limited to the field of psychoactive substance use and dependence, and WHO has given general consideration to these issues in the context of genetic counselling. For instance, "proposed ethical guidelines for genetic screening and testing" (WHO, 1998) provide that "results should not be disclosed to employers, insurers, schools or others without the individual's consent, in order to avoid possible discrimination". However, as the genetic research improves its predictive power, the stigmatization of and discrimination often associated with psychoactive substance use make it a particularly urgent issue that requires action beyond such general guidelines, as the genetic research improves its predictive power.

As discussed in Chapter 5, the use of immunotherapies and other neurological interventions, especially to the extent that they are irreversible, would raise difficult ethical issues. The neuroscience findings that the use of psychoactive substances shares many pathways in the brain with other human activities raise the question of what other pleasures or activities might be adversely affected by such interventions. The application of genetic modifications, particularly if heritable, would raise many of the same ethical issues currently being discussed in the context of human cloning.

The main ethical issues concerning therapies which interfere with the psychoactive effects of substance use, or which are aversive, are the requirement for patient consent to treatment, the patient's ability to give it, and the ethics of coerced treatment (see Chapter 7). The medications or other biological interventions at issue here are only one aspect of the means by which societies or groups coerce individuals regarding unwanted behaviours, and all such means are subject to similar ethical considerations. One additional consideration for prescription medications and medical procedures is the special ethical injunctions and constraints by which the medical profession and other health professions are guided (e.g. Declaration of Helsinki, see Box 7.1). Moreover, any treatment modality which is coerced should presumably have been shown to be effective.

Substitution therapy—using a medicine that is pharmacologically related to the dependence-producing substance—has often been controversial, with the argument stated in ethical terms. On the one hand, it is stated to be unethical for the state, or a treatment professional, to contribute to the continuation of the dependence, even if on a substitute regime. On the other hand, the counter-arguments of the demonstrated reductions in harm to society (e.g. criminal activity) or to the individual (e.g. HIV infection) from the substitute therapy are also ethical at their core. The general acceptance of nicotine replacement therapy might be regarded as indicating a gradual shift away from regarding the dependence itself as the harm, and towards a public health focus on the health and social harm which come from the use, whether dependent or not.

It should be noted that the topics discussed here and in Chapter 7 do not exhaust the range of ethical issues around psychoactive substances in the context of health practice and research. For instance, special ethical problems arise when psychoactive medications are used to treat behavioural problems in children; this may set up lifelong problems (i.e. predisposing them to later problematic drug use) and may reflect over-prescription of these substances. Another example is the ethics of "wash-out" studies to study psychoactive medications, in which patients in treatment facilities are entered into trials in which they are first taken off all the psychoactive medications they have been taking (whether as self-medication or by prescription), to evaluate their "baseline" condition.

A number of conceptual and policy issues might be addressed by scientific organizations and intergovernmental agencies in light of these developments in neuro-scientific and other research. These include such matters as the conceptual basis and empirical findings relevant to definitions of dependence and other substance use disorders in the International Classification of Diseases (ICD-10) and the Diagnostic and Statistical Manual of Mental Disorders (DSM-IV); the effectiveness of treatments for substance use disorders, and their place in systems of health and social services; and in particular the effectiveness, availability, and ethics of the use of medications and other biomedical interventions in treatment. As discussed earlier in this chapter, each such therapy which is currently in effect or still on the horizon, carries its own set of ethical issues, and these should be considered in the context of developing international standards for human rights in health services.

WHO already plays the role of a scientific arbiter on "scientific and medical" aspects in the classification of controlled substances under the international drug control treaties (Bruun, Pan & Rexed, 1975; Bayer & Ghodse, 1999). It exercises this role primarily through an Expert Committee on Drug Dependence, which meets every two years. As the intergovernmental agency with primary responsibility for global public health, WHO has responsibilities and interests concerning psychoactive substances which extend beyond the scope of the international treaties. One means for addressing these wider responsibilities has been to expand the scope of the Expert Committee, at least in some years (WHO, 1993), in order to cover the whole range of psychoactive substances and to consider a broader public health approach. However, reaching an expert judgement and building a global response concerning these matters will require other resources and expertise alongside the existing mechanism of the WHO Expert Committee.

Implications for public health policy

A substantial portion of the global burden of disease and disability is attributable to psychoactive substance use. In turn, a substantial portion of the burden attributable to substance use is associated with dependence. Tobacco and alcohol use are particularly prominent contributors to the total burden. Measures to reduce the harm from tobacco, alcohol and other psychoactive substances are thus an important part of health policy.

Neuroscience is a fast growing field of scientific research. Though the knowledge base is far from complete, there is a considerable amount of useful data with enormous potential for influencing policies to reduce the burden of disease and disability associated with substance use. The following recommendations are made to facilitate greater openness and assist all stakeholders in mobilizing action:

- All psychoactive substances can be harmful to health, depending on how they are taken, in which amounts and how frequently. The harm differs between substances and the public health response to substance use should be proportional to the health-related harm that they cause.

- Use of psychoactive substances is to be expected because of their pleasurable effects as well as peer pressure and the social context of their use. Experimentation does not necessarily lead to dependence but the greater the frequency and amount of substance used, the higher the risk of becoming dependent.

- Harm to society is not only caused by individuals with substance dependence. Significant harm also comes from non-dependent individuals, stemming from acute intoxication and overdose, and from the form of administration (e.g. through unsafe injections). There are, however, effective public health policies and programmes which can be implemented and which will lead to a significant reduction in the overall burden related to substance use.

- Substance dependence is a complex disorder with biological mechanisms affecting the brain and its capacity to control substance use. It is not only determined by biological and genetic factors, but psychological, social, cultural and environmental factors as well. Currently, there are no means of identifying those who will become dependent, either before or after they start using drugs.

- Substance dependence is not a failure of will or of strength of character but a medical disorder that could affect any human being. Dependence is a chronic and relapsing disorder, often co-occurring with other physical and mental conditions.

- There is significant comorbidity of substance dependence with various other mental illnesses; assessment, treatment and research would be most effective if an integrated approach were adopted. Treatment and prevention insights from other mental illnesses or substance dependence can be used to inform treatment and prevention strategies in the domain of the other. Attention to comorbidity of substance use disorders and other mental disorders is thus required as an element of good practice in treating or intervening in either mental illness or substance dependence.

- Treatment for substance dependence is not only aimed at stopping drug use—it is a therapeutic process that involves behaviour changes, psychosocial interventions and often, the use of substitute psychotropic drugs. Dependence can be treated and managed cost-effectively, saving lives, improving the health of affected individuals and their families, and reducing costs to society.

- Treatment must be accessible to all in need. Effective interventions exist and can be integrated into health systems, including primary health care. The health care sector needs to provide the most cost-effective treatments.

- One of the main barriers to treatment and care of people with substance dependence and related problems is the stigma and discrimination against them. Regardless of the level of substance use and which substance an individual takes, they have the same rights to health, education, work opportunities and reintegration into society, as does any other individual.

- Investments in neuroscience research must continue and expand to include investments in social science, prevention, treatment and policy research. The reduction in the burden from substance use and related disorders must rely on evidence-based policies and programmes which are the result of research and its application.

Conclusion

This report has summarized the advances in our understanding of the neuroscience of psychoactive substance use and dependence in recent decades, and has considered some of the ethical issues which are connected with these advances. The developments in neuroscience have greatly increased our knowledge about substance use and dependence, and the new knowledge poses substantial challenges for us to make ethical choices in applying the fruits of this knowledge, both globally and locally. Relevant organizational and professional bodies should play a leading role in meeting these challenges at global and regional levels.

References

Bayer I, Ghodse H (1999) Evolution of international drug control, 1945–1995. *Bulletin on Narcotics*, **51**:1–17.

Bruun K, Pan L, Rexed I (1975) *The Gentlemen's Club: international control of drugs and alcohol.* Chicago, University of Chicago Press.

Husak D (2002) *Legalize this! The case for decriminalizing drugs.* London, Verso.

Room R et al. (2001) Cross-cultural views on stigma, valuation, parity and societal values towards disability. In: Üstün TB et al., eds. *Disability and culture: universalism and diversity.* Seattle, WA, Hogrefe & Huber:247–291.

WHO (1993) *WHO Expert Committee on Drug Dependence. Twenty-eighth report.* Geneva, World Health Organization (WHO Technical Report Series, No. 836).

WHO (1998) *Proposed international guidelines on ethical issues in medical genetics and genetic services: report of a WHO Meeting on Ethical Issues in Medical Genetics, Geneva, 15–16 December 1997.* Geneva, World Health Organization (document WHO/HGN/GL/ETH/98.1; available from the Internet at http://www.who.int/ncd/hgn/hgnethic.htm).

Index

Note: bold page numbers denote material in figures, tables and boxes.

Acamprosate, and alcohol abuse 72
Acetylcholine 33
Action potential **29**, 30
ADHD, *see* Attention deficit hyperactivity disorder
Adoption studies 127
Alcohol dehydrogenase 135
Alcohol use 69–73, **107**
   adaptations to prolonged use 72
   behavioural effects 69–70
   and depression 183–184
   flushing/sensitivity response **134**
   genetic studies 132–136
      ALDH2 134–135
      combined risk with other psychoactive substances 138–147
      CYP2E1 135–136, 139
      linkage 133–134
      twinning 132–133
   mechanism of action 70
   prevalence of abuse 169
      abstention/consumption rates **8**
      mortality **17**
      selected countries 5–8, **6**
   schizophrenia 176
   and smoking, linkage studies 139
   tolerance and withdrawal 70–72
   treatment of dependence 72–73
Alcohol-metabolizing enzyme CYP2E1 135–136, 139
Aldehyde dehydrogenase 134
Amphetamines 93–96, **108**
   acute vs chronic use 175–176
   adaptations to prolonged use 96
   dependence, and schizophrenia 174–175
   development of tolerance 54

dopamine levels in frontal cortex 178
epidemic of amphetamine-type stimulant use **98**
mechanism of action 95
synthetic, *see* Ecstasy
tolerance and withdrawal 54, 95–96
gamma-Aminobutyric acid (GABA) 33
and alcohol abuse 70–72
and benzodiazepines 74
GABA-A receptors 31–33, 140–141
GABAergic systems 140–141
Anandamides 86
Animal models
ethical issues 209, 218–219
genetics 128–130
Antidepressants
placebo in smoking studies 181
reduction in cocaine use 182
SSRIs 185–186
Antipsychotic drugs
and dopamine receptor D2 174
typical/atypical, and schizophrenia 173
Antisocial personality disorder (ASPD) **189**
Atropine 104–105
Attention deficit hyperactivity disorder (ADHD), amphetamine treatment 94,
95, 96
Autonomy, ethical issues 216
Axon 28

Barbiturates, *see* Sedatives and hypnotics
Basal ganglia **24**
Behavioural processes underlying dependence 43–65
conditioning
classical/pavlovian 44–45
instrumental/operant 46–47
defined **56–57**
incentive 46–47
incentive–motivational responding 48
individual differences 55
motivation 48
reinforcement 47
reward 46
Beneficence, biomedical ethics 217
Benzodiazepines, *see* Sedatives and hypnotics
Brain anatomy and organization 19–25

Buprenorphine, treatment of opioid dependence 82, **83**
Bupropion, placebo in smoking studies 181

Candidate gene studies 128, 140–147
   conflicting results 149–9 ?????
   confounding issues 147–148
   dopaminergic system 141–145
Cannabinoids 84–88, **108**
   adaptations to prolonged use 88
   behavioural effects 85–6
   CB1 receptor 86–87
   mechanism of action 86–87
   therapeutic potential **85**
   tolerance and withdrawal 87–88
Catechol-*O*-methyltransferase polymorphisms 144–145
Cathinone, khat *(Catha edulis)* **94**
Caudate 23, **24**
Cerebral cortex 22
Cerebral hemispheres 22–25
Chloride channels (*see also* Ion channels) 74
Cholecystokinin, interactions with dopamine 147
Clinical trials, ethical issues 210–211, 225–227
   pharmacological treatments 225–227
      conflicts of interests 226–227
      distributive justice 217, 226
      trial design 225
   pharmacotherapy of prevention 211
Clozapine, schizophrenia 175–176
Co-morbidity 169–207
   hypotheses 170–176
Cocaine 89–93, **108**
   adaptations to prolonged use 91
   behavioural effects 89
   dependence, and schizophrenia 174–175
   dopamine levels in frontal cortex 178
   mechanism of action 89–90
   prevention studies, immunotherapy 229–231
   reduction in use with antidepressants 182
   tolerance and withdrawal 91
      development of tolerance 54
   treatment of dependence 92–93
   vaccines 92–93
Coercion, legal, treatment 232–235
Cognition, defined 56

Cognitive behavioural therapies **60**
Concurrent disorders
Conditioning
    classical/pavlovian 44–45
    definitions **56**
    instrumental/operant 46–47
Confidentiality, ethical issues 221–222, 230
Contingency management **60**
Controlled substances, illicit use 9–10
CREB, *see* Cyclic AMP response element binding protein
CREB-regulated pathways 37
Cyclic AMP response element binding protein (CREB) 37
CYP2A6 139
    gene frequency 75
CYP2D6 138
CYP2E1 135–136, 139

Declaration of Helsinki **212–216**
Delta receptor agonists 79
Dendrites 26–28
Dependence (*see also* Behavioural processes underlying dependence)
    43–65, 242
    candidate gene studies 128, 140–147
    criteria (DSM-IV) **14**
    criteria (ICD-10) **13**
    defined **13–15**, 15, 56, 58–59, 242
    and depression 182–183
    individual differences 55
    linkage studies 139
    models, ethical issues 231–232
    prevention studies, ethical issues 227–231
    reward and dependence issues 48–49
    with/without withdrawal 50
Dependence-producing drugs, *see* Psychoactive substances
Depressants (*see also* Antidepressants)
    behavioural effects **110**
Depression 180–188
    alcohol use 183–184
    effects of psychoactive substances 184–185
    limbic structures and substance dependence 187–188
    peptide systems 186–187
    psychostimulant dependence 182–183
    serotonin 185–186
    and tobacco smoking 181–182

Desmethylimipramine, reduction in cocaine use 182
Diencephalon **21**
Dimethoxy-4-methylamphetamine (DOM) 104
Dimethyltryptamine (DMT) 104
Distributive justice 217, 226
Disulfiram, and alcohol abuse 72–73
DMT, *see* Dimethyltryptamine
DOM, *see* Dimethoxy-4-methylamphetamine
Dopamine (*see also* Nucleus accumbens) 34
    cannabinoid binding sites 87
    and incentive sensitization 52–55
    interactions with cholecystokinin 147
    psychostimulant-induced levels in frontal cortex 178
    and reinforcement learning 50–52
    volatile solvent use 102–103
Dopamine beta hydroxylase (DBH) genotype 144
Dopamine receptors
    antagonists 177
    DRD1 142
    DRD2 142, 174
    DRD3 142–143
    DRD4 137, 143
    DRD5 143
Dopamine transporter 143
Dopaminergic system 141–145
    candidate genes for dependence 141–145
    dopamine (limbic) pathway 44, 106
Doxepin, placebo in smoking studies 181
Drug immunotherapies, prevention studies 229–231
DSM-IV, substance dependence criteria **14**

Ecstasy (MDMA) 96–100, **108**
    adaptations to prolonged use 100
    behavioural effects 99
    half-life in plasma 99
    mechanism of action 99
    tolerance and withdrawal 100
Electroencephalography (EEG) 40
Endocannabinoid system 86
Enkephalins 79
Entactogen, defined 97
Ephedrine, *see* Amphetamines
Epidemiological research, ethical issues 209–210, 224–225
Ethical issues 209–240, 244–247
    animal studies 209, 218–219

biomedical research on human subjects 210, 216–217, 219–222
  beneficence 217
  distributive justice 217, 226
  independent ethical review of risks and benefits 219
  informed consent 220
  non-maleficence 216–217
  privacy and confidentiality 221–222, 230
  recruitment of subjects 220–221
  respect for autonomy 216
clinical trials 210–211, 225–227
conflicts of interests 226–227
Declaration of Helsinki **212–216**
epidemiological research 209–210, 224–225
ethical analysis studies 211–218
models of dependence 231–232
prevention studies 227–231
provocation studies 223–224
public health policy 244–247
treatment studies 232–235
  access to treatment 232
  legally coerced treatment 232–235
types of research 209–211
vulnerable persons 222–223
  identification and definition 222–223

Fluoxetine, placebo in smoking studies 181
Fos, transcriptional regulator 37–38
Frontal cortex, psychostimulant-induced levels of dopamine 178

GBR-12909 92
Genes/genetics 35–36, 125–152
  alcohol use 132–136
  animal models 128–130
    transgenic animals 128–129
  candidate gene studies 128, 140–147
    confounding issues 147–148
  combined risk, psychoactive substances 138–147
  future directions 149–150
  heritability
    defined 126
    estimations 127
    selected substances **152**
  linkage studies 125, 127–128, 139
    confounding issues 147–148

opioid dependence 136–138
prevention studies 243–244
quantitative trait loci (QTL) 129–130
social and cultural aspects 150–151
tobacco dependence 130–132
Global use of psychoactive drugs 4–10
Globus pallidus 23
Glutamate 33–34
Glutamate transporter EAAT2 147
Glutamatergic afferents
in schizophrenia 177, 178–179
ventral tegmental area (VTA) 179

Habit, habituation, defined 56–57
Hallucinogens (*see also* Cannabis; Ecstasy) 104–106, **109**
adaptations to prolonged use 106
behavioural effects 105, **110**
mechanism of action 105
tolerance and withdrawal 105–106
Health issues 16–17
Helsinki Declaration **212–216**
Heritability
defined 126
dependence 138–139
estimations of 127
Heroin, treatment of heroin dependence **84**
Human rights, ethical issues 217–218
Hyoscyamine 104–105
Hypnotics, *see* Sedatives and hypnotics
Hypothalamus 21–22

ICD-10, substance dependence criteria **13**
Illicit drugs, *see* Psychoactive drugs, classification of use
Imipramine, reduction in cocaine use 182
Immunotherapy, prevention of cocaine use 229–231
Incentive 46–47
Incentive sensitization and dopamine 52–55
acquisition of drug use 55
and drug reward 53–54
psychomotor sensitization 53
and tolerance 54–55
Incentive–motivation 48, 57
Indolealkylamines 104
Informed consent 220
biomedical ethics 220

provocation studies 224
Ion channels 30, 31
IPC-1010, cocaine vaccine 92

Justice, distributive, biomedical ethics 217, 226

Kappa receptors 80, 137
Ketamine 104, 178–179
Khat *(Catha edulis)*, cathinone **94**

Legal coercion, treatment studies, ethical issues 232–235
Limbic system **25**
    dopamine pathway **44**, 106
    mesolimbic system and VTA 174–175
    and substance dependence 187–188
Linkage studies 125, 127–128
    dependence 139
d-Lysergic acid amine (LSA) 104
    serotonin autoreceptor agonist **109**
Lysergic acid diethylamide (LSD) 104–106

Magnetic resonance imaging (MRI) **39–40**
MAOI, *see* Monoamine oxidase inhibitor
MDMA, *see* 3,4-Methylenedioxymethamphetamine
Mental illness, and psychoactive substance use 169–207
Mescaline 104
Mesencephalon 21
Methadone
    treatment of opioid dependence 81–84
        substitution therapy **82**
Methamphetamine *(see also* Amphetamines)
    development of tolerance 54
N-Methyl-*D*-aspartate (NMDA), glutamate receptor antagonist, phency-
    clidine (PCP) **109**, 178–179
Methylenedioxyamphetamine (MDA) 104
3,4-Methylenedioxymethamphetamine (MDMA) *(see also* Ecstacy) 96–100
    behavioural effects 97–99
Methylphenidate, *see* Amphetamines
Models of dependence 231–232
    animal studies 219
        ethical issues 209, 218–219
Monoamine oxidase A 144
Monoamine oxidase inhibitor (MAOI), placebo in smoking studies 181
Motivation 48
Motivational enhancement therapy **60**

MRI, *see* Magnetic resonance imaging
Mu opioid receptor 137
Mu receptor agonists 79

Naloxone, treatment of opioid dependence 83–84
Naltrexone
    and alcohol abuse 72
    treatment of opioid dependence 83–84
Narcolepsy, amphetamine treatment 94, 96
Neurobiology, shared hypothesis of substance use 170–171, 188–191
Neuroimaging **39–40**
Neuroleptics
    and dopamine function 175
    dopamine receptor antagonists 177
    schizophrenia
        clozapine 175–176
        side-effects 172
Neuron anatomy and organization 25–29
Neuropeptide Y, neurotransmission in depression 187
Neurotransmission 29–31
Neurotransmitters 32–35
    defined 32
    examples 33–35
    release 30–31
Nicotine (*see also* Tobacco) **107**
    dopamine levels in frontal cortex 178
    half-life 75
    mechanism of action 76–77
    metabolism 131–132
Nicotinic receptors
    acetylcholine alpha-7 179–180
    beta-2 131
NMDA, *see* N-Methyl-D-aspartate
NMDA glutamate receptor antagonist, phencyclidine (PCP) **109**, 178–179
Norepinephrine 34
Nucleus accumbens (*see also* Dopamine) 24, 177
    dopamine receptors, DRD3 142–143
    "shell" region 51, 87

Opioid metabolizing enzymes 138
Opioid receptors 147
    kappa receptor 80, 137
    mu receptor 137
Opioids 79–84, **107**
    adaptations to prolonged use 81

behavioural effects 79–80, **110**
genetic studies 136–138
   combined risk with other psychoactive substances 138–147
   susceptibility 138
mechanism of action 80
opiate peptides 79
tolerance and withdrawal 80–81
treatment of dependence 81–84
   substitution therapy **82**

Paramethoxyamphetamine (PMA) 104
Parkinsonism, side-effect in schizophrenia 172
Pavlovian incentive learning 44–45, 51
PCP, *see* Phencyclidine
Pemoline, *see* Amphetamines
Peptide neurotransmitters 35
Peptide systems, depression 186–187
PET, *see* Positron emission tomography
Phencyclidine (PCP) 104
  NMDA glutamate receptor antagonist **109**, 178–179
Phenylethylamine drugs 104
PMA, *see* Paramethoxyamphetamine
Pons 20
Positron emission tomography (PET) 40
Prevention studies
  ethical issues 227–231
   drug immunotherapies 229–231
   early intervention studies 227–228
   pharmacotherapy, clinical trials 211
  genetics 243–244
Privacy and confidentiality, ethical issues 221–222, 230
Prodynorphin 137
Prosencephalon 20
Protein synthesis **27**
Provocation studies, ethical issues 223–224
Pseudoephedrine, *see* Amphetamines
Psilocybin 104
Psychoactive substances (*see also* Dependence; *specific substances*)
  adverse effects 10–12
  behavioural effects **110**
  cellular effects 36–38
  classification of use 2
  craving, defined 56
  definitions **15**

dependence
  criteria **13**
  and depression 182–183
  reward and dependence issues 46, 48–49, 53–54
and depression 184–185
development of antisocial personality disorder (ASPD) **189**
global use 4–10
heritability **152**
neuronal effects 38–39
and neuroscience 12–15
prevalence of use **9**
psychopharmacology 67–69
shared neurobiology hypothesis 170–171, 188–191
sociolegal status 1–4
as surrogates of conventional reinforcers 51–52
total global mortality **17**
treatment, ethical issues 232–235
withdrawal, with/without dependence 50
Psychotherapies **60**
Public health policy 241–249
  advances in neuroscience 241–244
  ethical issues 244–247
  recommendations 247–248

Quantitative trait loci (QTL) 129–130

Receptors 31–32
  targeting by drugs 38
Recruitment of subjects for research, ethical issues 220–221
Reinforcement 47, 57
  and dopamine 50–52
  drugs as surrogates of conventional reinforcers 51–52
Relapse prevention **60**
Research, *see* Ethical issues
Reward stimulus 46
  drug reward, and dependence 48–49
  incentive sensitization and dopamine 53–54
Rhombencephalon 20

Schizophrenia 171–180
  alcohol use 176
  clozapine 175–176
  high incidence of smoking 172–174
  positive/negative symptoms 173

psychostimulant use 175
    dependence 174–175
    neurobiological interactions 176–180
  side-effects, neuroleptic-induced 172
  tobacco smoking 171–174
Scopolamine 104–105
Sedatives and hypnotics 73–75, **107**
  adaptations to prolonged use 75
  behavioural effects 73
  mechanism of action 74
  tolerance and withdrawal 74–75
Sensitization (*see also* Incentive sensitization and dopamine; Tolerance)
  defined 57
  neural, persistence 58
Serotonergic systems 145–146
Serotonin 35
  and depression 185–186
Serotonin autoreceptor agonist, LSA **109**
Serotonin receptors 145–146
  5HT1B variant 145–146
Serotonin transporter 146
Shared neurobiology hypothesis, psychoactive substance use 170–171, 188–191
Signal transduction 31–32
Single photon emission computed tomography (SPECT) 40
Smoking, *see* Tobacco
Sociocultural factors, genetics 150–151
Sociolegal status of psychoactive substances 1–4
Solvents, *see* Volatile solvents
Somatostatin, neurotransmission in depression 187
SPECT, *see* Single photon emission computed tomography
Stimulants, behavioural effects **110**
Substance use, *see* Psychoactive substances
Substitution therapy 246
  treatment of opioid dependence **82**
Synapse
  chemical **31**
  structure and organization **28–29**
Synaptic plasticity 38
Synaptic structure, alterations, substance use 38–39

TA-CD, cocaine vaccine 92–93
Tardive dyskinesia, side-effect in schizophrenia 172
Telencephalon 22
Terminal buttons 28–29

Thalamus 24
TMA, *see* Trimethoxyamphetamine
Tobacco (*see also* Nicotine) 4–5, 75–78, **107**
    and alcohol use, linkage studies 139
    behavioural effects 75–76
    and depression 181–182
    genetic studies 130–132
        combined risk with other psychoactive substances 138–147
    mechanism of action 76–77
    PAHs in, hepatic enzyme induction 172
    placebo, bupropion 181
    prevalence of smoking
        mortality **17**
        and schizophrenia 172–174
        selected countries **5**
    tolerance and withdrawal 77–78
    treatment of dependence 78
Tolerance (*see also Specific substances*)
    defined 54–55, 57
    development 54–55
    and incentive sensitization 54–55
Tranquillizers, *see* Sedatives and hypnotics
Transcriptional regulator Fos 37–38
Transgenic animals 128–129
Treatment studies, ethical issues 232–235
    access to treatment 232
    legally coerced treatment 232
Trimethoxyamphetamine (TMA) 104
Tryptophan hydroxylase 146
Twinning and adoption studies 127, 132–133
Tyrosine hydroxylase 145

United Nations, drug control conventions **3**
Universal Declaration of Human Rights 217–218

Vaccines, treatment of dependence, cocaine 92–93
Ventral tegmental area (VTA) 21
    glutamatergic afferents 179
    and mesolimbic system 174–175
Volatile solvents 100–104, **109**
    behavioural effects 101–102
    environmental exposure 104
    mechanism of action 102–103
    tolerance and withdrawal 103
    use **101–102**

VTA, *see* Ventral tegmental area
Vulnerable persons, identification and definition 222–223

WHO, Expert Committee 246–247
Withdrawal of drugs (*see also Specific substances*)
    defined 57
    and depression 184–185
    with/without dependence 50